Diagnosis and Management of Sleep Disorders

Diagnosis and Management of Sleep Disorders

Edited by Destiny Lockhart

AMERICAN
MEDICAL PUBLISHERS
www.americanmedicalpublishers.com

American Medical Publishers,
41 Flatbush Avenue,
1st Floor, New York,
NY 11217, USA

Visit us on the World Wide Web at:
www.americanmedicalpublishers.com

ISBN: 978-1-63927-090-3

Cataloging-in-Publication Data

Diagnosis and management of sleep disorders / edited by Destiny Lockhart.
p. cm.
Includes bibliographical references and index.
ISBN 978-1-63927-090-3
1. Sleep disorders. 2. Nervous system--Diseases. 3. Sleep disorders--Diagnosis.
4. Sleep disorders--Treatment. I. Lockhart, Destiny.
RC547 .D53 2022
616.849 8--dc23

Table of Contents

Preface

The disorders that affect the sleep pattern of a person are referred to as sleep disorders. They negatively affect the normal physical, mental, social and emotional functioning of the person. Some of the common sleep disorders are bruxism, catathrenia, delayed sleep face disorder, hypopnea syndrome and idiopathic hypersomnia. The patient experiences involuntary grinding and clenching of teeth while sleeping in bruxism. Catathrenia causes nighttime groaning during exhalation. Delayed sleep phase disorder is an inability to awake and fall asleep at socially acceptable times. Sleep disorders are commonly diagnosed with the help of tests such as polysomnography and actigraphy. The treatment of sleep disorders depends on the diagnosis, the patient's medical and psychiatric history as well as the patient's preference. This book provides comprehensive insights into the field of sleep disorders. It presents researches and studies performed by experts across the globe. Those in search of information to further their knowledge will be greatly assisted by this book.

This book has been the outcome of endless efforts put in by authors and researchers on various issues and topics within the field. The book is a comprehensive collection of significant researches that are addressed in a variety of chapters. It will surely enhance the knowledge of the field among readers across the globe.

It gives us an immense pleasure to thank our researchers and authors for their efforts to submit their piece of writing before the deadlines. Finally in the end, I would like to thank my family and colleagues who have been a great source of inspiration and support.

Editor

Age and Gender Related Differences in Patient Awareness of Conditions Associated with Untreated Obstructive Sleep Apnea

Jeffrey J Stanley[1,2*], John Palmisano[1,3], Steven Hoshal[1], Lizabeth Binns[1] and Louise O'Brien[1,3,4]

[1]*Department of Neurology, Michael S. Aldrich Sleep Disorders Center, University of Michigan, Ann Arbor, Michigan, USA*

[2]*Department of Otolaryngology, Head and Neck Surgery, University of Michigan, Ann Arbor, Michigan, USA*

[3]*Department of Oral & Maxillofacial Surgery, University of Michigan, Ann Arbor, Michigan, USA*

[4]*Department of Obstetrics & Gynecology, University of Michigan, Ann Arbor, Michigan, USA*

[*]**Corresponding author:** Jeffrey J. Stanley, University of Michigan, Otolaryngology-Head and Neck Surger 1904 Taubman Center, 1500 E. Medical Center Drive, Ann Arbor, MI 48109-5312, E-mail: jjst@umich.edu

Abstract

Introduction: Patient education has been shown to improve continuous positive airway pressure (CPAP) compliance in the treatment of obstructive sleep apnea (OSA). This is facilitated by improving patient awareness of both the goals of treatment, proper use of the device and consequences of inadequate treatment. The most obvious outcome of successful therapy is an improvement in excessive daytime sleepiness. However, it is hypothesized that the long-term benefits of disease prevention and lessening the severity of conditions known to be associated with untreated OSA are less well recognized by patients. The purpose of this study was to document the degree of patient awareness of conditions associated with OSA. It is anticipated that a lack of knowledge exists in some patient subgroups; that if educated more intensely about these associations might be more diligent in participating in the treatment of their OSA.

Methods: This study was a cross-sectional survey of patients who had been prescribed positive airway pressure (PAP) therapy for OSA. This survey assessed patient knowledge of co-morbid medical conditions associated with untreated OSA.

Results: The vast majority of participants failed to recognize all of the most common co-morbid conditions. Significant differences in awareness were noted between different age groups and genders.

Conclusions: Patient education is important in achieving CPAP compliance. Patient education, as demonstrated by a relative lack of knowledge of associated co-morbidities, appears to be inadequate. Greater efforts at patient education during each and every patient encounter in the sleep disorders clinic are recommended.

Keywords: Obstructive sleep apnea; Continuous positive airway pressure; Patient knowledge; Age; Gender

Introduction

Conditions associated with untreated obstructive sleep apnea (OSA) include hypertension, congestive heart failure, coronary artery disease, cardiac arrhythmias, stroke, diabetes, neurocognitive impairment, depression, decreased quality of life and increased risk of motor vehicle accidents (MVA) [1-10]. These conditions contribute to increased age adjusted mortality rates in patients with OSA. The prevalence of these comorbid conditions and their association with OSA has been well documented. Sleep medicine providers routinely share information regarding these associated conditions with patients to both increase awareness of the potential sequelae of untreated OSA and to provide motivation to those striving to comply with medical treatment of their disease.

It is hypothesized that many of these comorbidities associated with OSA go unrecognized by patients with OSA. In part this occurs because of the vast array of new information presented at the time of diagnosis. This includes the introduction of new medical terminology, a review of treatment options and potential sequelae of untreated disease. In addition, there may be deficiencies in the educational programs available to patients with OSA. Nevertheless, many clinicians may expect that patients using CPAP would have acquired a high degree of familiarity with the consequences of inadequate treatment since this group has typically completed multiple encounters with their sleep medicine practitioner; sleep facility, and durable medical equipment company. There is a paucity of literature on patient knowledge of comorbidities associated with OSA. The purpose of this study was to determine the degree of patient awareness of conditions associated with OSA.

Methods

Participants

A de-identified cross-sectional survey was undertaken of 669 patients, age 18 years or older, who had been prescribed positive airway pressure (PAP) therapy for OSA. Positive airway pressure therapy included treatment with any form of positive airway pressure; continuous positive airway pressure (CPAP), bi-level positive airway pressure (Bi-Level PAP), or auto-titrating positive airway pressure (Auto PAP). Recruitment occurred over a consecutive 365 day period from March 2010 to March 2011 at the University of Michigan Sleep Disorders Center, accredited by the American Academy of Sleep Medicine. Patients attending a follow up clinic visit regarding their PAP therapy, ranging from 3 to 6 months following their initial diagnosis, were recruited to participate in a de-identified survey. All patients had been provided verbal counseling regarding short term and long term consequences of untreated OSA in categories of cardiovascular risk, neurocognitive effects, quality of life and risk of MVA during a sleep clinic visit following their initial diagnosis of OSA. Counseling was consistent across groups and was documented in the medical record. There were no exclusion criteria. No compensation was offered for participation.

Questionnaire

This survey assessed patient knowledge of conditions associated with untreated OSA including hypertension, congestive heart failure, coronary artery disease, cardiac arrhythmias, stroke, diabetes, neurocognitive impairment, depression, decreased quality of life and increased risk of motor vehicle accidents. Each comorbidity was listed as it appears in Table 1. Each patient was instructed to circle any or all conditions they believed to be associated with OSA. No additional description of each condition was provided. In addition, information regarding gender, age, preexisting medical conditions and self-reported duration of nightly PAP therapy use were also tabulated.

Medical Conditions	Female	Male
Arrhythmia	42%	43%
Congestive Heart Failure	51%	55%
Depression	72%	
Diabetes Mellitus	35%	29%
Hypertension	63%	59%
Myocardial Infarction	38%	29% (p=0.02)
Myocardial Ischemia	28%	20%
Motor Vehicle Accident	68%	64%
Stroke	46%	40%
Quality of Life	81%	80%

Table 1: Recognition of Conditions Associated with OSA by Gender.

Statistical analysis

All data were sequentially entered into a Microsoft Access database (Microsoft). Data were then analyzed using SPSS software (version 19, IBM, Armonk NY). Group differences were assessed by Chi Square tests for proportional data. A p-value of <0.05 was considered statistically significant.

Results

General results

Surveys were collected from 669 participants; 371 (55.4%) were male, 278 (41.6%) were female and 20 (3%) patients did not disclose their gender. Among the study participants 12% were 21-40 years of age, 54% were 41-60 years of age and 34% were 61 years of age or older. Eighty four percent of study participants reported CPAP use of greater than four hours/night.

Recognition of co-morbid conditions

The vast majority of participants failed to recognize every associated condition. In fact, only 8% of participants recognized all ten presented conditions known to be associated with untreated obstructive sleep apnea. Just over half of study participants recognized at least 50% of the associated conditions. The most recognized comorbid condition was diminished quality of life (80%) followed by increased risk of motor vehicle accident (65%), depression (64%), congestive heart failure (53%) and hypertension (50%). The least recognized co-morbid conditions were myocardial ischemia (23%), diabetes mellitus (31%), myocardial infarction (32%), stroke (43%) and cardiac arrhythmias (43%).

Gender differences

Two major differences in gender responses were noted. Women identified the association between depression and OSA more often than men (72% *vs.* 50%, p=0.001) as well as myocardial infarction (72% *vs.* 59%, p=0.02), (Table 1). Both men and women identified the association between decreased quality of life and OSA most frequently, at 80% and 81% respectively.

Age differences

The youngest age group (age 18-40 years) recognized the association of OSA and increased risk of motor vehicle accident, quality of life and depression as co-morbid conditions most frequently (81%, 78% and 71%, respectively), (Table 2). Both younger and middle aged (41-60 years) participants were significantly more likely than older aged (61 years or older) participants to recognize the association of OSA with depression (71% for age 18-40 years, 68% for age 41-60 years and 56% for age > 61 years, p<0.0001). Participants in the youngest age group were unlikely to recognize the association of untreated OSA with myocardial infarction and myocardial ischemia, (26% and 21%, respectively).

Middle aged participants were most likely to identify decreased quality of life, increased risk of motor vehicle accident, depression, hypertension and risk of myocardial infarction as conditions associated with OSA (82%, 70%, 68%, 63% and 59%, respectively). This age group was least likely to identify diabetes, 33%, and myocardial ischemia, 24%, as potential co-morbidities. Middle aged participants were more likely to recognize the association of OSA and myocardial infarction compared to younger study participants (59% *vs.* 26%, p=0.007) and they were slightly more likely than older patients to recognize this association (59% *vs.* 35%, p=0.07). The middle age group recognized the association between increased risk of MVA and untreated OSA more frequently than the oldest age group (p=0.03). Although the youngest participants (age 18-40 years) were slightly more likely to recognize this association than the middle age group, this difference did not reach statistical significance (p=0.06).

Participants older than 61 years of age were most knowledgeable of the association of OSA with impaired quality of life, increased risk of motor vehicle accident, hypertension, depression and congestive heart failure, with recognition rates of 77%, 61%, 59%, 56% and 53%, respectively. This age group was least likely to recognize myocardial infarction (35%), diabetes (28%) and myocardial ischemia (23%) as co-morbidities associated with OSA.

Medical Conditions	18-40 years	41-60 years	>61 years
Arrhythmia	42%	44%	43%
Congestive Heart Failure	51%	53%	53%
Depression	71%*	68%	56%* (*p<0.0001)
Diabetes Mellitus	36%	33%	28%
Hypertension	60%	63%	59%
Myocardial Infarction	26%*	59%*,**	35%** (*p=0.007) (**p=0.07)
Myocardial Ischemia	21%	24%	23%
Motor Vehicle Accident	81%*	70%*,**	61%** (*p=0.06) (**p=0.03)
Stroke	38%	44%	45%
Quality of Life	78%	82%	77%

Table 2: Recognition of Conditions Associated with OSA by Age Group.

Patients with an underlying existing medical condition

Study participants with an underlying diagnosis of hypertension or diabetes mellitus were significantly more likely to recognize the association of these diseases as associated with OSA than those without these concomitant illnesses (p<0.001). Patients with a diagnosis of either hypertension or diabetes were significantly more likely to recognize the association of OSA with decreased quality of life (p<0.001 and p=0.003, respectively) and depression (p=0.05 and p=0.01) when compared to those without these coexisting illnesses. Study participants with a diagnosis of hypertension were unlikely to be aware of the association of untreated OSA and myocardial ischemia and myocardial infarction (22% and 30%, respectively). Participants with a diagnosis of diabetes were also unlikely to be aware of the association of untreated OSA and myocardial ischemia and myocardial infarction (24% and 29%, respectively).

Discussion

The effects of untreated OSA include both an increased risk of cardiovascular disease and neurocognitive sequelae that can have a significant impact on quality of life and patient survival. Following a diagnosis of obstructive sleep apnea at the author's institution, a thorough patient educational program includes a review of the pathophysiology of OSA, available treatment options and clinical consequences of inadequate treatment. This study demonstrates that despite recruitment of a mostly compliant group of PAP users, retention of the latter appears to be poor. Awareness of the relationship between untreated OSA and quality of life was most frequent (79%). This is likely reflective of the improvement in quality of life noted by the majority of patients successfully treated with CPAP. Significant improvement in disease specific quality of life following successful CPAP therapy, as assessed by the Functional Outcomes of Sleep Questionnaire (FOSQ), has been previously demonstrated [10,11].

Significant differences between genders were identified. Women were significantly more likely to recognize depression and myocardial infarction as co-morbidities associated with untreated OSA. The higher prevalence of diagnosed clinical depression in women may account for a higher rate of awareness of this comorbidity [12]. Historically, however, there has been a lower rate of awareness of coronary artery disease symptomatology and early detection in women compared to men. Of note, there have been recent efforts to promote awareness regarding the signs and symptoms of myocardial infarction in women via public service campaigns. These educational efforts may account, in part, for the gender differences noted in the current study.

There were significant age group differences for recognition of depression and risk of motor vehicle accident. Both awareness and recognition of depression may be more common in younger adults as there has been a gradual decrease in the stigmata associated with this form of mental illness during the past several decades. In addition, it is generally accepted that the rate of motor vehicle accidents is highest in younger adults. This may be reflected by a greater of awareness by younger adults of the increased risk of MVA associated with untreated OSA.

It may not be surprising that patients with a diagnosis of hypertension or diabetes were significantly more likely than those without to recognize these diseases as associated co-morbidities. This subset of patients also had an increased awareness of the relationship between OSA and quality of life. Decreased quality of life has been previously shown to be associated with both hypertension and diabetes [12,13]. Of concern, however, was that neither patients with a diagnosis of hypertension or diabetes, classical risk factors for the development of cardiovascular disease, were likely to be aware of the relationship between OSA and myocardial ischemia or infarction.

Improvement in excessive daytime sleepiness, cognitive function and quality of life following the use of CPAP may serve as positive reinforcement for many patients. However, even with subjective improvement in quality of life measures, CPAP compliance remains problematic. When compliance is defined as greater than 4 hours of nightly use, 29-83% of patients with OSA are considered to be non-compliant [14]. Furthermore, there is a subset of patients with OSA who do not experience a subjective improvement in symptoms despite their documented use of CPAP. For these patients, CPAP compliance may be even more problematic.

Hence, patient education regarding the potential late sequelae of untreated OSA in this subset of patients is crucial as it may serve as the primary motivation for PAP use. Increased attention to patient education has been shown to be effective at improving CPAP compliance [15]. A recent Cochrane Airways Group review of randomized parallel controlled trials reported that educational interventions significantly increased overall duration of CPAP use and improved compliance as measured defined by >4 hours nightly use.

One strength of the current study is that it assessed knowledge of a wide variety of co-morbidities associated with untreated OSA not just those most commonly reported, e.g. hypertension and heart disease. In addition, the anonymous nature of the survey used should help improve the accurate assessment of patient knowledge, without encouraging guessing as individual patients were not being graded. Another strength is that this large cohort had a roughly equal number of male and female participants. The majority of participants were middle age in keeping with the usual prevalence of OSA. One notable limitation of this study was that the vast majority of participants were PAP compliant, with 84% reporting an average PAP use of greater than four hours/night. Because of this, meaningful statistical analysis to assess if increased knowledge of co-morbidities correlated positively with PAP compliance was not possible.

In this study of patients using CPAP, patient education regarding co-morbidities associated with untreated OSA was provided at the time of initial diagnosis. However, it is clear from the aforementioned results that this information was not fully assimilated by the majority of patients. One potential weakness f this study is that patients were provided a list of medical conditions as opposed to an open-ended questionnaire. This format may have helped patients identify potential comorbid conditions and may have lead to an overestimation of study participant's knowledge. Those individuals who already had a pre-existing condition were more likely to identify this association with OSA. However, as CPAP use is important in disease prevention, it is critical that those patients without pre-existing comorbidities be made aware of the cardiovascular and neurocognitive sequelae of untreated OSA in order to encourage CPAP compliance. This may be of particular importance in younger patients in whom the long term deleterious effects of untreated OSA have not yet manifested and may be prevented or attenuated with adequate treatment.

As patient education was provided at the time of diagnosis, it is possible that the time period between diagnosis and questionnaire administration may have affected the retention of this knowledge. Another potential weakness of this study is that the patient's own educational level was not assessed. This factor may have affected the ability of study participants to retain and assimilate new information regarding comorbidities associated with OSA. It is also plausible that the neurocognitive effects of untreated OSA, including poor concentration and impaired memory, may hinder routine attempts at patient education prior to or shortly after initiation of treatment. Patients may struggle to assimilate the vast amount of information presented at the time of their initial evaluations in the sleep disorders clinic, as the volume of this information regarding diagnosis, pathogenesis, treatment options and sequelae of inadequate treatment may be overwhelming.

Patient education is important in improving CPAP compliance. Knowledge of comorbidities associated with OSA may serve as motivation for improving CPAP compliance. It appears that there is a relative lack of knowledge of conditions associated with untreated OSA by all patients receiving PAP therapy. In addition, significant age and gender differences in patient awareness exist. The responsibility for patient education lies largely with sleep medicine providers who are keenly aware of the potential consequences of untreated OSA. Greater efforts in patient education regarding these associated conditions, with particular attention to subgroups identified as having significant knowledge deficits, during each and every patient encounter in the sleep disorders clinic are recommended [16].

Acknowledgement:

This study was approved by the University of Michigan Internal Review Board at the University of Michigan (IRB# HUM00035078 March 2010).

References

1. Börgel J, Sanner BM, Keskin F, Bittlinsky A, Bartels NK, et al. (2004) Obstructive sleep apnea and blood pressure. Interaction between the blood pressure-lowering effects of positive airway pressure therapy and antihypertensive drugs. Am J Hypertens 17: 1081-1087.
2. Bradley TD, Floras JS (1996) Pathophysiologic and therapeutic implications of sleep apnea in congestive heart failure. J Card Fail 2: 223-240
3. Gottlieb DJ, Yenokyan G, Newman AB, O'Connor GT, Punjabi NM, et al. (2010) Prospective study of obstructive sleep apnea and incident coronary heart disease and heart failure: The sleep heart health study. Circulation 122: 352-360.
4. Shah N, Redline S, Yaggi HK, Wu R, Zhao CG, et al. (2013) Obstructive sleep apnea and acute myocardial infarction severity: Ischemic preconditioning? Sleep Breath 17: 819-826.
5. Oza N, Baveja S, Khayat R, Houmsse M (2014) Obstructive sleep apnea and atrial fibrillation: Understanding the connection. Expert Rev Cardiovasc Ther 12: 613-621.
6. Li M, Hou WS, Zhang XW, Tang ZY (2014) Obstructive sleep apnea and risk of stroke: A meta-analysis of prospective studies. Int J Cardiol 172: 466-469.
7. Reutrakul S, Van Cauter E (2014) Interactions between sleep, circadian function, and glucose metabolism: Implications for risk and severity of diabetes. Ann N Y Acad Sci 1311: 151-173.
8. Weaver TE, Laizner AM, Evans LK, Maislin G, Chugh DK, et al. (1997) An instrument to measure functional status outcomes for disorders of excessive sleepiness. Sleep 20: 835-843.
9. Ejaz SM, Khawaja IS, Bhatia S, Hurwitz TD (2011) Obstructive sleep apnea and depression: A review. Innov Clin Neurosci 8: 17-25.
10. Ellen RL, Marshall SC, Palayew M, Molnar FJ, Wilson KG, et al. (2006) Systematic review of motor vehicle crash risk in persons with sleep apnea. J Clin Sleep Med 2: 193-200.
11. Moyer CA, Sonnad SS, Garetz SL, Helman JI, Chervin RD (2001) Quality of life in obstructive sleep apnea: A systematic review of the literature. Sleep Med 2: 477-491.
12. Piccinelli M, Wilkinson G (2000) Gender differences in depression. Critical review. Br J Psychiatry 177: 486-492.
13. Trevisol DJ, Moreira LB, Kerkhoff A, Fuchs SC, Fuchs FD (2011) Health-related quality of life and hypertension: A systematic review and meta-analysis of observational studies. J Hypertens 29: 179-188.

Does Type D personality Increase Perchance for CPAP Non-Adherence in Patients with OSA?

Monika Sharma and Samhita Panda*

Department of Sleep Medicine, Sir Ganga Ram Hospital, New Delhi, India

***Corresponding author:** Samhita Panda, Department of Sleep Medicine, Sir Ganga Ram Hospital, Delhi, India, E-mail: samhitapanda@yahoo.com

Abstract

Introduction: Adherence to Continuous Positive Airway Pressure (CPAP) therapy in patients with Obstructive Sleep Apnea (OSA) has been inconclusively linked to gender, age, disease severity, sleepiness and socioeconomic status. This study aimed to examine the association between distressed personality and CPAP adherence in Indian patients with OSA.

Method: This was a single center, prospective study conducted at a tertiary-care hospital in Delhi, India. Patients diagnosed as OSA by polysomnography (PSG) (and underwent CPAP titration), who completed the questionnaires and returned for follow-up were recruited. Demographic data, clinical and PSG variables were collected. DS14 for Type D personality was administered. Subjects were followed for minimum 30 days of CPAP treatment for adherence verification. Good CPAP compliance was defined as CPAP use >4 hours/night at least 5 days/week.

Result: Sixty-nine patients with OSA (age: 52.23 ± 12.28 years, 76% male) were enrolled. 73% (n=50) had severe OSA while 73.9% had Type D personality (n=51). Although 79.7% (n=55) agreed to CPAP use and 75.4% (n=52) actually initiated therapy, only 43% (n=30) had good CPAP compliance. Therefore, majority (57%, n=39) of patients had poor compliance with CPAP. There was no association between age, gender, marital status and degree of OSA with distressed personality. Interestingly, overall 90% (n=36) of patients having poor acceptance and/or compliance possessed Type D personality as compared to 10% (n=3) non-type D CPAP users ($p<0.000$).

Conclusion: Distressed personality possibly contributes towards poor CPAP adherence in Indian OSA patients. A multi-dimensional approach including intensive screening for personality profiles, use of patient education and behavior modifications at time of prescription of CPAP may help improve CPAP adherence.

Keywords: Obstructive sleep apnea; Continuous positive airway pressure; Non-compliance; Adherence; Type D personality

Introduction

Sleep apnea is known to be significantly associated with medical, metabolic and cardiovascular diseases, as well as psychological and mood disturbances. Obstructive sleep apnea (OSA), that is associated with repeated episodes of complete or partial blockage of upper airway during sleep, can lead to serious health consequences, including metabolic, cardiovascular comorbidities, marked psychological distress and poor quality of life [1-5].

Approximately one in five adults suffers from mild OSA, 1 in 15 moderate OSA and 1 of 20 have severe OSA [6]. The prevalence of OSA in Indian population varies from 13 to 18% [7,8]. Prevalence of OSA in middle-aged urban Indian population is 9.3% [7] and it is three-fold higher in men as compared to women. The prevalence of OSA increases with age, though age is not an independent risk factor for the OSA.

Among the various treatment options available, continuous positive airway pressure (CPAP) is the first line of therapy especially for moderate to severe OSA. CPAP treatment improves neuro-cognitive deficits including impairment in higher mental processes such as concentration, memory, and executive function, affect in patients with severe depression, behavioral morbidity like excessive daytime sleepiness (EDS), and possibly reduces an increased chance of accidents [9].

Adherence is defined as 'the extent to which a person's behavior-taking medications, following a diet and/or executing lifestyle changes, corresponds with agreed recommendations from a health care provider'. This definition given by Haynes and Rand has been adopted by World Health Organization [10]. Compliance with CPAP remains a major drawback. Although this treatment is more successful than other modalities, adherence to CPAP for OSA has been problematic.

The problem is further magnified due to concern regarding its side effects. The rate of adherence failure ranges from 5% to 89% in the first week to 6 months [11,12]. Previous studies made attempts to examine the predictors of non-compliance with CPAP therapy and found significant relationships with gender, age, severity of disease, symptoms of sleepiness and socioeconomic status, though the findings are inconsistent [13,14].

Other studies made an attempt to answer this question by examining personality changes and its association with CPAP adherence [15] Depression may also reduce adherence to CPAP [16].

No individual factor has been found to be consistently predictive of adherence.

Type D personality is defined as a combination of negative affectivity (NA) or a tendency to experience negative emotions and social inhibition (SI) or a tendency to inhibit the expression of emotions to others because of insecurity and tension [17].

Studies from the general population of Denmark and Belgium have shown that type D was present in 28% and 21% of patients with CAD [17,18]. Type D is an independent predictor of negative outcomes such as poor health status, (recurrent) myocardial infarction and increased risk of mortality in cardiovascular patients [18-20].

Several studies have demonstrated that the effect of Type D personality on adverse outcomes is independent of biomedical risk factors [21]. Results of earlier studies showed that the prevalence of type D among cardiovascular patients is 27%-31% compared to 13%-24% in normative population [22].

Other studies examined non-cardiovascular population like sleep apnea [15], melanoma [23], mild brain injury [24] and vertigo [25]. In these studies, type D was found to be associated with increased report of anxiety and depression, health complaints, adverse health related behaviors and poor compliance to treatment [15,23-25].

The present study aimed to examine 1) the prevalence of distressed personality in Indian patients with OSA therapy, and 2) the association of distressed personality in Indian patients with OSA and CPAP non-adherence.

Method

This was a single center, prospective study conducted at a tertiary care hospital in New Delhi, India. The study was approved by the institutional ethics committee. All individuals attending the Sleep clinic at the hospital and suspected to have OSA were scheduled for level 1 Polysomnography (PSG) at the hospital.

Patients, who were diagnosed as having OSA after PSG, were recommended to undergo CPAP titration. Those patients fulfilling the criteria below and returning for follow-up were recruited for the study.

Inclusion criteria

Those who complained of snoring, sleep apnea, or EDS and were found by the sleep physician to have OSA and gave informed consent were recruited.

Exclusion criteria

Subjects suffering from 1) anemia 2) liver and kidney disease 3) neuro-psychiatric disorders 4) cardiac failure 5) spine disorder 6) on multiple drugs 7) any other significant medical disorder contributing to poor sleep were excluded.

Demographic data

Demographic data was collected from the patients regarding age, gender, clinical, sleep variables and personality profile. Data was achieved by two questionnaires: DS14 for Type D personality and Epworth Sleepiness Scale (ESS).

Subjects were followed up for minimum 30 days of CPAP treatment for adherence verification. All information was obtained through face to face interview and psychometric testing conducted by sleep medicine expert and sleep psychologist respectively.

Parameters measured

Severity of OSA: PSG was performed in the hospital-based sleep laboratory. The channels included electroencephalography, electro-oculography, and electromyography of chin and tibialis anterior, electrocardiography, measurement of respiratory flow, thoracic or abdominal movements and arterial oxygen saturation.

Apnea was defined as cessation of airflow for at least 10 seconds and hypopnea was defined as blood oxygen desaturation of 4% or greater and 30% reduction in airflow for more than 10 seconds. The apnea-hypopnea index (AHI) was the number of apneas and hypopneas per hour of sleep. OSA syndrome was diagnosed when a patient had an AHI greater than 5 with symptoms of excessive daytime sleepiness, or an AHI greater than 15 regardless of daytime symptoms, in line with the recommendations of the American Academy of Sleep Medicine [6].

Severity of OSA was judged from AHI, and graded as mild OSA ($5 \leq AHI < 15$/hour), moderate OSA ($15 \leq AHI < 30$/hour), and severe OSA ($AHI \geq 30$/hour). Patients with OSA who decided to use CPAP therapy were subjected to CPAP titration the following night. Optimal pressures for CPAP were determined by manual titration.

Distressed personality: DS-14 was used to measure negative affect (NA), social inhibition (SI) and Type D personality [17]. The questionnaire containing 14 items and a 5-point Likert-type scale ranging from 0=false to 4=true, was used to evaluate for distressed personality. The 14 items of the whole scale, as well as the seven items on each of the NA and SI scales, can be summarized. A score of 10 and more on both of the subscales indicates that the person has a Type D personality.

Excessive daytime sleepiness: The ESS is widely used in the field of sleep medicine as a subjective measure of a patient's sleepiness [26]. The test is a list of eight situations in which one rates the tendency to become sleepy on a scale of 0-no chance of dozing, to 3-high chance of dozing. The maximum total score is 24.

Adherence: Adherence to CPAP therapy was defined on the basis of the extent of CPAP use. Good compliance with CPAP therapy was defined as use of CPAP for more than 4 hours per night for at least 5 days per week. The data collected was split into two groups and subjected to statistical analysis. Group A comprised of patients with OSA possessing distressed personality whereas Group B had non-type D personality.

Statistical analysis

Statistical analyses were performed using a statistical software package (SPSS version 17.0). Continuous variables were summarized as mean ± SD or median and categorical variables as proportions.

Differences between groups were assessed for categorical variables with Chi-square or Fisher's exact test. ANOVA were used for comparison of continuous variables between groups. All tests were two sided and a p value less than 0.05 was considered statistically significant.

Results

Study population

One hundred and eight individuals at risk for OSA were scheduled for level 1 PSG at the hospital. Out of these, 76 underwent PSG (Figure 1). A total of 69 patients with confirmed OSA completing the questionnaires and returning for follow up were recruited for the study.

The final sample included 53 men (76%) and 16 women (24%). The mean age of the study population was 52.23 ± 12.28 years (range=20-69 years). Majority of the subjects were married (n=66) and suffered from severe degree of OSA (n=50).

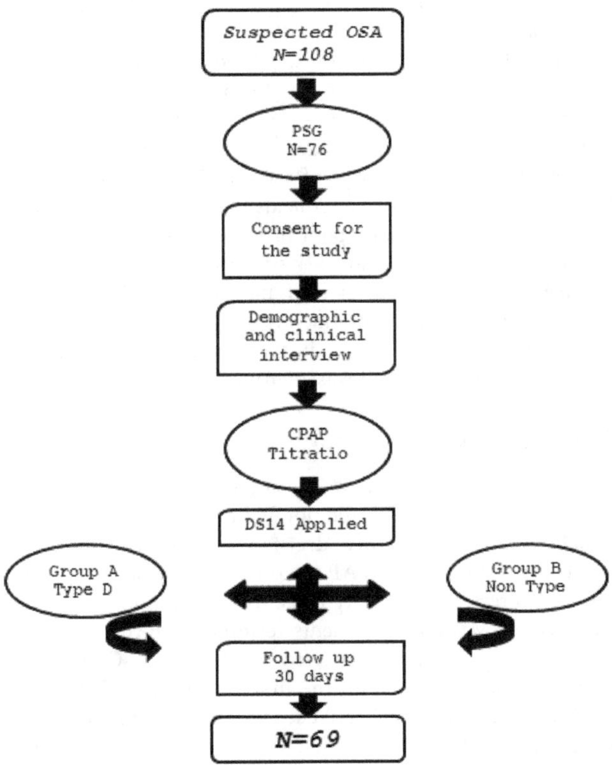

Figure 1: Flow chart showing recruitment of patients into the study.

	Group A	Group B	Total	P value
	n=51 [73 %]	n=18 (27%)	n=69 (%)	
Age				
Mean (±S.D)	53.78 (12.736)	47.83 (9.901)	52.23 (12.82)	0.08
Male gender	37 (72.5%)	16 (88.9%)	53	0.2
Married	48 (94.1%)	18 (100%)	66	0.6
SI				
Mean (±S.D)	15.24 (4.942)	6.28 (2.845)	12.89	0
NA				
Mean (±S.D)	16.06 (4.149)	9.72 (3.801)	14.4	0
ESS [Mean(±S.D)]	12.49 (5.815)	13.72 (5.367)	12.85 (8.48)	0.4
Degree of OSA in participants				
Mild	4 [7.8]	2 [11.1]	6 [8.7]	
Moderate	9 [17.6]	4 [22.2]	13 [18.8]	0.8
Severe	38 [74.5]	12 [66.7]	50 [72.5]	
Patients with OSA who agreed for CPAP therapy				
Agreed	40 [78.4]	15 [83.3]	55 [79.7]	0.7
Disagreed	11 [21.6]	3 [16.7]	14 [20.3]	
Patients who started CPAP therapy				
Yes	37 [72.5]	15 [83.3]	52 [75.4]	0.5
No	14[27.5]	3 [16.7]	17 [24.6]	
Overall acceptance and/or CPAP compliance.				
Good	15 [29.4]	15 [83.3]	30 [43.5%]	0
Poor	36 [70.6]	3 [16.7]	39 [56.5%]	

Table 1: Comparison of demographic and sleep variables between patients having OSA with and without Type D personality. NA: Negative Affect; SI: Social Inhibition; ESS: Epworth Sleepiness Scale; OSA: Obstructive Sleep Apnea; CPAP: Continuous Positive Airway Pressure.

Psychological variables

Distressed personality was measured with the help of DS14 and showed that 73% (n=51) of patients with OSA had Type D personality. Approximately 73% men and 27% women possessed Type D personality.

Comparison between Group A (patients with Type D) and Group B (patients with non-Type D personality) showed no difference in gender and marital status (p=0.2 and 0.6 respectively) whereas average age did marginally differ statistically between the groups (p=0.08).

The two facets of DS14, NA and SI were looked at independently. The mean score of NA and SI was higher in Type D OSA subjects than non-type D OSA subjects with statistically significant difference (p=0.0) (Table 1).

Sleep-related variables

The average score of ESS in the study population was 12.85. Though the ESS score was more in non-type D patients, the difference was statistically insignificant (Table 1). Further analysis of polysomnography revealed that 7.2% had mild OSA, 18.8% had moderate OSA and 72.5% subjects had severe OSA (Table 1).

CPAP is the gold standard treatment for OSA and was offered to all patients after diagnosis. Although 79.7% (n=55) subjects agreed to CPAP usage, 75.4% (n=52) actually initiated therapy. Only 43.5% (n=30) of the entire sample (n=69) were identified as having a good compliance indicating poor adherence to therapy in the majority.

Though a comparable number of patients in both groups initially agreed to use CPAP, 83.3% non-Type D patients started using CPAP after recommendation compared with 72.5% of Type D OSA patients

(Table 1). All non-Type D OSA patients (15/15) agreed for CPAP therapy actually started therapy compared to 92.5% (37/40) Type D OSA patients. Among the total CPAP users (n=52), 42.3% (n=22) had poor CPAP compliance while 30 patients had good CPAP compliance. Interestingly, all 22 non-compliant patients had Type D personality while all 15 non-Type D patients who accepted CPAP were compliant. This exhibits lack of self-care behavior in type D patients. Finally, 56.5% (n=39) of all OSA patients (n=69) had poor CPAP acceptability and/or compliance of which 92.3% (n=36) had Type D personality. Type D OSA patients had a higher tendency to reject CPAP use and be non-complaint if initially accepting CPAP (70.6%) compared to 16.7% non-type D CPAP users (p=0.0). Therefore, overall, Type D personality was significantly associated with poor acceptance and/or compliance of CPAP (p<0.0).

Discussion

The present study found that there is a high prevalence of distressed personality in Indian patients with OSA. Additionally, distressed personality is associated with poor acceptability of CPAP therapy and subsequent CPAP adherence. Factors influencing CPAP adherence are varied and no individual factor has been found to have a consistent causal relationship with CPAP adherence [11-15]. At the present time, there are no studies conducted in Indian subcontinent throwing light on prevalence of type D in general population and/or patients with specific diseases. This study highlights the high frequency of distressed personality in OSA and associated poor CPAP compliance.

Type D across age, gender and marital status

Significant age difference was found across the two groups. It was seen that majority of the distressed personality patients were older than non-distressed patients (p=0.08). No statistically significant difference was found in gender and marital status indicating that type D personality affects both genders in a similar manner irrespective of marital status. Although our results are in accordance with Brostrom et al. [15] it is difficult to draw conclusions because of lack of literature on Indian population.

Distressed personality in Indian patients with OSA

The present study indicates a positive association between distressed personality and OSA. We found that approximately three-fourth of OSA patients examined possessed distressed personality. These results are consistent with prevalence data for other medical conditions such as cardiovascular disease [27]. Brostrom et al. from Sweden found 30% incidence of type D personality in OSA patients [15]. This highlights a much higher rate of prevalence of distressed personality in Indian patients with OSA as compared to other populations. Possible mechanisms of this higher prevalence rate can be attributed to the higher prevalence of psychiatric disorders with prominent somatic and emotional features, and sleeplessness arising from stressful, mechanical and sedentary lifestyle of people in the metropolis. Most importantly, this problem is magnified with the present status of sleep medicine in India. It is still an emerging branch of medicine where sleep disorders largely remaining un-diagnosed and undertreated and the general population has poor health seeking behaviors [8].

Type D and clinical outcomes

A positive correlation between distressed personality and severe negative clinical outcomes has been reported in a number of studies [21-25]. Various studies on possible mechanisms behind type D personality have given birth to the understanding that Type D not only increases vulnerability for negative clinical outcomes in cardiovascular patients but also negatively affect the prognosis of other medical conditions like melanoma, mild brain injury and vertigo [23-25]. Studies on Type D among cardiovascular patients have shown that Type D is an independent predictor of negative outcomes such as poor health status, (recurrent) myocardial infarction and increased risk of mortality [19]. Our study supports these findings as majority of OSA patients had distressed personality, more so in the subgroup found to have non-compliance.

Type D and self-care behavior

We found that 79.7% (n=55) OSA patients examined, agreed for CPAP therapy whereas 14 (20.3%) decided against it (p=0.747). Further analysis revealed that 75.4% (n=52) actually initiated the treatment and the number for those who did not start the treatment, increased to 17 (24.6%). Majority (n=14) of these patients belonged to type D group though the difference was statistically insignificant (Table 1). However, this finding is considered important as it throws light on the pattern of self-management of these patients. Lack of motivation and display of avoidance behavior leads to self-neglected medical care, adverse clinical outcomes and poor prognosis. Behavioral mechanisms attached with distressed personality such as an unhealthy lifestyle and reluctance to consult medical staff may be directly linked to this behavior pattern and consequently negative clinical outcomes. Findings from this study are in sync with previous studies on cardiovascular and non-cardiovascular population [28-30].

Refusal rate for CPAP therapy

In our study, we found that 79.7% patients diagnosed with OSA, agreed for CPAP therapy. We did not find any significant role of type D personality in making this decision. However, 24.6% patients subsequently did not start CPAP treatment. All those rejecting therapy possessed distressed personality while those with non-type D accepted CPAP therapy. Many OSA patients terminate CPAP treatment at an earlier stage. Rolfe et al. reported that 90% of CPAP treatment interruptions happened within the first 4 months [31]. Weaver et al. showed that the pattern of CPAP use is determined in the first week of treatment and remains stable after that time [32]. Patients skipping nights of treatment also use CPAP for shorter nightly duration [12]. The rate of rejection of CPAP therapy amongst OSA patients in our study is in accordance with an earlier study which observed that 5-50% rejected CPAP before or during titration [33].

Association of type D and CPAP adherence

Our study revealed that at the end of follow up, 30 participants were CPAP compliant (15 in both groups) whereas 22 failed to use CPAP for minimum of 4 hrs/d for atleast 5 days/week. All 22 CPAP non-compliant patients possessed type D personality. These findings are in accordance with that in previous studies [23]. Brostrom et al. showed that patients with Type D personality had significantly higher complaints of adverse events with CPAP therapy and reported a higher rate of continued sleepiness than non-type D personalities, despite comparable level of disease severity. Results showed 50% of patients with type D personality used their CPAP less than 4 hours per night compared to 16% of non-type D patients tested [14]. This amounted to a significantly lower objective adherence (p<0.001) for OSA patients with Type D than those without Type D, both with respect to mean use of 4 hours per night and 85% self-rated sleep time per night [14].

Limitation

This prospective exploratory study does not allow us to confer a causal relationship but provides us a preliminary understanding of distressed personality and CPAP compliance. The enrolment of consecutive cases visiting a tertiary care hospital in the National Capital Region of India and predominantly including middle to high socioeconomic status patients could have led to a selection bias. Other potential factors for CPAP noncompliance such as mask discomfort were not studied as the study only focused on distressed personality. It is difficult to establish a clear relationship between distressed personality and CPAP adherence because of the influence of pre-existing medical or other psychological conditions because of the scope of the study. Also, the bed partner's preference and perceived benefits were not taken into consideration.

Conclusion

Despite CPAP being the treatment of choice in most cases of OSA, treatment adherence rates are low. The present study suggests the benefits of evaluating for psychological variables like patients' personality, understanding of illness, attitudes and beliefs towards their medical condition. As depression is also known to be associated with poor compliance, assessment for psychological disorders, especially depression and anxiety at the initiation of treatment can be beneficial. Apart from this, behavioral modification, counselling and early patient and partner education regarding knowledge about OSA and CPAP, its benefits and expectations can be useful. Also, regular follow ups with the psychologist and sleep specialists with telemonitoring if possible can be effective for identifying treatment problems and adherence early in the course. This would facilitate screening of non-complaint patients as also enable to formulate an individualized approach aimed at helping the patient adapt to this demanding treatment before and after the initiation of CPAP therapy and consequently, increase the likelihood of treatment adherence.

Acknowledgement

We would like to thank all the participants for their cooperation.

References

1. Peppard PE, Young T, Palta M, Skatrud J (2000) Prospective study of the association between sleep disordered breathing and hypertension. N Eng J Med 342: 1378-1384.
2. Coughlin SR, Mawdsley L, Mugarza JA, Calverley PM, Wilding JP (2004) Obstructive sleep apnea is independently associated with an increased prevalence of metabolic syndrome. Eur Heart J 25: 735-741.
3. Shahar E, Whitney CW, Redline S, Lee ET, Newman AB, et al. (2001) Sleep –disordered breathing and cardiovascular disease: cross sectional results of the sleep heart health study. Am J Resp Crit Care Med 163: 19-25.
4. Sharafkhaneh A, Giray N, Richardson P, Young T, Hirshkowitz M (2005) Association of psychiatric disorders and sleep apnea in a large cohort. Sleep 28: 1405-1411.
5. Ohayon MM (2003) The effects of breathing-related sleep disorders on mood disturbances in the general population. J Clin Psychiatry 64: 1195-1200.
6. American Academy of Sleep Medicine Task Force (1999) Sleep-related breathing disorders in adults: Recommendation for syndrome definition and measurement techniques in clinical research. Sleep 22: 667-689.
7. Reddy EV, Kadhiravan T, Mishra HK, Sreenivas V, Handa KK, et al. (2009) Prevalence and risk factors of obstructive sleep apnea among middle-aged urban Indians: a community-based study. Sleep Med 10: 913-918.
8. Panda S, Taly AB, Sinha S, Gururaj G, Girish N, et al. (2012) Sleep related disorders among healthy population in South India. Neurology India 60: 68-74.
9. D'Ambrosio C, Bowman T, Mohsenin V (1999) Quality of life in patients with obstructive sleep apnea: effect of nasal continuous airway pressure-a prospective study. Chest 115: 123-129.
10. Sabate, E (2003) Adherence to Long-Term Therapies: Evidence for Action. WHO Publications, Geneva.
11. Haniffa M, Lasserson T, Smith I (2004) Interventions to improve compliance with continuous positive airway pressure for obstructive sleep apnoea. Cochrane Database Syst 18: CD003531.
12. Weaver TE, Grunstein RR (2008) Adherence to Continuous Positive Airway Pressure Therapy. The challenges to effective treatment. Proc Am Thorac Soc 5: 173-178.
13. Gay P, Weaver T, Loube D, Iber C (2006) Positive Airway Pressure Task Force; Standards of Practice Committee; American Academy of SleepMedicine. Evaluation of positive airway pressure treatment for sleep related breathing disorders in adults. Sleep 29: 381-401.
14. Budhiraja R, Parthasarathy S, Drake CL (2007) Early CPAP use identifies subsequent adherence to CPAP therapy. Sleep 30: 320-324.
15. Brostrom A, Stromberg A, Martensson J, Ulander M, Harder L, et al. (2007) Association of Type D personality to perceived side effects and adherence in CPAP-treated patients with OSAS. J Sleep Res 16: 439-447.
16. Law M, Naughton M, Ho S, Roebuck T, Dabscheck E (2014) Depression may reduce adherence during CPAP titration trial. J Clin Sleep Med 10: 163-169.
17. Denollet J (2005) DS14: standard assessment of negative affectivity, social inhibition, and Type D personality. Psychosom. Med 67: 89-97.
18. Denollet J, Vaes J, Brutsaert DL (2000) Inadequate response to treatment in coronary heart disease: adverse effects of Type D personality and younger age on 5-year prognosis and quality of life. Circulation 102: 630-635.
19. Martens EJ, Mols F, Burg MM, Denollet J (2009) Type D personality predicts clinical events after myocardial infarction, above and beyond disease severity and depression. J Clin Psychiatry 71: 778-783.
20. Pedersen SS, Denollet J (2006) Is Type D personality here to stay? Emerging evidence across cardiovascular disease patient groups. Curr Cardiol Rev 2: 205-213.
21. Denollet J, Schiffer AA, Spek V (2010) A general propensity to psychological distress affects cardiovascular outcomes: evidence from research on the Type D (distressed) personality profile. Circ Cardiovasc Qual Outcomes 3: 546-557.
22. Pedersen SS, Denollet J (2004) Validity of the Type D personality construct in Danish post-MI patients and healthy controls. J Psychosom Res 57: 265-272.
23. Mols F, Holterhues C, Nijsten T, Van de Poll-Franse LV (2010) Personality is associated with health status and impact of cancer among melanoma survivors. Eur J Cancer 46: 573-580.
24. Stulemeijer M, Andriessen TM, Brauer JM, Vos PE, Van Der Werf S (2007) Cognitive performance after mild traumatic brain injury: the impact of poor effort on test results and its relation to distress, personality and litigation. Brain Inj 21: 309-318.
25. De Valck CFJ, Denollet J, Wuyts FL, van de Heyning PH (2007) Increased handicap in vertigo patients with a Type D personality. Audiological Medicine 5: 169-175.
26. Johns MW (1991) A new method for measuring daytime sleepiness: The Epworth Sleepiness Scale. Sleep 14: 540-545.

6. Ipsiroglu OS, McKellin WH, Carey N, Loock C (2013) "They silently live in terrorâ€¦" why sleep problems and night-time related quality-of-life are missed in children with a fetal alcohol spectrum disorder. Soc Sci Med 79: 76-83.
7. Clark CP, Gillin JC, Golshan S, Demodena A, Smith TL, et al. (1998) Increased REM sleep density at admission predicts relapse by three months in primary alcoholics with a lifetime diagnosis of secondary depression. Biol Psychiatry 43:601-607.
8. Brower KJ (2003) Insomnia, alcoholism and relapse. Sleep Med Rev 7: 523-539.
9. Manni R, Ratti PL, Terzaghi M (2011) Secondary "incidental" REM sleep behavior disorder: do we ever think of it? Sleep Med 12 Suppl 2: S50-53.
10. Nettleton S, Neale J, Pickering L (2011) Techniques and transitions: a sociological analysis of sleeping practices amongst recovering heroin users. Soc Sci Med 72: 1367-1373.
11. Pud D, Zlotnick C, Lawental E (2012) Pain depression and sleep disorders among methadone maintenance treatment patients. Addict Behav 37: 1205-1210.
12. Matuskey D, Pittman B, Forselius E, Malison RT, Morgan PT (2011) A multistudy analysis of the effects of early cocaine abstinence on sleep. Drug Alcohol Depend 115: 62-66.
13. Morgan PT, Malison RT (2007) Cocaine and sleep: early abstinence. ScientificWorldJournal 7: 223-230.
14. Boscolo-Berto R, Viel G, Montagnese S, Raduazzo DI, Ferrara SD, et al. (2012) Narcolepsy and effectiveness of gamma-hydroxybutyrate (GHB): a systematic review and meta-analysis of randomized controlled trials. Sleep Med Rev 16: 431-443.
15. Reyes-Vázquez C, Prieto-Gómez B, Dafny N (2012) Interferon modulates central nervous system function. Brain Res 1442: 76-89.
16. Lauer CJ, Krieg JC (1998) Slow-wave sleep and ventricular size: a comparative study in schizophrenia and major depression. Biol Psychiatry 44: 121-128.
17. Wu JC, Gillin JC, Buchsbaum MS, Schachat C, Darnall LA, et al. (2008) Sleep deprivation PET correlations of Hamilton symptom improvement ratings with changes in relative glucose metabolism in patients with depression. J Affect Disord 107: 181-186.
18. Schouw ML, Gevers S, Caan MW, Majoie CB, Booij J, et al. (2012) Mapping serotonergic dysfunction in MDMA (ecstasy) users using pharmacological MRI. Eur Neuropsychopharmacol 22: 537-545.
19. Cox SM, Benkelfat C, Dagher A, Delaney JS, Durand F, et al. (2011). Effects of lowered serotonin transmission on cocaine-induced striataldopamine response: PET [^{11}C]raclopride study in humans.Br J Psychiatry 199:391-397.
20. Hvolby A, Jørgensen JI, Bilenberg N (2005) [Sleeping disorders can imitate attention deficit/hyperactivity disorder]. Ugeskr Laeger 167: 3893-3894.
21. Khurshid KA, Khan AA (2009) Delayed sleep phase disorder and attention deficit and hyperactivity symptoms in a teenager. Atten Defic Hyperact Disord 1: 211-213.
22. Holst SC, Bersagliere A, Bachmann V, Berger W, Achermann P, et al. (2014) Dopaminergic role in regulating neurophysiological markers of sleep homeostasis in humans. J Neurosci 34: 566-573.
23. Landolt HP (2011) Genetic determination of sleep EEG profiles in healthy humans. Prog Brain Res 193: 51-61.
24. Guindalini C, Martins RC, Andersen ML, Tufik S (2010) Influence of genotype on dopamine transporter availability in human striatum and sleep architecture. Psychiatry Res 179: 238-240.
25. Bodenmann S, Rusterholz T, Dürr R, Stoll C, Bachmann V, et al. (2009) The functional Val158Met polymorphism of COMT predicts interindividual differences in brain alpha oscillations in young men. J Neurosci 29: 10855-10862.
26. Benedetti F, Barbini B, Bernasconi A, Fulgosi MC, Dallaspezia S, et al. (2010) Acute antidepressant response to sleep deprivation combined with light therapy is influenced by the catechol-O-methyltransferase Val(108/158)Metpolymorphism. J Affect Disord 121:68-72.
27. Brummett BH, Krystal AD, Siegler IC, Kuhn C, Surwit RS, et al. (2007) Associations of a regulatory polymorphism of monoamine oxidase-A gene promoter (MAOA-uVNTR) with symptoms of depression and sleep quality. Psychosom Med 69: 396-401.
28. Darlington TM, Ehringer MA, Larson C, Phang TL, Radcliffe RA (2013) Transcriptome analysis of Inbred Long Sleep and Inbred Short Sleep mice. Genes Brain Behav 12: 263-274.
29. Mendlewicz J (2009) Disruption of the circadian timing systems: molecular mechanisms in mood disorders. CNS Drugs 23 Suppl 2: 15-26.
30. Yang HS, Shimomura K, Vitaterna MH, Turek FW (2012) High-resolution mapping of a novel genetic locus regulating voluntary physical activity in mice. Genes Brain Behav 11: 113-124.
31. Xie L, Kang H, Xu Q, Chen MJ, Liao Y, et al. (2013) Sleep drives metabolite clearance from the adult brain. Science 342: 373-377.

3

Effect of Continuous Positive Airway Pressure Treatment on Hemograms of Patients with Severe Obstructive Sleep Apnea in the Lack of Comorbidities

Ozge oral Tapan*, Begum Gorgulu, Kemal Can Tertemiz, Aylin Ozgen Alpaydin, Ibrahim Oztura, Oya Itil and Baris Baklan

Department of Chest Disease, Dokuz Eylul Universitesi Tip Fakultesi, Turkey

***Corresponding author:** Ozge oral Tapan, Department of Chest Disease, Dokuz Eylul Universitesi Tip Fakultesi, Turkey, E-mail: ozgeeoral@hotmail.com

Abstract

In this study, we aimed to evaluate the effect of CPAP treatment on hemograms of patients with severe OSA in the lack of comorbidities which might affect the real values of hematological parameters.

This retrospective cohort study patients selected from those whose polysomnography reports were compatible with severe OSAS and who underwent PAP titration in our sleep medicine department. 49 patients were enrolled to the study. The baseline hemograms of the participants were collected from one of the patients' visits before they started to use CPAP devices. The control hemograms were evaluated from one of the control visits in the first six months of treatment. We examined the red cell distribution width (RDW), mean platelet volume (MPV), hemotocrit (Hct) and platelet (Plt) count from the hemograms.

The mean age was 58.2 years ± 11.3 years, 38.8% were female and 61.2% were male. 69.4% were non-smokers and 30.6% were ex-smokers. The mean body mass index (BMI) was 31.6 ± 5.8 while the mean apnea hypopnea index (AHI) was 50.2 ± 29. The mean duration of CPAP therapy was 4.8 months ± 3.3 months. The mean RDW, MPV, Hct and Plt count values before CPAP treatment were in normal ranges of laboratory tests. All of the values reduced after CPAP therapy but only the decrease in MPV was statistically significant.

The reduced values supported that CPAP treatment helped to control hypercoagulability and prevented from cardiovascular disorders in OSAS. Hemogram may be a cheap and easily found laboratory test for monitoring the response to CPAP therapy.

Keywords: Continuous positive airway pressure; Hemograms; Severe obstructive sleep apnea

Introduction

Obstructive sleep apnea syndrome (OSAS) is characterized by repetitive episodes of total or partial upper airway obstruction that occur during sleep, usually associated with a reduction in blood oxygen saturation and arousals from sleep. Intermittent hypoxemia, sympathetic nervous system hyperactivity, oxidative stress, vascular endothelial dysfunction and metabolic dysregulation cause the systemic inflammation that underlies OSAS and its complications. Cardiovascular disorders are the most important cause of morbidity and mortality in OSAS [1]. Hypercoagulability was reported to be associated with cardiovascular complications [2,3]. Mean platelet volume (MPV) indicates platelet activation but does not notice any spesific disease [4]. It was found to be significantly higher in patients with severe OSAS [5]. MPV may increase in other diseases such as hypercholesterolemia, diabetes mellitus, hypertension, ischemic stroke, myocardial infarction and smoking [6-8]. Red blood cell distribution width (RDW) is a laboratory measure of size variability and heterogeneity of erythrocytes. Also RDW contributes to platelet activation [9]. In several studies the association between hematological parameters such as RDW, MPV and platelet distribution width (PDW) and OSAS severity has been investigated [10-13]. Since continuous positive airway pressure (CPAP) is accepted as the gold standard therapy for OSAS, the effect of CPAP treatment on these hematological parameters in OSAS was demonstrated in some studies [14,15]. To our knowledge the comorbidities that might affect the real value of hematological parameters have not been excluded in these recent studies.

In this study, we aimed to evaluate the effect of CPAP treatment on hemograms of patients with severe OSA in the lack of comorbidities which might affect the real values of hematological parameters. In the other hand we tried to find out if a simple and a cheap test as hemogram could be used for monitoring the regular use of CPAP devices in severe OSA patients.

Methods

This retrospective cohort study protocol was approved by the institutional review committee on clinical research of the Dokuz Eylul University Faculty of Medicine, Turkey. Patients selected from those whose polysomnography reports were compatible with severe OSAS (AHI>30) and who underwent PAP titration in our sleep medicine department. We used the polysomnography and CPAP titration reports which were scored according to the American Academy of Sleep Medicine (AASM). The major inclusion criteria for this study was using the CPAP device for >4 h/day and >5 days/week during at least 1 month. Patients who were non-smokers or ex-smokers for at least 12 months included. Patients with comorbidities such as hypertension, diabetes mellitus, hypercholesterolemia, hematological diseases, chronic obstructive pulmonary disease and asthma were excluded. We reached the data of 94 severe OSA patients. 35 had several comorbidities. 7 were active smoker. 3 had to use antiagreagans for a while. 49 patients were enrolled to the study. Hematological parameters of the patients were collected from the laboratory records of our hospital. The baseline hemograms of the participants were collected from one of the patients' visits before they started to use CPAP devices. The control hemograms of the subjects were evaluated from one of the control visits in the first six months of CPAP treatment. We examined the red cell distribution width (RDW), mean platelet volume (MPV), hemotocrit (Hct) and platelet (Plt) count from the hemograms. We called the patients one by one to be sure if they used their CPAP devices regularly and did not use any drugs such as acetyl salicylic acid, clopidogrel, dipiradamol, heparin, aminophylline, verapamil, nonsteroidal anti-inflammatory drugs, corticosteroids, furosemide, and antibiotics which may affect the platelet function.

Statistical analyses were performed with the Statistical Package for the Social Sciences (SPSS Inc., Chicago, IL, USA) version 22 software package. All the values were calculated as the mean ± standard deviation. We used paired sample t-test to compare the pre- and post-treatment data of the study group.

Results

Of all the participants, the mean age was 58.2 years ± 11.3 years, 38.8% (n=19) were female and 61.2% (n=40) were male. 69.4% (n=34) were non-smokers and 30.6% (n=15) were ex-smokers. The mean pack years of cigarette smoking was 30.4 ± 15.8 in ex-smokers. The mean body mass index (BMI) was 31.6 ± 5.8 while the mean apnea hypopnea index (AHI) was 50.2 ± 29.1 and the mean minimum oxygen saturation (Min. SpO_2) was 74.2 ± 9.8. The mean duration of CPAP therapy was 4.8 months ± 3.3 months. Demographic and polisomnographic characteristics of the patients are summarized in Table 1.

Variables	n=49 (%)
Age, years (mean ± SD)	58.2 ± 11.3
Gender	
Female	19 (38.8)
Male	30 (61.2)
BMI, kg/m^2 (mean ± SD)	31.6 ± 5.8
Non-smoker	34 (69.4)
Ex-smoker	15 (30.6)
Pack years of cigarette smoking (mean ± SD)	30.4 ± 15.8
AHI, event/h (mean ± SD)	50.2 ± 29.1
Lowest SpO_2, % (mean ± SD)	74.2 ± 9.8
Duration of CPAP therapy, months (mean ± SD)	5.8 ± 3.3

SD: standard deviation; BMI: body mass index;
AHI: apnea hypopnea index; Lowest SpO_2: minimum oxygen saturation

Table 1: Demographic and polisomnographic characteristics of patients.

The mean RDW, MPV, Hct and Plt count values before CPAP treatment were in normal ranges of laboratory tests. As known, normal range values of Hct between female and male are declared differently in hemograms. Mean Hct values were 39.7% ± 5.6% (36% to 46%) in female, 41.9% ± 3.7% (41% to 53%) in male. The mean Hct and Plt values did not show any significant change after CPAP treatment ($p>0.05$). Normal range values of RDW (11.8% to 14.3 %), MPV (6.9fl to 10.8 fl) and Plt (15610^3/μl to 373 10^3/μl) were the same for female and male. Of all patients the mean RDW and MPV values were 14.6% ± 1.5%, 9.15 fl ± 1.2 fl before CPAP while the mean RDW and MPV values were 14.4% ± 1.6%, 8.9 fl ± 1.3 fl after CPAP. Mean RDW, MPV, Hct and Plt count values reduced after CPAP therapy but only the decrease in MPV was statistically significant ($p<0.05$). Results of comparison of patients' hematological parameters before and after CPAP treatment are presented in Table 2.

	Before CPAP	After CPAP	p
RDW, % (mean ± SD)	14.6 ± 1.5	14.4 ± 1.6	0.37
MPV, fl (mean ± SD)	9.15 ± 1.2	8.9 ± 1.3	0.02
Hct, % (mean ± SD)	41.4 ± 4.5	41.3 ± 4.2	0.35
Plt count, 10^3/μl (mean ± SD)	243.8 ± 56.8	241.8 ± 65.4	0.76

CPAP: continuous positive airway pressure; RDW: red cell distribution width; SD: standard deviation, MPV: mean platelet volume; Hct: hemotocrit; Plt: platelet

Table 2: Hematological data of patients before and after CPAP.

Discussion

In this study, the hematological parameters related to hypercoagulability such as RDW, MPV, Hct and Plt of severe OSA patients without any comorbidity were in normal range values before CPAP treatment. We demonstrated that RDW, MPV (p: 0.02), Hct and Plt count parameters reduced in the first 6 months of CPAP therapy. The reduced values supported that CPAP treatment helped to control hypercoagulability and prevented from cardiovascular disorders in OSAS.

The importance of sleep to health and cardiovascular disease is well known. In several studies it has been shown that repetitive episodes of hypoxia and reoxygenation during sleep provoked platelet activation and/or systemic inflammation and platelet activation might lead to hypercoagulability and cardiovascular disease in OSAS [10,16-19]. Platelets with high volume are metabolically and enzymatically more active and secrete more mediators [20,21]. Varol et al. [5] reported an increasement in MPV levels of OSA patients and Erden et al. [13] claimed a positive correlation between MPV and AHI. But Kurt et al. [10] did not found any correlation between MPV and the severity of OSAS. It has been shown that smoking activated platelet function [22]. Also Topcuoglu et al. [23] showed that MPV did not indicate OSAS severity in the absence of comorbidities. Similarly, we did not found an abnormality in the mean MPV of our severe OSA patients without any comorbidity which were claimed to affect platelet activation.

Oxidative stress and inflammation were shown to be linked to RDW [24]. Inflammation is related to ineffective erythropoiesis. Inflammatory cytokine production desensities bone marrow erythroid progenitors to erythropoiesis, inhibits red blood cell maturation and promotes anisocytosis [25]. Several studies tried to explain the association between RDW and the severity of inflamatory diseases such as cardiovascular and pulmonary diseases [26,27]. Ozsu et al. [11] demonstrated that RDW values of OSA patients were higher than controls and they found an association between RDW and severity of OSAS. They reported that RDW associated with cardiovascular disorders in OSA patients. However, Kurt and Yildiz [10] did not show any correlation between RDW and AHI. The mean RDW of our severe OSA patients without comorbidities was in the normal range value before treatment. Our finding supports that the RDW levels increase in the OSA patients with cardiovascular disorders.

Saygin et al. [28] found a significant increase in Plt count with the severity of OSAS. In their study the Plt value correlated with AHI in the patients <40 years old with cardiovascular disease and in the patients ≥ 40 years old without cardiovascular comorbidities. Their patients with cardiovascular diseases had higher hematocrit correlated with the severity of OSAS. Hct is expressed as the per cent of a blood sample occupied by intact red blood cell. It affects blood viscosity and platelet aggregation.

Hct may be an indicator of inflammation and oxidative stress in OSAS. Karakas et al. [29] did not found any correlations between AHI and Hct. But the mechanisms of Plt activation in patients with OSAS may be the chronic intermittent hypoxia and high levels of catecholamines which is a result of sympathetic activity [30-32]. Minogluchi et al. [33] reported that the levels of sCD40L and sP-selectin which were known as Plt activation markers increased in patients with moderate and severe OSAS. Hui at al. [19] found a positive correlation between Plt and AHI. The mean values of Hct and Plt count were in normal range in our severe OSA patients. These results might change if they have been compared with a healty control group. This was one of the limitations of our study.

CPAP therapy is still the most effective treatment for patients with OSAS. CPAP relieves airway obstruction and reduces hypoxia and inflammation [34]. CPAP treatment decreases platelet aggregability [35]. Several studies demonstrated the increase in blood viscosity before and the decrease after CPAP treatment [36,37]. Varol et al. [38] showed that 6 months of CPAP therapy reduced MPV values of severe OSA patients but they found platelet counts higher than baseline. Sokucu et al. [14] reported that 6 months of CPAP therapy significantly decreased MPV value but increased RDW. Feliciano et al. [39] showed that RDW significantly decreased after PAP treatment. We also found a decrease in the mean RDW value of our patients after treatment. Sokucu et al. [14] did not find any significant difference in platelet count between OSA group and controls after 6 months of CPAP treatment. Feliciano et al. [39] also reported a significant decrease in platelet count of 48 male OSA patients (18 mild, 5 moderate, 25 severe) after 6 months of CPAP therapy. Similar to Feliciano at al. the mean platelet count value of our study patients decreased after CPAP treatment but this was not statistically significant. The severity of OSAS is associated with increased Hct but it does not present as polycythemia [40]. Khan et al. [41] showed a significant increase in Hct after 1 year of CPAP therapy in elderly OSA patients. Their claim was that hypoxic stimulation of erythropoiesis might obscure anemia of aging in OSA patients over 65 years, and CPAP treatment restored this anemia. In our patient's avarage age 58.2, Hct values decreased in the first 6 months of CPAP treatment but it was not at the anemia limit.

There are some limitations of our study such as small sample size and the lack of control group. It was a retrospective study and we observed the hemograms that were analyzed in the first 6 months visit after CPAP treatment initiation. We standardized the CPAP treatment period at least 1 month.

Conclusion

The reducements in both MPV and blood viscosity with CPAP may protect from cardiovascular complications associated with OSAS. Hemogram may be a cheap and easily found laboratory test for monitoring the response to CPAP therapy of OSA patients. Further prospective cohort studies with large sample sizes will help to use hemograms in routine controls for CPAP therapy compliance.

References

1. American Academy of Sleep Medicine (2005) International classification of sleep disorders, version 2: Diagnostic coding manual.
2. E Solh AA, Akinnusi ME, Baddoura FH, Mankowski CR (2007) Endothelial cell apoptosis in obstructive sleep apnea: A link to endothelial dysfunction. Am J Respir Crit Care Med 175: 1186-1191.
3. Jelic S, Padeletti M, Kawut SM, Higgins C, Canfield SM, et al. (2008) Inflammation, oxidative stress, and repair capacity of the vascular endothelium in obstructive sleep apnea. Circulation 117: 2270-2278.
4. Vagdatli E, Gounari E, Lazaridou E, Katsibouurlia E, Tsikopoulou F, at al. (2010) Platelet distribution width: A simple, practical and spesific marker of activation of coagulation. Hippokratia 14: 28-32.
5. Varol E, Ozturk O, Gonca T, Has M, Ozaydin M, et al. (2010) Mean platelet volume is increased in patients with severe obstructive sleep apnea. Scand J Clin Lab Invest 70: 497-502.
6. Yazici A, Kaya A, Kaya Y, Albayrak S, Cinemre H, et al. (2009) Lifestyle modification decreases the mean platelet volume in prehypertensive patients. Platelets 20: 58-63.
7. Bath PM, Butterworth RJ (1996) Platelet size: Measurement, physiology and vascular disease. Blood Coagul Fibrinolysis 7: 157-161.
8. Hekimsoy Z, Payzin B, Ornek T, KandoÄŸan G (2004) Mean platelet volume in Type 2 diabetic patients. J Diabetes Complications 18: 173-176.
9. Patel KV, Ferrucci L, Ershler WB, Longo DL, Guralnik JM (2009) Red blood cell distribution width and the risk of death in middle-aged and older adults. Arch Intern Med 169: 515-523.
10. Kurt OK, Yildiz N (2013) The importance of laboratory parameters in patients with obstructive sleep apnea syndrome. Blood Coagul Fibrinol 24: 371-374.
11. Ozsu S, Abul Y, Gulsoy A, Bulbul Y, Yaman S, et al. (2012) Red cell distribution width in patients with obstructive sleep apnea syndrome. Lung 190: 319-326.
12. Sökücü SN, Karasulu L, Dalar L, Seyhan EC, Altın S (2012) Can red blood cell distribution width predict severity of obstructive sleep apnea syndrome? J Clin Sleep Med 8: 521-525.
13. Erden ES, Yengil E, Tuncel E, Kayim Bilgic H, Demirkose M, et al. (2013) Investigation of the relationship between mean platelet volume and obstructive sleep apnea syndrome. JCEI 4: 492-496.
14. Sokucu SN, Ozdemir C, Dalar L, Karasulu L, Aydin S, et al. (2014) Complete blood count alterations after six months of continuous positive airway pressure treatment in patients with severe obstructive sleep apnea. J Clin Sleep Med 10: 873-878.
15. Cortuk M, Simsek G, Kiraz K, Haytoglu S, Zitouni B, et al. (2016) Effect of Continuous Positive Airway Pressure Treatment on Mean Platelet Distribution Width in Patients with Sleep Apnea Syndrome. Eurasian J Pulmonol 18: 85-89.
16. Rahangdale S, Yeh SY, Novack V, Stevenson K, Barnard MR, et al. (2011) The influence of intermittent hypoxemia on platelet activation in obese patients with obstructive sleep apnea. J Clin Sleep Med 7: 172-178.
17. Waters KA, Mast BT, Vella S, O'Brien LM, Bailey S, et al. (2007) Structural equation modelling of sleep apnea, inflammation, and metabolic dysfunction in children. J Sleep Res 16: 388-395.

18. Geiser T, Buck F, Meyer BJ, Bassetti C, Haeberli A, et al. (2002) In vivo platelet activation is increased during sleep in patients with obstructive sleep apnea syndrome. Respiration 69: 229-234.
19. Hui DS, Ko FW, Fok JP (2004) The effects of nasal continuous positive airway pressure on platelet activation in obstructive sleep apnea syndrome. Chest 125: 1768-1775.
20. Karpatkin S (1969) Heterogeneity of human platelets. II. Functional evidence suggestive of young and old platelets. J Clin Invest 48: 1083-1087.
21. Gawaz M, Langer H, May AE (2005) Platelets in inflammation and atherogenesis. J Clin Invest 115: 3378-3384.
22. Varol E, Icli A, Kocyigit S, Erdogan D, Ozaydin M, et al. (2013) Effect of smoking cessation on mean platelet volume. Clin Appl Thromb Hemost 19: 315-319.
23. Topcuoglu OB, Cetintas G, Sarac S, Oruc O, Kuyucu T (2016) In the absence of co-morbidities mean platelet volume is not a severity indicator in OSAS. Eur J Gen Med 12: 134-138.
24. Kalay N, Aytekin M, Kaya MG, Ozbek K, KarayakalÄ M, et al. (2011) The relationship between inflammation and slow coronary flow: increased red cell distribution width and serum uric acid levels. Turk Kardiyol Dern Ars 39: 463-468.
25. Lattimore JD, Celermajer DS, Wilcox I (2003) Obstructive sleep apnea and cardiovascular disease. J Am Coll Cardiol 41: 1429-1437.
26. Isik T, Uyarel H, Tanboga IH, Kurt M, Ekinci M, et al. (2012) Relation of red cell distribution width with the presence, severity, and complexity of coronary artery disease. Coron Artery Dis 23: 51-56.
27. Hampole CV, Mehrotra AK, Thenappan T, Gomberg-Maitland M, Shah SJ (2009) Usefulness of red cell distribution width as a prognostic marker in pulmonary hypertension. Am J Cardiol 104: 868-872.
28. Saygin M, Ozturk O, Ozguner MF, Akkaya A, Varol E (2016) Hematological parameters as predictors of cardiovascular disease in obstructive sleep apnea syndrome patients. Angiology 67: 461-470.
29. Karakas MS, Altekin RE, Baktir AO, Ucar M, Altekin RE, et al. (2013) Association between mean platelet volume and severity of disease in patients with obstructive sleep apnea syndrome without risk factors for cardiovascular disease. Turk Kardiyol Dern Ars 41: 14-20.
30. Ziegler MG, Nelesen R, Mills P, Ancoli-Israel, Kennedy B, et al. (1997) Sleep apnea, norepinephrine release rate, and day-time hypertension. Sleep 20: 224-231.
31. Somers VK, Dyken ME, Clary MP, Abboud FM (1995) Sympathetic neural mechanisms in obstructive sleep apnea. J Clin Invest 96: 1897-1904.
32. von Känel R, Dimsdale JE (2000) Effects of sympathetic activation by adrenergic infusions on hemostasis in vivo. Eur J Haematol 65: 357-369.
33. Minoguchi K, Yokoe T, Tazaki T, Minoguchi H, Oda N, et al. (2007) Silent brain infarction and platelet activation in obstructive sleep apnea. Am J Respir Crit Care Med 175: 612-617.
34. KaramanlÄ H, Äzol D, Ugur KS, Yıldırım Z, Armutçu F, et al. (2014) Influence of CPAP treatment on airway and systemic inflammation in OSAS patients. Sleep Breath 18: 251-256.
35. Oga T, Chin K, Tabuchi A, Kawato M, Morimoto T, et al. (2009) Effects of obstructive sleep apnea with intermittent hypoxia on platelet aggregability. J Atheroscler Thromb 16: 862-869.
36. Dikmenoglu N, Ciftci B, Ileri E, Guven SF, Seringec N, at al. (2006) Erythrocyte deformability, plasma viscosity and oxidative status in patients with severe obstructive sleep apnea syndrome. Sleep Med 7: 255-261.
37. Tazbirek M, Slowinska L, Skoczynski S, Pierzchala W (2009) Short-term continuous positive airway pressure therapy reverses the pathological influence of obstructive sleep apnea on blood rheology parameters. Clin Hemorheol Microcirc 41: 241-249.
38. Varol E, Ozturk O, Yucel H, Gonca T, Has M, et al. (2011) The effects of continuous positive airway pressure therapy on mean platelet volume in patients with obstructive sleep apnea. Platelets 22: 552-556.
39. Feliciano A, Linhas A, Marçoa R, Cysneiros A, Martinho C, et al. (2017) Hematological evaluation in males with obstructive sleep apnea before and after positive airway pressure. Rev Port Pneumol 23: 71-78.
40. Choi JB, Loredo JS, Norman D, Mills PJ, Ancoli-Israel S, et al. (2006) Does obstructive sleep apnea increase hematocrit? Sleep Breath 10: 155-160.
41. Khan AM, Ashizawa S, Hlebowicz V, Appel DW (2011) Anemia of aging and obstructive sleep apnea. Sleep Breath 15: 29-34.

4

Electrophysiological Difference in Obstructive Sleep Apnea with and without REM sleep Behavior Disorder: Cardiopulmonary Coupling Analysis

Yun Kyung Park[1], **Su Jung Choi**[2] **and Eun Yeon Joo**[2,3*]

[1]*Department of Neurology, College of Medicine, Konyang University Hospital, Korea*
[2]*Department of Neurology, Neuroscience Center, Samsung Biomedical Research Institute, Samsung Medical Center, Sungkyunkwan University School of Medicine, Seoul, Korea*
[3]*Department of Health Sciences and Technology, SAIHST, Sungkyunkwan University, Seoul, Korea*

Abstract

Objectives: Although rapid eye movement behavior disorder (RBD) and obstructive sleep apnea syndrome (OSA) have different pathophysiology, RBD patients with OSA appeared to have more stable sleep compared to patients with OSA and to verify it by cardiopulmonary coupling (CPC) method.

Methods: The polysomnography (PSG) data of 138 subjects with OSA (AHI ≥ 15), RBD with OSA (AHI ≥ 15), RBD, normal control (N=32, 26, 29, 51, respectively) were collected. For conducting case control study between RBD with OSA and patients with OSA only, a total of 32 OSA controls, matched for age, AHI and BMI were recruited. CPC parameters were obtained using CPC analyzer in Rem Logic. Sleep spectrogram by CPC analyses revealed the percentage of stable tidal volume [high-frequency coupling (HFC), 0.1–0.4 Hz] and fluctuation tidal volume [low-frequency coupling (LFC), 0.01 Hz to 0.1 Hz)] during sleep.

Results: Although there was no significant Apnea-Hypopnea index (AHI) difference between RBD with OSA and OSA group (AHI 29.1 ± 15.6/hr *vs.* 34.1 ± 18.9, p=0.332), there was significant difference in CPC measurements. In RBD-OSA group showed lower LFC (35.9 ± 16.8 *vs.* 49.7 ± 21.3, p=0.010) than OSA group. Unlike higher AHI in RBD with OSA than RBD group (29.1 ± 15.6/hr *vs.* 3.2 ± 1.6, p<0.001), there was no significant difference in CPC study. Both OSA group and RBD with OSA group showed higher LFC (OSA *vs.* normal: 49.7 ± 21.3 *vs.* 28.4 ± 13.3, p<0.001, RBD with OSA *vs.* normal: 35.9 ± 16.8 *vs.* 28.4 ± 13.2 p=0.035) and lower HFC (OSA *vs.* normal: 37.5 ± 20.0 *vs.* 56.2 ± 16.2, p<0.001, RBD with OSA *vs.* normal: 46.8 ± 20.8 *vs.* 56.2 ± 16.2, p=0.031) when compared with normal control group, respectively.

Conclusions: In terms of autonomic-respiratory interaction, RBD with OSA showed similar CPC profile (higher LFC and lower HFC than normal) to OSA group but less severe than pure OSA group. It suggests that RBD may have a protective effect on OSA.

Keywords: Rapid eye movement behavior disorder; Obstructive sleep apnea syndrome; Cardiopulmonary coupling analysis

Introduction

Rapid eye movement sleep behavior disorder (RBD) is characterized by loss of normal skeletal muscle atonia during rapid eye movement (REM) sleep, in association with abnormal motor behavior while dreaming. Patients with RBD exhibit increased phasic or tonic muscle activity seen on electromyogram channels during polysomnography [1]. The prevalence of RBD has not been well researched yet, but previous epidemiological studies of RBD suggested that RBD is not rare in the elderly, with prevalence estimates of 0.38% to 2.01% in the elderly population [2,3]. However, these dream-enacting behaviors can also occur in other sleep disorders, a clinical situation termed as "pseudo-RBD" [4]. Abnormal sleep behavior can occur in patients with obstructive sleep apnea (OSA), Iranzo et al. described a group of 16 patients with severe OSA who reported harmful dream-enacting behaviors resembling RBD, but in whom PSG failed to demonstrate REM sleep without atonia [5]. OSA is a highly prevalent disease characterized by recurrent episodes of upper airway obstruction that result in recurrent arousals and episodic oxyhemoglobin desaturation during sleep. OSA and RBD have different pathophysiologic substrates. While RBD is thought to reflect dysfunction of the brainstem structures that modulate REM sleep, OSA is caused by various factors such as impaired upper airway anatomy and pharyngeal dilator muscle activity, neural control of the pharyngeal muscles, respiratory arousal threshold and stability of the respiratory control system [1,6,7]. There were several studies dealt with RBD and OSA, mostly severe OSA as a disguiser of pseudo-RBD [5,8]. But there were few studies to assess if the sum of conflicting reaction resulted in lower severity of OSA, considering the opposite action on muscle activity. Huang et al. reported that patients with RBD and OSA presented shorter duration of apneas and hypopneas during REM than NREM sleep [9]. Although the previous study revealed excessive EMG activity associated with RBD probably protected from long apneas shorter respiratory events and less REM sleep-related exacerbation, could not disclose the impact of RBD with OSA on overall sleep stability. Cardiopulmonary coupling (CPC) analysis is an uncomplicated and inexpensive method, which is ECG-based method to assess sleep stability and phenotype of sleep apnea based solely on the continuous electrocardiogram (ECG) [10]. Previous studies about sleep apnea [11], fibromyalgia [12], and

***Corresponding author:** Eun Yeon Joo, Department of Neurology, Neuroscience Center, Samsung Biomedical Research Institute, Samsung Medical Center, Sungkyunkwan University School of Medicine, Seoul, Korea; E-mail: eunyeon1220.joo@samsung.com

depression [13] revealed the association between the CPC indices and the sleep quality. CPC signals are known have two basic patterns: high frequency coupling (HFC), representing breath-to breath stability of tidal volume or sinus arrhythmia; in contrary, low-frequency coupling (LFC) is known to associated with variation of fluctuating tidal volumes and heart rate [14].

In this study, we hypothesized that RBD with OSA is associated with better sleep quality relative to OSA in conditions with a similar degree of sleep-disordered breathing (apnea-hypopnea index). We tested this hypothesis by employing the CPC method to investigate and quantify physiologic sleep stability in each group.

Material and Method

Subjects

This study was conducted by retrospective review of subjects who performed PSG in university hospital from November, 2009 to October, 2014. We included the patients who visited sleep clinic with complaints of abnormal sleep behaviors. Diagnosis of RBD were based on the international classification of sleep disorder (ISCD) second or third edition, which included: 1) Presence of REM sleep without atonia on PSG; 2) sleep-related, injurious, potentially injurious, or disruptive behaviors by history (i.e., dream enactment behavior); 3) abnormal REM sleep behavior documented during polysomnographic monitoring [15]. We excluded subjects who had other sleep disorder (i.e., Parasomnia other than REM sleep behavior disorder), other neurologic disorder and acute medical illness which may affect PSG and CPC parameters. We also excluded pseudo-RBD; subjects who had severe OSA mimic the symptoms of RBD, after careful review of their sleep study. But in case of subject could be diagnosed both RBD and OSA, instead of excluding them, they were divided into two groups as RBD with OSA (n=26) or RBD only (n=29) group. All subjects were evaluated with overnight PSG and divided into two groups according to the apnea-hypopnea index (AHI). We designated patients with AHI lower than 5 as 'RBD only' group and with AHI higher than 15 as 'RBD with OSA (RBD-OSA)' group. Finally, fifty normal control subjects (AHI<5/h), without any specific sleep complaints and medical history, were also reviewed.

Case-control study

A case-control study was conducted to compare the characteristics of sleep-related respiratory events between RBD with OSA (RBD-OSA) and patients with OSA only (OSA controls). The inclusion criterion for RBD with OSA patients and OSA controls was apnea-hypopnea index (AHI) ≥ 15/h. Among fifty-five patients with RBD, 26 cases were designated as RBD-OSA and included for analysis. The total of 32 OSA control out of 236 OSA subjects, matched for age, AHI and BMI were recruited from patients who visited sleep clinic.

Overnight polysomnography

All patients underwent a PSG study by Embla N7000 & RemLogic (Embla Systems, Denver, CO, USA). The recordings included electroencephalogram (C3-A2, C4-A1, O1-A2, and O2-A1), bilateral electrooculograms and chin electromyogram to determine sleep stage and arousal events. Other devices included piezo bands to check chest and abdominal respiratory effort, finger pulse oximetry, singling lead electrocardiogram with the modified V2 lead, bilateral leg electromyograms, pre-tracheal microphone for snoring, and body position. Air-flow was monitored with thermistors and nasal-cannula pressure transducer. Sleep and arousal scoring were performed using standard criteria. The PSG were scored for sleep and sleep-disorders breathing events using the 2007 guidelines of the American Academy of Sleep Medicine [16-18]. RBD patients were closely monitored by technicians for any movement or vocalization. REM sleep without atonia (RSWA) was definded when following findings were detected. 1) sustained muscle activity in REM sleep with 50% of the epoch having increased chin EMG amplitude, and/or 2) excessive transient muscle activity, defined by the presence of 5 or more mini-epochs (a 30 second epoch is divided into ten 3-second mini-epochs) in an epoch having transient muscle activity lasting at least 0.5 seconds [17]. Other findings from PSG were amounts of each sleep stage, sleep latency, total sleep time (TST), sleep efficiency (SE), and wake after sleep onset (WASO).

Cardiopulmonary coupling analysis

Cardiopulmonary coupling analysis was performed with single-lead electrocardiography data extracted from the PSG by Rem Logic CPC analyzer. The analysis composed of five parameters: 1) high-frequency coupling (HFC, spectrogram peaks in the frequency range of 0.1 Hz to 0.5 Hz), which indicates stable sleep; 2) low-frequency coupling (LFC, spectrogram peaks in the frequency range of 0.01 Hz to 0.1 Hz), which indicates unstable sleep; 3) very-low-frequency coupling (VLFC, spectrogram peaks in the frequency range of 0.00391 Hz to 0.01 Hz), which indicates awake or REM sleep; 4) other (spectrogram peaks other than HFC, LFC, and VLFC, typically <1% to 2%); and 5) elevated low-frequency coupling (e-LFC, a subset of LFC with especially large low-frequency power), which is known to correlate with sleep fragmentation and sleep apnea [10,14].

Statistical analysis

Statistical analyses were performed with SPSS software (SPSS 18.0, SPSS Inc., Chicago, IL, USA). A p value of less than 0.05 was required for statistical significance. Independent t-test or Mann-Whitney U test was employed to compare the PSG characteristics and Apnea-related parameters between RBD-OSA patients and their OSA controls when Appropriate. Pearson's Chi-square test was used to compare categorical variables.. Between groups comparisons were performed with a one-way analysis of variance (ANOVA). Turkey's honest significant difference post hoc test was used to test the significance among groups. Partial Spearman correlations between CPC parameters and PSG data in each group were calculated after adjusting for age, BMI and AHI.

Results

Demographics

29 subjects were designated as RBD, 26 as RBD-OSA and 32 subjects as OSA control. Demographic data of subjects are presented in Table 1. There were no significant differences in age, sex and ESS score among those three groups. The proportion of males in each group was predominantly higher than female, but there was no significant difference between the groups. Each group had a similar degrees of neurodegenerative disease, diabetes and cerebrovascular accident prevalence rate, but the prevalence of hypertension was significantly higher in the OSA group (5/29(17.2%) *vs.* 4/26(15.4%) *vs.*16/32(50.0%) p=0.004 RBD only, RBD-OSA, OSA respectively). RBD group showed significant lower BMI compare to OSA group. (23.9 ± 2.5 *vs.* 25.4 ± 2.7 *vs.* 25.9 ± 3.5 p=0.042, RBD only, RBD-OSA, OSA respectively) RBD group and RBD-OSA group had higher periodic limb movement index (PLMI) than OSA group. (35.3 ± 50.4 *vs.* 20.2 ± 29.2 *vs.* 6.7 ± 10.1, p=0.006 RBD only, RBD-OSA, OSA respectively) Beck depression index (BDI) was reported higher in RBD-OSA as compared to OSA group (11.2 ± 7.6 *vs.* 14.4 ± 9.2 *vs.* 7.9 ± 7.5, p=0.019 RBD only, RBD-

Parameters	RBD (n=29)	RBD-OSA (n=26)	OSA (n=32)	*P* value
Demographic and clinical characteristics				
Age(years)	64.8 ± 8.5	64.9 ± 9.9	62.4 ± 9.7	0.51
Gender(male/female)	17-Dec	18-Aug	20-Dec	0.254†
BMI (kg/m²)	23.9 ± 2.5 [a]	25.4 ± 2.7 [a,b]	25.9 ± 3.5 [b]	**0.042**
ESS score	7.7 ± 3.9	8.0 ± 6.1	7.7 ± 5.9	0.97
BDI	11.2 ± 7.6 [a,b]	14.4 ± 9.2 [a]	7.9 ± 7.5 [b]	**0.019**
Neurodegenerative disease, n (%)	2 (6.9)	3 (11.5)	1(3.1)	0.454†
	(Idiopathic Parkinson's disease:2)	(Idiopathic Parkinson's disease:1, Multiple systemic atrophy:1 Vascular dementia:1)	(Alzheimer dementia:1)	
Hypertension, n (%)	5 (17.2) [a]	4 (15.4) [a]	16 (50.0)	**0.004†**
Diabetes, n (%)	4 (13.8)	1 (3.8)	2(6.3)	0.358†
Cerebrovascular accident, n (%)	6 (20.7)	3 (11.5)	4 (12.5)	0.565†
Polysomnographic features				
Total sleep time(min)	356.0 ± 62.8	353.4 ± 63.9	343.2 ± 47.2	0.658
Sleep efficiency (%)	77.9 ± 12.2	78.0 ± 12.5	78.1 ± 10.6	0.998
Sleep latency(min)	19.8 ± 17.7	22.4 ± 42.7	12.0 ± 11.2	0.285
REM (%)	21.7 ± 8.3	18.6 ± 7.6	18.5 ± 8.1	0.22
Stage 1(%)	18.9 ± 10.8 [a]	25.5 ± 11.4 [a,b]	27.8 ± 15.5 [b]	0.026
Stage 2(%)	54.6 ± 6.6	52.6 ± 14.4	50.5 ± 12.4	0.397
Slow wave sleep (%)	4.8 ± 7.6	1.7 ± 2.4	3.2 ± 5.1	0.121
Total AHI (/hour)	3.2 ± 1.6	29.1 ± 15.6 [a]	34.1 ± 18.9 [a]	<0.001
PLM index (/hour)	35.3 ± 50.4 [a]	20.2 ± 29.2 [a,b]	6.7 ± 10.1 [b]	0.006
Arousal index (/hour)	19.0 ± 9.4 [a]	26.6 ± 11.5 [a,b]	31.0 ± 15.7 [b]	0.002
WASO (%)	18.8 ± 11.7	18.0 ± 10.5	19.9 ± 10.0	0.796

Analysis of variance (ANOVA) on the average abundance Values in the same column followed by the same letter are not significantly different from each other at the 95% confidence interval using Tukey's post-hoc Honestly Significant Difference (HSD) test.
BMI, body mass index; WASO, wake after sleep onset; AHI, apnea hypopnea index; ESS, Epworth sleepiness scale; BDI, Beck Depression Index; PLMS, periodic limb movements during sleep.
†Fisher exact test.

Table 1: Sample characteristics of RBD, RBD-OSA and OSA controls.

OSA, OSA respectively). OSA and RBD-OSA group showed higher arousal index in comparison with RBD group (19.0 ± 9.4 *vs.* 26.6 ± 11.5 *vs.* 31.0 ± 15.7, p=0.002 RBD only, RBD-OSA, OSA respectively).

Comparison of respiratory-related and CPC parameters between RBD-OSA, OSA control

Table 2 depicts the comparison of OSA severity variables. Although the basal SpO_2 levels were similar (96.0 ± 0.9 *vs.* 95.1 ± 2.1, p=0.154), RBD-OSA group demonstrated higher nadir SpO_2 during sleep (85.6 ± 5.2 *vs.* 80.9 ± 7.2, p=0.003) shorter maximum apnea duration (34.4 ± 22.2 *vs.* 48.8 ± 28.5, p=0.028) and mean apnea duration (18.4 ± 8.5 *vs.* 23.7 ± 11.8, p=0.023) than OSA controls. The comparison of CPC parameters of both OSA-RBD and OSA control groups are presented in Table 3. Although there was no significant Apnea-Hypopnea index (AHI) difference between RBD-OSA and OSA group (AHI 29.1 ± 15.6/hr *vs.* 34.1 ± 18.9, p=0.332), there was significant difference in CPC measurements. In RBD-OSA group showed lower LFC (35.9 ± 16.8 *vs.* 49.7 ± 21.3 p=0.010) than OSA group. RBD-OSA group showed higher HFC than OSA group (46.7 ± 20.8 *vs.* 37.5 ± 20.0, p=0.069), but this difference was not statistically significant. Unlike higher AHI in RBD-OSA than RBD group (29.1 ± 15.6/hr *vs.* 3.2 ± 1.6, p<0.001), there was no significant difference in CPC study. RBD-OSA group showed higher LFC values than RBD group (35.9±16.8 *vs.* 28.5±18.8, p=0.086), but statistically insignificant. Both OSA group and RBD-OSA group showed higher LFC (OSA *vs.* normal: 49.7 ± 21.3 *vs.* 28.4 ± 13.3, p<0.001, RBD-OSA *vs.* normal: 35.9 ± 16.8 *vs.* 28.4 ± 13.2, p=0.035) and lower HFC (OSA *vs.* normal: 37.5 ± 20.0 *vs.* 56.2 ± 16.2, p<0.001, RBD with OSA vs. normal: 46.8 ± 20.8 *vs.* 56.2 ± 16.2, p=0.031) when compared with normal control group, respectively. Table 4 demonstrated comparison of demographic, PSG parameters and CPC parameters of RBD *vs.*

Parameters	RBD-OSA (N=26)	OSA control (N=32)	*P* value‡
Total AHI	29.1 ± 15.6	34.1 ± 18.9	0.332
REM AHI	27.4 ± 15.1	33.0 ± 19.3	0.303
NREM AHI	28.1 ± 17.2	30.7 ± 19.5	0.415
Basal SpO_2 (%)	96.0 ± 0.9	95.1 ± 2.1	0.154
lowest SpO_2 during sleep (%)	85.6 ± 5.2	80.9 ± 7.2	**0.003**
O_2 desaturation index	24.7 ± 15.1	31.2 ± 18.8	0.226
Mean apnea duration(sec)	18.4 ± 8.5	23.7 ± 11.8	**0.023**
Maximum apnea duration(sec)	34.4 ± 22.2	48.8 ± 28.5	**0.028**
Mean hypopnea duration(sec)	26.8 ± 7.3	28.8±6.1	0.159
Maximum hypopnea duration(sec)	63.1±17.2	71.9 ± 26.2	0.179
Obstructive Apnea index	8.5 ± 13.4	8.4 ± 11.2	0.057
Central Apnea index	0.1 ± 0.2	0.2 ± 0.6	0.095
Mixed Apnea index	1.9 ± 4.2	4.0 ± 6.0	0.166
F hypopnea	71.6 ± 26.3	63.6 ± 27.2	0.663

AHI: Apnea Hypopnea Index; SpO_2 Oxygen Saturation Measured by Pulse Oximeter;
F hypopnea: Fraction of Events that were Hypopneas.
‡ Mann-Whitney U test.

Table 2: Comparison of respiratory-related parameters between RBD-OSA and OSA.

Parameters	RBD-OSA	OSA	*P* value‡
HFC duration (%)	46.7 ± 20.8	37.5 ± 20.0	0.069
LFC duration (%)	35.9 ± 16.8	49.7 ± 21.3	**0.01**
vLFC duration (%)	15.9 ± 7.1	12.3 ± 5.7	0.084
eLFC	18.0 ± 16.5	30.9 ± 18.6	**0.012**

HFC: High Frequency Coupling; LFC: Low Frequency Coupling; vLFC: Very Low Frequency Coupling; eLFC.
‡ Mann-Whitney U test.

Table 3: CPC characteristics of RBD-OSA *vs.* OSA controls.

Parameters	RBD (n=29)	Normal control (n=51)	*P* value
Demographic and clinical characteristics			
Age (years)	64.8 ± 8.5	47.9 ± 5.9	**<0.001**
Gender (male/female)	17-Dec	24/27	0.320†
BMI (kg/m²)	23.9 ± 2.5	22.6 ± 1.8	**0.005**
ESS score	7.7 ± 3.9	6.9 ± 4.1	0.412
BDI	11.2 ± 7.6	7.1 ± 6.3	**0.019**
Polysomnographic features			
Total sleep time(min)	356.0 ± 62.8	388.7 ± 47.5	**0.019**
Sleep efficiency (%)	77.9 ± 12.2	90.1 ± 11.1	**<0.001**
Sleep latency (min)	19.8 ± 17.7	8.4 ± 6.8	**0.002**
REM (%)	21.7 ± 8.3	22.8 ± 5.0	0.525
Stage1 (%)	18.9 ± 10.8	13.5 ± 4.9	**0.016**
Stage 2(%)	54.6 ± 6.6	58.0 ± 6.2	**0.025**
Slow wave sleep (%)	4.8 ± 7.6	5.7 ± 5.6	0.538
Total AHI (/hour)	3.2 ± 1.6	2.2 ± 2.2	**0.027**
PLM index (/hour)	35.3 ± 50.4	4.8 ± 8.6	**0.003**
Arousal index (/hour)	19.0 ± 9.4	14.6 ± 6.0	**0.027**
WASO (%)	18.8 ± 11.7	9.8 ± 6.8	**<0.001**

BMI: Body Mass Index; WASO: Wake After Sleep Onset; AHI: Apnea Hypopnea Index; ESS: Epworth Sleepiness Scale; BDI: Beck Depression Index; PLMS: Periodic Limb Movements during Sleep.
†Fisher exact test.

Table 4: Sample characteristics of RBD and normal controls.

normal control. RBD group was significantly older than normal control (64.8 ± 8.5 *vs.* 47.9 ± 5.9, p<0.001) and showed higher BMI (23.9 ± 2.5 *vs.* 22.6 ± 1.8, p=0.005) and BDI score (11.2 ± 7.6 *vs.* 7.1 ± 6.3, p=0.019). PSG parameter showed poor sleep efficiency (77.9 ± 12.2 *vs.* 90.1 ± 11.1, p<0.001), delayed sleep latency (19.8 ± 17.7 *vs.* 8.4 ± 6.8, p=0.002), increased PLMI (35.3 ± 50.4 *vs.* 4.8 ± 8.6, p=0.003), higher arousal index (19.0 ± 9.4 *vs.* 14.6 ± 6.0, p=0.027) and longer wakefulness after sleep onset (WASO) (18.8 ± 11.7 *vs.* 9.8 ± 6.8, p<0.001) in RBD compared to normal control. Overall, these results suggested that normal control had better PSG parameters than those of RBD group, but there was no significant difference in CPC parameters (Table 5).

Correlation analysis between PSG parameters and CPC parameters

In OSA group, the correlations between PSG parameters and CPC parameters analyzed by Spearman's correlation analysis model, was presented in Table 6. HFC was negatively correlated with AI, AHI (rho=-0.626, p<0.001, rho=-0.633, p<0.001), positively correlated lowest SaO_2 (rho=0.504, p=0.003) and did not show significant correlation with TST, sleep latency, SE, WASO and PLM index. LFC and e-LFC showed positive correlation with AI, AHI (rho=0.635, p<0.001 and rho=0.651, p<0.001 in LFC, rho=0.60, p<0.001 and rho=0.587, p<0.001 in e-LFC), and negative correlation with lowest O_2 saturation (rho=-0.507, p=0.003 and rho=-0.462, p=0.003). LFC and e-LFC did not show significant correlation with TST, sleep latency, SE, WASO and PLM index, either. VLFC did not show correlation with all PSG parameters. Unlike PSG

Parameters	RBD	Normal	*P* value‡
HFC duration (%)	52.3 ± 23.0	56.2 ± 16.2	0.545
LFC duration (%)	28.5 ± 18.8	28.4 ± 13.3	0.535
vLFC duration (%)	17.5 ± 8.1	14.8 ± 5.3	0.104
eLFC	13.6 ± 14.8	13.7 ± 10.1	0.426

HFC: High Frequency Coupling; LFC: Low Frequency Coupling; vLFC: Very Low Frequency Coupling; eLFC.
‡ Mann-Whitney U test.

Table 5: Sample characteristics of RBD and normal controls.

parameters showed good correlation with CPC parameters in OSA group, RBD-OSA group demonstrated positive correlation between HFC and lowest O_2 saturation (rho=0.507, p=0.008) and weak positive correlation with HFC and sleep latency (rho=0.49, p=0.033) (Table 7). LFC showed weak negative correlation with lowest O_2 saturation (rho=-0.414, p=0.035). Other than that, there was no significant correlation with TST, SE, WASO and PLM index.

Discussion

The key findings of this study, based on the CPC analysis, include the followings:

1) Despite a similar degree of AHI, reduced unstable sleep was found in RBD-OSA group compared with OSA controls.

2) In spite of the findings suggesting poor sleep quality in polysomnography, there was no significant difference in CPC results between RBD group and normal control group.

Quality sleep is defined as normal sleep architecture with lack of fragmentation and an absence of sleep disordered breathing. The CPC analysis is an automated measure of sleep physiology and complements traditional sleep-scoring system used to assess sleep stability/quality because it objectively contains features of physiological dynamics not accounted by EEG-based techniques [13]. Among the CPC parameters, the HFC is a physiologic marker of stable and consolidated sleep. On the other hand, the LFC is related to breath-to-breath fluctuation of tidal volumes and cyclic variations in a heart rate, reflecting unstable and fragmented sleep [14]. The VLFC is associated with wake or rapid eye movement (REM) period, and elevated LFC (e-LFC) is associated with probable apneas or hypopneas [14].

Several previous CPC studies consistently demonstrated that decreased HFC and increased LFC in OSA [14,19-21]. The same results were obtained in this study, both RBD-OSA and OSA group showed higher HFC and lower LFC than normal control. The tendency in CPC feature of obstructive sleep apnea was maintained, but RBD-OSA group had lesser unstable sleep than OSA group. In the previous study, increased muscle activities during REM sleep, apnea related parameters such as nadir SpO_2, maximum oxygen desaturation duration and apnea/hypopnea duration were less severe in RBD-OSA patients than their OSA controls [9]. The study provided the evidence to support that hypothesis quantitatively, by measuring REM-related EMG activity (REMREEA), suggested that increased REMREEA was associated with lower severity of OSA in RBD patients [9]. As shown in the previous study, our study also demonstrated that RBD-OSA group had higher nadir SpO_2, shorter maximum and mean apnea duration during sleep than OSA controls. According to recent various insights into sleep apnea pathogenesis, the neural control of muscles also contributing to OSA phathogenesis [7]. In the transcranial magnetic stimulation (TMS) studies in OSA, decreased moter excitatory potential (MEP) suggesting enhanced depression of the cortical motor neuron activity

Parameters	TST	SL	SE	AI	AHI	Lowest SpO_2	WASO (%)	PLMI
HFC	0.081	0.31	-0.096	-0.626**	-0.633**	0.504**	0.013	-0.068
LFC	-0.023	-0.249	0.149	0.635**	0.651**	-0.507**	-0.066	0.039
vLFC	-0.14	-0.104	-0.217	-0.107	-0.192	0.163	0.185	0.207
e-LFC	-0.014	-0.3	0.153	0.600**	0.587**	-0.462**	-0.059	0.126

TST: Total Sleep Time; SL, Sleep Latency; SE: Sleep Efficiency; AI: Arousal Index; AHI: Apnea-Hypopnea Index; WASO: Wakefulness After Sleep Onset; PLMI: Periodic Limb Movement Index; HFC: High Frequency Coupling; LFC: Low Frequency Coupling; vLFC: Very Low Frequency Coupling; eLFC.
Spearmans rho values are presented. * $p<0.05$ ** $p<0.01$

Table 6: Partial Spearman correlation analysis between PSG parameters and CPC parameters after adjustment of age, gender and BMI in patients of OSA only (n=32).

Parameters	TST	SL	SE	AI	AHI	Lowest SpO_2	WASO	PLMI
HFC	-0.036	0.419*	-0.077	-0.197	-0.091	0.507**	-0.02	0.07
LFC	0.046	-0.264	0.022	0.334	0.271	-0.414*	0.094	-0.233
vLFC	-0.016	-0.376	0.081	-0.239	-0.302	-0.343	-0.087	0.154
e-LFC	0.139	-0.163	0.078	0.265	0.266	-0.233	0.016	-0.226

TST: Total Sleep Time; SL, Sleep Latency; SE: Sleep Efficiency; AI: Arousal Index; AHI: Apnea-Hypopnea Index; WASO: Wakefulness After Sleep Onset; PLMI: Periodic Limb Movement Index; HFC: High Frequency Coupling; LFC: Low Frequency Coupling; vLFC: Very Low Frequency Coupling; eLFC.
Spearmans rho values are presented. * $p<0.05$ ** $p<0.01$

Table 7: Partial Spearman correlation analysis between PSG parameters and CPC parameters after adjustment of age, gender and BMI in patients of RBD with OSA (n=26).

was observed. Those abnormality were outside of the pharyngeal district which means wide spread dysfunction of the cortical-spinal system in OSA [22]. The pathogenesis of RBD is assumed that involvement of several brainstem structures, such as cholinergic pedunculopontine nucleus (PPN) which activates the muscle tone inhibitory system [23]. The dysfunction of GABAergic basal ganglia output which controls postural muscle tone by modulating PPN neuron may contribute to muscular atonia of REM sleep [24]. In terms of dysfunctional neural control of both diseases, it is possible that modulation of neural activity to increased muscular tone for lowering the severity of OSA. There was one case report of resolved OSA after implanting subthalamic nucleus deep brain stimulation [25]. Other non-anatomical traits, such as a low respiratory arousal threshold (awaken easily), is also important for many patients [7]. Premature awakening may prevent accumulation of respiratory stimuli to upper-airway dilator muscle activation as well as the resulting stabilization of sleep and breathing [26]. Sommerauer et al. reported that cortical arousability in response to respiratory and motor event is significantly attenuated in Parkinson's disease (PD) patients. They suggested that loss of multiple arousal promoting nuclei, such as the PPN, the locus coeruleus(LC) and the dorsal raphe neucleus, was responsible for the low arousability in PD [27]. Given that RBD also related to PPN and LC lesions, increased arousal threshold might also have contributed to reduce unstable sleep in RBD-OSA group. PSG and CPC parameters showed HFC, LFC had significant correlation with AI, AHI and nadir SpO_2 during sleep in OSA group, which was consistent with previous study [21]. But RBD-OSA group showed no correlation between PSG and CPC parameters except for lowest Oxygen saturation during sleep and HFC. One possible explanation for this discrepancy is that CPC showed a closer relationship with CAP/non-CAP rather than conventional NREM-stage scoring [10]. CPC is not a sleep-stage or respiratory event detector but does provide a dynamic measure of cardiopulmonary coupling during sleep. Therefore, tight correlations with visually scored sleep states would not be expected [10]. Those explanations also could be applied to the discrepancy between PSG and CPC parameters in RBD *vs.* normal control. In spite RBD group showed poor sleep quality indicators including lower SE, higher AI, PLMI and WASO, CPC revealed that there was no significant difference to normal control. Regarding the CPC finding of RBD and RBD-OSA, LFC was higher in RBD-OSA without statistical significance. Although AHI was higher in the group of RBD-OSA, both groups had poor sleep quality with lower sleep efficiency and higher arousal index on PSG and it might reduce the effect of sleep-disordered breathing on CPC profiles.

There were several findings which reflect the characteristics of each group. In this study, there were more males in all groups. OSA [28] and RBD [2,29,30] both are male and elderly predominant disorder and thought to be naturally reflected in our study. In RBD group showed high PLMI which is very common in idiopathic RBD, occurring in all stages of sleep, especially during REM sleep [31]. Another intriguing finding was that RBD-OSA patients showed significantly higher BDI score than OSA controls. Considering greater prevalence of depression in patients with RBD when compared to those without in early PD patient [32], they might share common pathophysiology. It perhaps explained by the proximity of the serotoninergic raphe and other brainstem nuclei to the nuclei implemented in the pathophysiology of RBD [33]. Several strengths worth to note in this study. To our knowledge, this is the first study investigating CPC analysis in RBD patient. In addition, we investigate CPC in four well-characterized group which were RBD only, RBD with OSA, OSA only and normal control. By comparing those four groups in terms of demographics, PSG parameters and CPC parameters, this study provided new evidence of protective effect of RBD on OSA. We confirmed our initial findings of the correlation study that RBD patients had less severe apnea-related parameters by case-control study. Lastly, as previous study revealed that decreased heart rate variability in patients with RBD [34], simultaneous incorporating both cardiac interbeat(R-R) and ECG-derived respiration (EDR) investigation of this study minimized the limitation in cardiopulmonary coupling analysis of possible autonomic dysfunction subjects.

However, several limitations should also be noted in this study. First, separated CPC analysis according to REM *vs.* NREM sleep was not available. Since the time window of assessment of CPC is 8 minutes, unlike 30 seconds in PSG. This study showed RBD with OSA had more stable sleep than OSA control group. But we did not reveal the mechanism of the effect of RBD on OSA. Further studies with documentation of various factors developing OSA such as anatomical change, neuromuscular aspect and respiratory arousal threshold in each group are warranted to confirm our findings.

Another limitation was significant age difference between normal group and the other groups (RBD, RBD-OSA, and OSA). Aging itself is associated with changes in sleep architecture, decreased sleep efficiency and increased arousal. The prevalence of sleep disorders increases with age (e.g. Insomnia, RBD, and OSA) [35]. Also coexistent illness or medication use which might effect on sleep is very common among elderly people. We had difficulty with recruit normal control of similar age with RBD and OSA group for those reasons.

Lastly, RBD is known to a precursor of PD or dementia and also related to cognitive impairment even in idiopathic RBD [23]. Since OSA is also known to cause cognitive dysfunction [36,37], measuring objective score related to neurodegeneration might help us understating various aspects of those two diseases. Since pure RBD showed similar profile to normal control in terms of CPC analysis, it could be used as screening test for patients with RBD whether pure RBD or other complicating sleep disorder which require further investigation. If RBD patient showed poor quality of sleep measured by CPC, concomitant disease (e.g. insomnia, depression, fibromyalgia) or pseudo-RBD should be considered. In this regard, our study suggested that the differences of the CPC between RBD and OSA could also help differentiate the ambiguous cases.

Conclusion

In conclusions, our study demonstrated that OSA patients with RBD showed more stable sleep than patients with OSA without RBD patients, which was proven by CPC parameters. It suggests that RBD probably has a positive impact on OSA, and this raises the need for further study to investigate the mechanism of RBD and OSA.

Acknowledgments

This research was supported by Basic Science Research Program through the National Research Foundation of Korea funded by the Ministry of Science, ICT & Future Planning, Republic of Korea (No. 2014 R1A1A3049510) and by Samsung Biomedical Research Institute grant (#SMO116).

References

1. Boeve BF (2010) REM sleep behavior disorder: Updated review of the core features, the REM sleep behavior disorder-neurodegenerative disease association, evolving concepts, controversies, and future directions. Ann N Y Acad Sci 1184:15-54.
2. Kang SH, Yoon IY, Lee SD, Han JW, Kim TH, et al. (2013) REM sleep behavior disorder in the Korean elderly population: prevalence and clinical characteristics. Sleep 36: 1147-1152.
3. Chiu HF, Wing YK, Lam LC, Li SW, Lum CM, et al. (2000) Sleep-related injury in the elderly--an epidemiological study in Hong Kong. Sleep 23: 513-517.
4. Schenck CH, Mahowald MW (2002) REM sleep behavior disorder: clinical, developmental, and neuroscience perspectives 16 years after its formal identification in SLEEP. Sleep 25: 120-138.
5. Iranzo A, Santamaria J (2005) Severe obstructive sleep apnea/hypopnea mimicking REM sleep behavior disorder. Sleep 28: 203-206.
6. Patil SP, Schneider H, Schwartz AR, Smith PL (2007) Adult obstructive sleep apnea: pathophysiology and diagnosis. Chest 132: 325-337.
7. Edwards BA, Eckert DJ, Jordan AS (2017) Obstructive sleep apnoea pathogenesis from mild to severe: Is it all the same? Respirology 22: 33-42.
8. Henriques-Filho PS, Pratesi R (2008) Sleep apnea and REM sleep behavior disorder in patients with Chiari malformations. Arq Neuropsiquiatr 66: 344-349.
9. Huang J, Zhang J, Lam SP, Li SX, Ho CK, et al. (2011) Amelioration of obstructive sleep apnea in REM sleep behavior disorder: implications for the neuromuscular control of OSA. Sleep 34: 909-915.
10. Thomas RJ, Mietus JE, Peng CK, Goldberger AL (2005) An electrocardiogram-based technique to assess cardiopulmonary coupling during sleep. Sleep 28: 1151-1161.
11. Harrington J, Schramm PJ, Davies CR, Lee-Chiong TL, (2013) An electrocardiogram-based analysis evaluating sleep quality in patients with obstructive sleep apnea. Sleep Breath 17: 1071-1078.
12. Thomas RJ, Mietus JE, Peng CK, Goldberger AL, Crofford LJ, et al. (2010) Impaired sleep quality in fibromyalgia: Detection and quantification with ECG-based cardiopulmonary coupling spectrograms. Sleep medicine 11: 497-498.
13. Yang AC, Yang CH, Hong CJ, Tsai SJ, Kuo CH, et al. (2011) Sleep state instabilities in major depressive disorder: Detection and quantification with electrocardiogram-based cardiopulmonary coupling analysis. Psychophysiology 48: 285-291.
14. Thomas RJ, Mietus JE, Peng CK, Gilmartin G, Daly RW, et al. (2007) Differentiating obstructive from central and complex sleep apnea using an automated electrocardiogram-based method. Sleep 30: 1756-1769.
15. Medicine AAoS (2005) International Classification of Sleep Disorders: Diagnostic and Coding Manual. 2nd Westchester.
16. Rechtschaffen KA (1968) A manual of standardized terminology, techniques and scoring systems for sleep stages of human subjects. Washington DC: Brain Information Service/Brain Research Institute, University of California
17. Iber CA-IS, Chesson AL, Quan SF (2007) The AASM Manual for the scoring of sleep and associated events: rules, terminology and technical specifications. Westchester, IL: American Academy of Sleep Medicine
18. Task Force of the American Sleep Disorders Association (1992) EEG arousals: scoring rules and examples: a preliminary report from the Sleep Disorders Atlas. Sleep 15:173-184.
19. Lee WH, Ahn JC, We J, Rhee CS, Lee CH, et al. (2014) Cardiopulmonary coupling analysis: changes before and after treatment with a mandibular advancement device. Sleep Breath 18: 891-896.
20. Guo D, Peng CK, Wu HL, Mietus JE, Liu Y, et al. (2011) ECG-derived cardiopulmonary analysis of pediatric sleep-disordered breathing. Sleep medicine 12: 384-389.
21. Hea RP, Eun YJ, Seung BH (2015) Electrophysiological characteristics of obstructive sleep apnea syndrome with insomnia: polysomnography and cardiopulmonary coupling analysis. J Sleep Med 12: 53-58.
22. Lanza G, Lanuzza B, Arico D, Cantone M, Cosentino FI, et al. (2015) Direct comparison of cortical excitability to transcranial magnetic stimulation in obstructive sleep apnea syndrome and restless legs syndrome. Sleep med 16: 138-142.
23. Nardone R, Bergmann J, Kunz A, Christova M, Brigo F, et al. (2012) Cortical afferent inhibition is reduced in patients with idiopathic REM sleep behavior disorder and cognitive impairment: a TMS study. Sleep med 13: 919-25.
24. Takakusaki K, Obara K, Nozu T, Okumura T (2011) Modulatory effects of the GABAergic basal ganglia neurons on the PPN and the muscle tone inhibitory system in cats. Arch Ital Biol 149: 385-405.
25. Margarida D, Ana A (2014) Effect of Deep Brain Stimulation on a Patient With Obstructive Sleep Apnea and Parkinson Disease: A Case Report. Chest 145: 570A.
26. Eckert DJ, Owens RL, Kehlmann GB, Wellman A, Rahangdale S, et al. (2011) Eszopiclone increases the respiratory arousal threshold and lowers the apnoea/hypopnoea index in obstructive sleep apnea patients with a low arousal threshold. Clinical science 120: 505-514.
27. Sommerauer M, Imbach LL, Jarallah M, Baumann CR, Valko PO (2015) Diminished event-related cortical arousals and altered heart rate response in Parkinson's disease. Movement disorders 30: 866-870.
28. Sforza E, Chouchou F, Collet P, Pichot V, Barthelemy JC, et al. (2011) Sex differences in obstructive sleep apnea in an elderly French population. The Eur respir j 37: 1137-1143.

29. Schenck CH, Hurwitz TD, Mahowald MW (1993) Symposium: Normal and abnormal REM sleep regulation: REM sleep behaviour disorder: an update on a series of 96 patients and a review of the world literature. J sleep res 2: 224-231.

30. Olson EJ, Boeve BF, Silber MH (2000) Rapid eye movement sleep behaviour disorder: demographic, clinical and laboratory findings in 93 cases. Brain 123: 331-339.

31. Fantini ML, Michaud M, Gosselin N, Lavigne G, Montplaisir J (2002) Periodic leg movements in REM sleep behavior disorder and related autonomic and EEG activation. Neurology 59: 1889-1894.

32. Savica R, Rocca WA, Ahlskog JE (2010) When does Parkinson disease start? Arch Neurol 67: 798-801.

33. Rolinski M, Szewczyk-Krolikowski K, Tomlinson PR, Nithi K, Talbot K, et al. (2014) REM sleep behaviour disorder is associated with worse quality of life and other non-motor features in early Parkinson's disease. J Neurol Neurosurg Psychiatry 85: 560-566.

34. Boeve BF, Silber MH, Saper CB, Ferman TJ, Dickson DW, et al. (2007) Pathophysiology of REM sleep behaviour disorder and relevance to neurodegenerative disease. Brain 130: 2770-2788.

35. Lanfranchi PA, Fradette L, Gagnon JF, Colombo R, Montplaisir J (2007) Cardiac autonomic regulation during sleep in idiopathic REM sleep behavior disorder. Sleep 30: 1019-1025.

36. Wolkove N, Elkholy O, Baltzan M, Palayew M (2007) Sleep and aging: 1. Sleep disorders commonly found in older people. CMAJ 176: 1299-1304.

37. Kielb SA, Ancoli-Israel S, Rebok GW, Spira AP (2012) Cognition in obstructive sleep apnea-hypopnea syndrome (OSAS): Current clinical knowledge and the impact of treatment. NeuroMolecular Med 14: 180-193.

5

Evaluating and Managing Insomnia: Non-pharmacological Treatments

Sharon Valente[*]

Greater Los Angeles Healthcare System, Los Angeles, CA, USA

***Corresponding author:** Sharon Valente, Greater Los Angeles Healthcare System, Los Angeles, CA, USA, E-mail: sharon.valente@va.gov

Abstract

For about 40% of Americans, Insomnia is a major health issue that often leads to fatigue, reduced immunity, and dangerous driving. A good night sleep is essential for functioning and performance. It also influences mood, cognition, concentration, fatigue, and healing. Insomnia may be related to medical and psychiatric disorders, shift work, stimulants, travel, anxiety, pain, and other problems (e.g., poor sleep environment). People with insomnia (e.g., difficulty falling asleep, frequent awakenings and daytime drowsiness) tend to rely on alcohol, drugs, and other remedies. Insomnia may reflect sleep apnea or other medical or mental health disorders that require evaluation as well as poor sleep hygiene. Insomnia can be brief, episodic or chronic. Unfortunately, many people assume that insomnia is normal and do not report it to the nurse or seek treatment. Sleep deprivation impairs the person's physical, mental, and cardiac functioning. Often insomnia is treated with medications which may have side effectives or be habit forming. Individuals with insomnia need evaluation of the precipitants of insomnia, education about sleep hygiene, and information about non-pharmacological treatments. In clinic and hospital settings, nurses are in a pivotal position to identify sleep problems, educate patients, and refer them for follow up.

Keywords: Insomnia; Complementary therapies; Non-pharmacological treatments

Introduction

Insomnia is a major health issue in the United States; about 50 million Americans report a sleep disturbance within the past year and 33-40% report insomnia nearly every night [1,2]. It is common among the elderly who use a large percentage of sleep medications and people with mental health or medical disorders, asthma, heart failure, chronic fatigue, pain, and anxiety and those who work nights. Transient insomnia lasts less than a week; short-term insomnia continues from 1-3 weeks, and chronic insomnia (more than 3 weeks) occurs in about 10-15% of cases. Insomnia may be defined as difficulty falling asleep, difficulty maintaining sleep, early morning awakening, or non-restorative sleep. Insomnia creates excess sleepiness which can be hazardous when you drive a car or operate machinery. People self-medicate with over the counter remedies, drugs or alcohol and would benefit from non-pharmacological options and may avoid medications which can be addictive. However, insomnia is rarely reported [3] and so most insomnia remains untreated.

Although most people know what insomnia is, many assume it is normal. Few seek advice from their health care provider and do not know the available non-pharmacological treatments. Whether in a clinical or hospital setting, nurses are in a pivotal position to identify sleep problems, educate patients about interventions, and refer them for follow up. Sleep deprivation impairs the immune system, white blood count, brain function and heart variability [1]. It impacts mood, cognition, and fatigue and delays recovery and healing. Disturbed sleep can also suggest medical or neurological problems that require evaluation (e.g., heart failure, osteoarthritis, Parkinson's disease) [3,4]. (see Figure 1 case example).

The purpose of this article is to review the basic concepts regarding sleep, assessment, management and non-pharmacological treatments.

The nurse will have effective approaches to evaluate, educate, and refer people with insomnia and to recommend non-pharmacological treatments (e.g., relaxation, mindfulness, acupressure).

Normal Sleep

While the specific functions of sleep are debated, it plays an essential role in the health -it is restorative, enhances energy conservation and yet sleep needs vary with age and activity. Sleep is a dynamic process involving brain activity. The functions of sleep impact the brain, immune system, and nerves. Sleep progresses from four stages of Non-Rapid Eye Movement (NREM) that progress to Rapid Eye Movement (REM). In stage 1 or the transitional stage, wakefulness moves to the early stage of sleep (e.g., physiology is altered, peristalsis slows, core body temperature drops and sensory awareness lessens) (Reinoso-Suarez, 2011). Stage 2 is the longest stage and Stages 3-4 are deep restorative sleep. During REM sleep blood pressure and respiratory rates fluctuate and respirations become shallow and dreams can be remembered. REM appears important in memory and potentially sustaining life [5].

A sleep cycle lasts between 1½ to 2 hours as stage 2 and REM increase. The sleep/wake cycle is circadian. As daylight turns to night, melatonin, a natural sedative, is secreted. Aging changes the sleep cycle as time in Stage 3 and REM decrease and stages 1 and 2 increase. The hours of sleep required decrease from 7-8 hours to 6-6 ½ for older adults. Natural remedies that improve sleep include foods with tryptophan, cherry juice, seaweed, kiwi fruit, melatonin and valerian. The DSM V includes diagnoses of insomnia disorder, narcolepsy, breathing related sleep disorders (e.g., apnea and hypoventilation), circadian sleep-wake disorders, REM behavior disorder and restless legs syndrome [2,4].

Case Example:

Ms. J was a delightful well nourished and well developed 58 year old woman with hypertension, pre diabetes, arthritis, and bipolar disorder. She was hospitalized for pneumonia. The nurse observed that she had difficulty falling asleep, staying asleep and complained of feeling tired. She said the hospital was noisy and the nurse provided ear plugs.

Ms. J confirmed that she has had difficulty falling and staying asleep for a couple of weeks, is fatigued, and takes day time naps. She has no nightmares, apnea, or restlessness. She worries about many things. She has taken over the counter pills for sleep. She often drank 1-2 glasses of wine before bed and takes an over the counter (OTC) pill for sleep. During hospitalization the nurse recommended she try sleep hygiene, chamomile tea, progressive relaxation, mindfulness and some of the other CAM interventions. Ms J was interested in hypnosis and cognitive behavioral therapy after discharge. The nurse also recommended reducing alcohol before bedtime.

Course of Treatment

Mrs. J was diagnosed with hypertension, short-term insomnia, arthritis and bipolar disorder and was hospitalized for treatment of pneumonia. She was encouraged to try complimentary/alternative medicine (CAM) strategies during hospitalization and use ear plugs. She found progressive relaxation and mindfulness very useful and she liked chamomile tea. Her pneumonia resolved. However, gall stones were identified on xray and she was scheduled for surgery a month later. After discharge she agreed to: try melatonin or at night for sleep, follow healthy sleep habits, and use a 2 week sleep diary.

She takes Metoprolol 50 po at bedtime for hypertension.

Metformin for prediabetes

Aspirin prn for arthritis.

She also agreed to consult her mental health provider about cognitive behavioral therapy (CBT) for anxiety and insomnia treatment

Psychosocial Data: Mrs. J lives at home and her family are in other states. She exercises with walking, going to the gym and golf. She volunteers in her community. She does not keep regular sleep hours and often eats a heavy meal with wine before bed. She watches TV in her bedroom and reads a lot. She worries about family members and their medical illnesses and their financial needs. She does not smoke, rarely exercises, and does not drink coffee. She drinks 1-2 glasses of wine before bed. She denies any other drug use.

Figure 1: Case example: Vignette of Mrs. J.

Screening and Assessment

A Nursing assessment of sleep rests on sleep quality and patterns, medical, substance and psychiatric history. Assessment includes a risk factors and sleep history (e.g., usual sleep patterns, sleep onset and duration, time to fall asleep, frequency of awakenings, and difficulty returning to sleep) (See Case Example in Figure 1). Sometimes if pain, worry, or anxiety are triggering the insomnia, the nurse can recommend some relaxation or improved pain management. Risk factors for insomnia include: traveling, shift work, elderly, pregnancy, menopause, substance abuse, stimulants (e.g., caffeine, nicotine), medications, medical disorders, and pain.

Descriptions of sleep disruptions and self-management strategies are important (e.g., early morning awakening, nightmares, or restlessness). The nurse considers medical or psychological disorders, medications, or behaviors (e.g., snoring, alcohol, sleep apnea) that impair sleep. A sleep history (e.g., sleep schedule, habits, timing, quality, symptoms and sleep duration) assists evaluation. A description of the symptoms during the day and the consequences of insomnia are helpful in identifying precipitants (e.g., daytime sleepiness, fatigue, and irritability). With the assessment, the nurse may be able to resolve the sleep problems with interventions or may work with the health care team to conduct a more thorough assessment for other disorders such as sleep apnea.

Assessment can be improved by using standardized self-report instruments such as an Epworth Sleepiness Scale, Pittsburgh Sleep Quality Index, and Fatigue Severity Scale that provides objective data of sleep and sleep diaries or logs to track sleep wake patterns and daily variations [6]. The Epworth Sleepiness Scale is a self-report tool that rates daytime sleepiness and the chance of dozing or sleeping on a scale (0-never to 3 high chance) for various experiences: sitting and reading, watching TV, sitting inactive in a public place and 4 other activities). A score of 10 or more is sleepy and should suggest an evaluation or improved sleep hygiene, 18 is very sleepy [7]. The Pittsburgh Sleep Quality Index (PSQI) differentiates older adults' poor and good sleep by measuring sleep quality, latency, duration, disturbances, medication and daytime dysfunction. It uses a 0 to 3 scale (e=negative extreme) [8]. A sum of 5 or more indicates a poor sleeper. It includes items for a bed partner to complete. The Fatigue Severity Scale is a copyright self-rated measure of how fatigue affects motivation, exercise, physical functioning in various medical and neurologic conditions. It is a 9 item tool measured on a 7 point Likert scale (e.g., I am easily fatigued). A high score indicates agreement with the item. The score is the average of all items. People with depression alone score 4.5 but those with fatigue from a chronic disease average about 6.5.

Education and Management

Educating patients about healthy sleep and nonpharmacological interventions is important. Nurses should promote good sleep habits and offer non-pharmacological or behavioral interventions (e.g., relaxation, CAM, sleep restriction, stimulus control, relaxation) and pharmacology to promote sleep in conjunction with behavioral interventions.

Healthy Sleep Habits

Education on healthy sleep habits is an essential and includes a regular sleep/wake schedule, avoidance of stimulants, alcohol and caffeine 4-6 hours before bedtime, and sleep hygiene. Sleep hygiene includes lowering the core body temperature with a warm bath or socks is useful, reducing exposure to bright light before bedtime, and eliminating daytime naps. Recommendations include minimizing light and noise, maintaining a comfortable room temperature and using the bedroom only for sleep (e.g., removing TVs or computers). Sleep recommendations also include: sleep until you feel rested, exercise regularly 20 minutes/day; avoid stimulants, smoking, hunger before bed, reduce worries, and create a cool environment for sleeping [2]. Cognitive restructuring helps to counter any negative thoughts regarding sleep or sleep restriction. Cognitive behavioral therapy has been effective in 60% – 80% of cases.

Many patients prefer non-pharmacological interventions that may be natural, herbal, or behavioral and often without side effects. They may fear becoming addicted to sleep medications or not tolerate them well.

Nonpharmacologic Treatment

Resolve barriers to sleep (e.g., symptoms, medications, worry). If symptoms hinder sleep, treat the symptoms (e.g., headache or cough). Next, consider if medications that disrupt sleep can be withdrawn or replaced. If pain interrupts sleep, improve pain management. If noise is a problem (e.g. in hospitals), consider ear plugs or sound machines. Educate the patient about healthy sleep habits, regular exercise, and elimination of alcohol, caffeine and smoking before bedtime. Stress management or relaxation therapy is useful for reducing anxiety (12). Hypnosis tapes or self-hypnosis can improve sleep. Some people find herbal remedies (e.g., chamomile tea, valerian root, and melatonin) and essential oils (lavender) helpful. Others like warm milk and foods containing tryptophan such as peanuts that help them fall asleep. Literature and resources on healthy sleep habits are useful for many patients.

Progressive relaxation

About 23% of adults with insomnia use relaxation and breathing techniques (Bertisch, 2012). (see Case example in Figure 1) When anxiety or worry interferes with sleep, the patient can learn to use progressive relaxation - to tense and relax muscle groups to gradually relax. The nurse can teach these techniques and some patients will appreciate a book or DVD recording to guide relaxation. Often one starts at the top of the head and systematically focuses on that body part and briefly tenses and relaxes it. When this technique is used properly, it reduces tension and relaxes the patient and improves sleep. Research shows that relaxation improves falling asleep, the quality of sleep and restful sleep [9]. Researchers reported that use of progressive relaxation has led to an 80% decrease of sleep medications. This technique is for the nurse to teach and easy to learn and effectively reduces insomnia.

Mindfulness

Mindfulness (MBSR) is a state of consciousness that is growing in popularity as a method of reducing stress, insomnia and other conditions [10,11]. It focuses awareness in the present moment and focuses one's complete attention. It can combine mindfulness meditation and yoga and is easy to learn and use to reduce stress and thoughts that interfere with sleep quality. The mind is a powerful factor in stress and mindfulness can improve blood pressure and emotional reactivity and it offers a way to relate and take control over life. MBSR has improved sleep outcomes. The nurse can teach or the patient can learn mindfulness online, in books or DVDs.

Hypnosis

Hypnosis is focused attention that creates an inner calm, relaxation, and trance that can alleviate symptoms (e.g., insomnia, anxiety, fear and distress). A trance state naturally occurs when one becomes totally engrossed in a film or game and ignores time and the environment. During a hypnotic trance, suggestions can encourage relaxing and restful sleep and the ability to sleep soundly and ignore distractions. While its medical uses are not completely known, hypnosis offers benefits in insomnia, anxiety, pain relief, anesthesia, and fatigue [6,12]. Hypnosis led to a significant improvement in sleep for those with fibromyalgia [12]. Patients can learn to use self-hypnosis to control insomnia and anxiety. The National Institutes of Health have approved hypnosis as one relaxation method for insomnia. A skilled hypnotist, self-help instructions, and DVDs can provide education or guide hypnosis. Nurses can seek training in hypnosis or refer the patient to other educational resources.

Acupressure

Acupressure is an alternative technique where a finger or body pressure is applied to pressure points, meridians, or energy channels in the body to realign the chakras. Evidence supports the treatment of chronic insomnia with acupressure [13]. Some wrist bands exist for sale that offer pressure on this point. When meridians and the flow of energy become blocked, then imbalance or illness can occur. The goal is to restore health and balance by applying pressure to specific points. Individuals can learn the pressure points that are associated with insomnia or other imbalances and use gentle pressure on these points to relieve symptoms and improve well being. For example, the HT7 wrist, shimien acupressure point is located on the bottom of your foot. If you were to draw a line from both of your ankle bones to the sole of your foot, the point is where these lines overlap at the midline of the sole (just above the heel of the foot). It's the most tender spot in this area. Pressure on this point can alleviate insomnia. Various written and online instructions and classes exist to teach acupressure.

Cognitive behavioral therapy

Cognitive behavioral therapy (CBT) helps improve sleep by changing irrational thoughts, assumptions, and negative beliefs about sleep and negative thinking patterns and can be done online (e.g., I have to sleep soundly for 8 hours or I will be exhausted) [11,14]. CBT challenges negative beliefs and assumptions about sleep that trigger anxiety, fear, and worry that disrupt sleep. CBT can be used with other approaches (e.g., relaxation) to reduce sleep latency (time to get to sleep) and sleep efficiency. Cognitive restructuring uses guided discovery (e.g., keeping a neutral stance, not interpreting, using Socratic questioning, and allowing the patient to uncover the meaning in the situation) and to uncover core beliefs about sleep. Patients consider the advantages and disadvantages of the belief and asks if it works as a guiding strategy in life.

In this theory, a negative view of the world and automatic and negative thinking patterns (e.g., the future is bleak, the world is barren, and the self is worthless disrupt mood and normal functioning such as sleep) [15]. CBT can help the patient dispel an irrational fear can be so strong that it interferes with treatment and quality of life. After identifying the thoughts that preceded insomnia, patients can learn to control these thoughts by distraction, discussion, or relaxation. Cognitive treatment focuses on here-and-now, problem solving, and rational thinking and can help people meet psychological, educational, and social support needs. It may include homework assignments to identify their irrational thoughts and assumptions about sleep. In many settings, nurses can refer patients to psychology or social work for CBT classes or treatments.

Pharmacologic Treatment

Short term treatment often involves benzodiazepines Zolpidem (Ambien) 10 orally at bedtime and elderly patients typically start at a half dose or Zaleplon (Sonata) 5-10 mg orally at bedtime. Melatonin is produced in the dark hours and may be helpful. Benzodiazepines (e.g. temazepam (Restoril), flurazepam (Dalmane) VERY long acting, triazolam (Halcion), estazolam (ProSom, Eurodin), lorazepam (Ativan), and clonazepam (Klonopin) are commonly prescribed. Short acting benzodiazepines such as Halcion and used with caution as they are addictive. For long term treatment, antihistamines, sedating antidepressants (e.g., trazodone, mirtazapine (Remeron), paroxetine (Paxil) can be useful if the patient is also depressed. These medications are discontinued gradually to avoid rebound insomnia. Clinicians need to be mindful of the potential for tolerance, dependence, and withdrawal with benzodiazepines. If the patient has a history of substance abuse or mental illness, clinicians will be wise to consult with a psychiatrist. The nurse will want to educate patients about when to take the drugs, side effects, and the potential impact on gait and balance particularly for elderly patients. If the symptoms are secondary to a psychiatric disorder (e.g., mood disorder or anxiety) nurses can refer to a psychiatrist or advanced practice psychiatric nurse. Patients with sleep apnea (e.g. heavy snoring) require referral to a sleep specialist. Antihistamines are not usually helpful for long term treatment as people develop tolerance or have side effects drug.

Follow up appointments should be weekly for short term problems to monitor treatment effectiveness, compliance and tolerance potential. Side effects of these drugs require monitoring to see if the patient experiences any dizziness, impaired balance, fall risk, confusion, or other symptoms. Elderly patients should take these drugs starting at a half dose and before bedtime to avoid excessive daytime sleepiness. Fall risk is important so discuss this thoroughly and have the patient discontinue the drug if gait or balance is impaired.

If the insomnia occurs for longer than a month, consider consultation or referral. Nurses are well positioned to educate patients about healthy sleep habits and to recommend non-pharmacological strategies. In many clinical settings patients report difficulty sleeping and the nurse can help them improve sleep hygiene and understand the various treatments available. Untreated insomnia can lead to chronic fatigue or decreased activity and unmanaged sleep apnea can be fatal. Nurses can use the information about sleep hygiene and insomnia treatments to help their patients and themselves improve the quality of sleep.

Conclusion

Insomnia is a common problem for many Americans and can range from a brief to chronic disorder. It is a common problem for shift workers, travelers, and those with pain and anxiety. While many people self-medicate their insomnia with OTC pills, they need evaluation for medical or mental health causes of the problem and education about sleep hygiene and other non-pharmacological treatments available. Nurses who detect insomnia can evaluate the symptoms, educate the person about sleep hygiene and non-pharmacological treatments and refer the patient for further evaluation and management. Without treatment, insomnia can impair the quality of life and pose dangers if the person drives or operates machinery. Encouraging patients to try mindfulness or other complimentary therapies as well as CBT and sleep hygiene is helpful.

References

1. Buysse DJ (2013) Insomnia. JAMA 309: 706-716.
2. Kraus SS, Rabin LA (2012) Sleep America: managing the crisis of adult chronic insomnia and associated conditions. J Affect Disord 138: 192-212.
3. APA. (2013) Sleep Wake Disorders. In A. P. Association, Diagnostic and Statistical Manual of Mental Disorders DSM 5. American Psychiatric Association.
4. Grohol J (2013) DSM-5 Changes: Sleep-Wake Disorders. PsDSM-5-changes: Sleep Wake Disorders. Psych Central.
5. Reinoso-Suárez F, de Andrés I, Garzón M (2011) Functional anatomy of the sleep-wakefulness cycle: wakefulness. Adv Anat Embryol Cell Biol 208: 1-128.
6. Bell C, McLeod LD, Nelson LM, Fehnel SE, Zografos LJ, et al. (2011) Development and psychometric evaluation of a new patient-reported outcome instrument measuring the functional impact of insomnia. Qual Life Res 20: 1457-1468.
7. Martinez D, Breitenbach TC, Lumertz MS, Alcântara DL, da Rocha NS, et al. (2011) Repeating administration of Epworth Sleepiness Scale is clinically useful. Sleep Breath 15: 763-773.
8. Bush AA (2012) The Pittsburgh Sleep Quality Index in older primary care patients with generalized anxiety disorder: psychometrics and outcomes following cognitive behavioral therap. Psychiatry Research 199: 24-30.
9. Bertisch SM, Wells RE, Smith MT, McCarthy EP (2012) Use of relaxation techniques and complementary and alternative medicine by American adults with insomnia symptoms: results from a national survey. J Clin Sleep Med 8: 681-691.
10. Ong JC, Ulmer CS, Manber R (2012) Improving sleep with mindfulness and acceptance: a metacognitive model of insomnia. Behav Res Ther 50: 651-660.
11. Garland SC (2014) Mindfulness-based stress reduction compared with cognitive behavioral therapy for the treatment of insomnia comorbid with cancer: a randomized, partially blinded, noninferiority trial. J Clinical Oncology 32: 449-457.
12. Picard P, Jusseaume C, Boutet M, Dualé C, Mulliez A, et al. (2013) Hypnosis for management of fibromyalgia. Int J Clin Exp Hypn 61: 111-123.
13. Sarris J, Byrne GJ (2011) A systematic review of insomnia and complementary medicine. Sleep Med Rev 15: 99-106.
14. Cheng SD (2012) Computerised cognitive behavioural therapy for insomnia: a systematic review and meta-analysis. Psychotherapy & Psychosomatics 81: 206-216.
15. Falloon K, Arroll B, Elley CR, Fernando A 3rd (2011) The assessment and management of insomnia in primary care. BMJ 342: d2899.

6

Excessive Daytime Sleepiness in Patients with Depressive Symptoms in a Nigerian Family Practice Setting

Shittu RO[1]*, Issa BA[2], Olanrewaju GT[2], Odeigah LO[1], Sule AG[1], Sanni MA[3] and Aderibigbe SA[4]

[1]*Department of Family Medicine, Kwara State Specialist Hospital, Nigeria*
[2]*Department of Behavioral Sciences, University of Ilorin Teaching Hospital, Nigeria*
[3]*Department of Hematology, Kwara State Specialist Hospital, Nigeria*
[4]*Department of Epidemiology and Community Health, University of Ilorin Teaching Hospital, Nigeria*

Abstract

Objectives: Clinically significant Excessive Daytime Sleepiness (EDS) is frequently encountered among patients with depressive symptoms, and a significant association was observed between depression, body mass index and EDS. Incidentally this sleep disorder is often overlooked. The aim of this study was to examine the association between excessive daytime sleepiness, depressive symptoms, body mass index and blood pressure in a Nigerian family practice setting.

Methods: This was a hospital based cross sectional study. Systematic sampling method was used in recruiting the patients. The PHQ-9 was administered to the respondents to screen for depressive symptoms. EDS was evaluated using the Epworth Sleepiness Scale (ESS). The international classification of BMI was used. Classification of hypertension was made according to (JNC 7).

Results: One hundred and seventy eight (44.5%) were found to have one form of depression or the other. There was female preponderance. Depression was prominent in the age group 51-60 years, more among the married than the single, as well as those with low socio economic status. There was strong statistical association between age, sex, marital status, level of education, occupation and monthly income (p-values 0.008, 0.000, 0.000, 0.003, 0.000 and 0.001 respectively). Forty five (25.3%) were hypertensive. Fifty nine (33.1%) scored 10 or more on the ESS which was clinically significant sleepiness. Forty seven (26.4%) were obese constituting (23.7%) of the poor sleepers. Ninety three (52.2%) were poor sleepers, sleeping less than the normal 7 hours.

Conclusion: In this study, significant EDS was found with patients with depressive disorders and higher body mass index. Therefore patients with a complaint of EDS should be thoroughly assessed for depression and obesity.

Keywords: Excessive daytime sleepiness; Depressive symptoms; Nigerian; Family practice setting

Introduction

The impact of sleep on psychomotor performance varies with the degree of sleepiness.

Mild sleepiness produces only minor disruptions of daily functions. Moderate sleepiness is associated with sleepy episodes occurring during activities. Severe sleepiness may impair function, causing a broad range of neuropsychological deficits like depression [1].

One major cause of sleepiness is insufficient sleep. Sleep deprivation and the resultant daytime sleepiness can result in depression, anger and confusion. Acute sleep deprivation also affects daytime alertness and mood [2].

Poor sleepers experience more problems with daytime functioning than good sleepers and highly depressed poor sleepers report greater impairment in function during the day. Examination of level of sleepiness among people with insomnia complaints and found that different levels of sleepiness were related to nocturnal sleep latencies.

Sleep debt secondary to sleep deprivation is one of the cardinal causes of EDS [3]. Other common causes include narcolepsy, idiopathic hypersomnia and obstructive sleep apnea and drugs that have sedative/hypnotic properties [4]. Medical aetiology of EDS includes head trauma, cerebrovascular disease and brain tumors [5]. EDS and depressive symptoms may also be familial or hereditary.

The symptoms of EDS range from drowsiness and reduced performance to episodes of involuntary sleep in spite of efforts to remain awake [6]. Individuals who have EDS also have increased risk of motor vehicle crashes, industrial disasters and occupational errors [7-10]. EDS occurs among depressed individuals and is a predictor of and a risk factor for depression [11-14].

EDS is one of the main symptoms of depressive disorder [13]. Epidemiological studies have indicated a strong association between EDS and depression [11-13]. This sleep disturbance and others play a significant role as predictors of depression. They are indeed important when screening for depression onset. EDS frequently leads depressed patients to seek medical assistance, yet it is commonly under evaluated [15]. Therefore, the understanding and proper management of this sleep disturbance is required for proper clinical evaluation and eventual management of the patients.

There is paucity of data on EDS among depressed patients in Nigeria in particular and West Africa in general. The aim of this study

***Corresponding author:** Shittu RO, Department of Family Medicine, Kwara State Specialist Hospital, Sobi, Ilorin, Kwara State, Nigeria;
E-mail: oorelopehospital@gmail.com

was therefore to evaluate EDS in outpatients with depressive symptoms and to study its relationship with Body Mass Index (BMI). This will also create the awareness that is required by physicians in the family practice setting show that number of people with EDS who are mismanaged will be reduced.

Methodology

This study was carried out at the Family Medicine Department of the Kwara State Specialist Hospital, Sobi, Ilorin, Nigeria, from 30th October to 30th November, 2013. The Patients Health Questionnaire (PHQ-9) [16] (Appendix A) which is a brief, 9 item, patients self-report depression assessment tool that was derived from the interview-based PRIME-MD [17] was used. It was specifically developed for use, in primary care general medical settings. Many depression screening and severity tools have been used in primary care, with good results. The PHQ-9, however, offers several advantages, because it is easily understood and it has very high face validity for patients and clinicians in primary care. Many other instruments use a 1-week time frame, but the PHQ-9 uses a 2 week time frame, which conforms to DSM-4 criteria. It is the only tool that was specifically developed for use as a patient self-administered depression diagnostic tool, rather than as a severity or screening tool. It is the only short self-report tool that can reasonably be used both for diagnosis of DSM-4 major depression as well as for tracking of severity of major depression over time [18]. Psychometric evaluation of the PHQ-9 revealed a sensitivity ranging from 62%-92% and a specificity between 74%-88% [16-18]. All subjects were screened for depression using PHQ-9. Scoring and level of depression was assessed viz: (1-4) Minimal depression, (5-9) Mild depression, (10-14) Moderate depression, (15-19) moderately severe depression, and (20-27) severe depression. Some direct depression care, such as care support, coordination, case management, and treatment was embarked on. Using the systematic random sampling, the PHQ-9 was administered to all the respondents, to screen for depression, until the estimated sample size of 178 was obtained. Respondents who scored one and more were assessed clinically for depression. The severity of the depression was further classified as minimal, mild, moderate and severe [15-17].

EDS was evaluated in the patients using the English Language version of the Epworth Sleepiness Scale (ESS) (Appendix B). This is a self-administered, eight-item, well-validated [18] and widely used subjective sleepiness scale. The patients were asked to score the likelihood of falling asleep in eight different situations. Scores on the ESS range from 0 to 24, with higher scores indicating greater likelihood of sleepiness. This questionnaire measures the propensity of patients to sleep or doze during active and passive situations commonly encountered during the wake period. The metrics of the ESS ranges from 0 to 24. ESS scores <10 were considered as indicative of less severe sleepiness and scores > 10 were deemed clinically significant sleepiness [19].

Height and weight were measured according to standardized procedures. Body Mass Index (BMI) was calculated as weight in Kg divided by height in m^2 (kg/m^2). The international classification of BMI was used. The principal cut-off points were as follows: moderate thinness (16.00-16.99), mild thinness (17.00-18.49), normal (18.50-24.99), pre-obese (25.00-29.99), obese class I (30.00-34.99), obese class II (35.00-39.99), obese class III (>40.00) [20].

An Accosson Mercury sphygmomanometer was used to measure the resting blood pressure of the subjects. Blood pressure was measured 3 times in the sitting position by trained and certified technicians using a standard mercury sphygmomanometer. The onsets of the first-phase (systolic) and fifth-phase (diastolic) Korotkoff sounds were recorded. The mean of the second and third measurements were used in the analyses. Classification of hypertension was made according to the seventh report of the Joint National Committee on Prevention, Detection, Evaluation and Treatment of high blood pressure (JNC 7). The following classification of blood pressure for adults aged ≥18 years was used.

Normal	Systolic: <120 mm Hg	Diastolic: <80 mm Hg
Pre-hypertension	Systolic: 120-139 mm Hg	Diastolic: 80-89 mm Hg
Stage 1 hypertension	140-159 mm Hg	Diastolic: 90-99 mm Hg
Stage 2 hypertension	≥ 160 mm Hg	Diastolic: ≥ 100 mm Hg

Completed questionnaire and measurements were entered into a computer data base. The data were analyzed using the epidemiological information (Epi-info) 2005 software package of Center for Disease Control and Prevention (CDC). The 2 by 2 contingency tables were used to carry out Chi-square test and to find out the level of significance and values less than 0.05 were regarded as statistically significant.

Results

Table 1 shows the association between socio-demographic variables and depression. Majority were females, depression was prominent in the age group 51-60 years, more among the married than the single as well as those with low socio economic status. There was strong statistical association between age, sex, marital status, level of education and occupation, (p-values 0.008, 0.000, 0.000, 0.003, and 0.000 respectively).

Table 2 displays the Epworth Sleeping Scale used to determine the level of Daytime Sleepiness and Depression. Fifty nine (33.1%) scored 10 and more which was considered clinically significant sleepiness.

Table 3 shows the association between Excessive Daytime Sleepiness and Duration of Sleep. Ninety three (52.2%) were poor sleepers with less than the normal 7 hours of sleep.

Table 4 displays the association between Excessive Daytime Sleepiness and Body Mass Index (BMI). Forty seven (26.4%) were obese. While 14 (23.7%) were poor sleepers.

Table 5 shows the association between Excessive Daytime Sleepiness and Blood Pressure. Forty five (25.3%) were hypertensive, out of which 16 (5.5%) were poor sleepers.

Discussion

Most of the patients were low-income middle-aged women. These results compare favorably with a previous work carried out in a major public hospital [21]. Women were reported to have depressive symptoms more frequently than men [22], as well as elderly and middle-aged adults in relation to youngsters [23]. This result differs considerably from the study of Eldevik where it was reported that men were affected to a greater extent than women [24].

The results showed that almost half of the patients with depressive symptoms in this study experienced clinically significant EDS. These findings are consistent with previous reports of a strong association between daytime sleepiness and depression [11,25].

Many of the patients (33.1%) had EDS defined as ESS score of ≥ 10. This was comparable to the work of Chellappa and colleagues [26] who reported 42.8% and to the (44.8%) reported by Mume et al. [27] but lower than 57.2% reported by Chellappa [26]. This result was higher

Variables	DEPRESSION				Total	P-value
	Minimal Depression	Mild Depression	Moderate Depression	Severe Depression		
Age						
21-30	15	6	2	1	**24**	**0.008**
31-40	13	8	0	2	**23**	
41-50	36	11	0	0	**47**	
51-60	31	20	0	0	**51**	
≥ 61	24	9	0	0	**33**	
Total	**119**	**54**	**2**	**3**	**178**	
Sex						
Male	33	3	0	3	**39**	0.000
Female	86	51	2	0	**139**	
Total	**119**	**54**	**2**	**3**	**178**	
Ethnicity						
Hausa	116	51	2	3	**172**	**0.567**
Yoruba	3	1	0	0	**4**	
Igbo	0	2	0	0	**2**	
Others	0	2	0	0	**2**	
Total	**119**	**54**	**2**	**3**	**178**	
Religion						
Christianity	21	6	0	0	**27**	**0.541**
Islam	98	48	2	3	**151**	
Total	**119**	**54**	**2**	**3**	**178**	
Marital Status						
Married	73	27	2	0	**102**	**0.000**
Single	7	2	0	3	**12**	
Divorced	5	1	0	0	**6**	
Separated	6	6	0	0	**12**	
Widow	28	18	0	0	**46**	
Total	**119**	**54**	**2**	**3**	**178**	
Level of Education						
Non-formal	71	37	0	0	**108**	**0.003**
Primary	16	6	0	0	**22**	
Secondary	16	7	0	2	**25**	
Tertiary	16	4	2	1	**23**	
Total	**119**	**54**	**2**	**3**	**178**	
Occupation						
Trader	38	18	0	0	**56**	**0.000**
Civil servant	19	4	2	2	**27**	
Self employed	45	28	0	0	**73**	
Unemployed	15	4	0	0	**19**	
Student	2	0	0	1	**3**	
Total	**119**	**54**	**2**	**3**	**178**	

Table 1: Association between Socio-Demographic Variables and Depression.

EDS	Level of Depression				Total	p-value
	Minimal Depression	Mild Depression	Moderate Depression	Severe Depression		
≤ 10	88	29	2	0	**119**	**0.003**
≥ 10	31	25	0	3	**59**	
Total	**119**	**54**	**2**	**3**	**178**	

Table 2: Association between Excessive Daytime Sleepiness and Depression.

than that obtained from analysis of the Geolong Osteoporosis Study, where 13% of the 844 women surveyed were found to have EDS, as measured by the Epworth Sleepiness Scale. Some other studies also found a significant association between EDS and depression [11]. Hayley et al. [28] reported that EDS patients had an increased likelihood of experiencing current and/or a lifetime history of depressive disorders compared to those without EDS. Overall, sleepiness may be attributed to depressive disorder [29].

There is thus ample evidence that EDS is a red flag of depression. EDS and depression have some genes in common and may be familial [5]. EDS has also been found to be strongly associated with suicidal ideation in depressed patients [30]. It is therefore clear that for complete clinical evaluation of depressive symptoms, evaluation of EDS is paramount. The clinician must therefore have a high index of suspicion of depressive disorder in patients who present with features of EDS. Incidentally, there are no facilities for objective and subjective evaluation of sleep complaints in Nigeria, making it difficult to make a cast iron diagnosis. It is therefore imperative for the authorities to

EDS	DURATION OF SLEEP				Total	p-value
	≥ 7	6.1-7hours	5-6hours	<5hours		
≤ 10	65	13	26	16	**119**	**0.023**
≥ 10	20	5	25	9	**59**	
Total	**85**	**17**	**51**	**25**	**178**	

Table 3: Association between Excessive Daytime Sleepiness and Duration of Sleep.

EDS	Body Mass Index		Total	p-value
	≤ 10	≥ 10		
Moderate thinness	0	3	**3**	**0.029**
Mild thinness	4	3	**7**	
Normal	46	21	**67**	
Pre-Obese	36	18	**54**	
Obese Class 1	23	4	**27**	
Obese Class 2	7	5	**12**	
Obese Class 3	3	5	**8**	
Total	**119**	**59**	**178**	

Table 4: Association between Excessive Daytime Sleepiness and Body Mass Index (Bml).

EDS	BLOOD PRESSURE				Total	p-value
	Normal	Pre-HTN	Stage 1	Stage 2		
≤ 10	66	24	14	15	**119**	**0.776**
≥ 10	28	15	8	8	**59**	
Total	**94**	**39**	**22**	**23**	**178**	

Table 5: Association between Excessive Daytime Sleepiness and Blood Pressure.

provide enough facilities and personnel in the field of sleep medicine to assist in this regard. Clinicians should be aware of the magnitude of the problem of EDS, especially among depressed patients, and should adopt holistic approach to assist them.

The current study demonstrated a significant association between EDS and Body Mass Index. Previous researches have established that EDS in non-pathological populations is not necessarily attributable to BMI and/or obesity [31]. Hayley et al. [28] reported that EDS and depression were independent of BMI. Thus, despite the established link between EDS and depression [32] and BMI and depression, future research assessing the prevalence of EDS while controlling for BMI to assess the mechanisms of this relationship will deepen and broaden our knowledge in this field. It has further been suggested that EDS may be related to the weight gain which is from the use of both antidepressant medication and neuroleptic medications, or a combination of these [33]. There is new evidence that a preceding maladaptive lifestyle and health factors often associated with the development of depression, such as obesity [34] contribute to maintain negative lifestyle and health outcomes which are recognized to share pathology with EDS, such as sleep disturbances.

Forty five (25.3%) were hypertensive, out of which 16 (5.5%) were poor sleepers. No significant association was found between EDS and blood pressure, contrary to Cui et al. [35] where the prevalence of self-reported EDS and mean values of systolic and diastolic blood pressure levels were significant.

Conclusion

In the present study, clinically significant EDS was frequently encountered among patients with depressive symptoms, and a significant association was observed between depression and EDS. Thus, careful investigation of daytime sleepiness in depressed patients is advised during clinical evaluation.

Incidentally, there are no facilities in Nigeria for proper evaluation of sleep complaints. Concerted effort should be made by appropriate authorities to establish facilities for dealing with sleep complaints. Besides, enough personnel in the field of sleep medicine in the country should be encouraged. It is expected that with adequate and proper facilities in place, the number of personnel in this field will gradually increase. In the meantime, clinicians should be aware of the magnitude of the problem of EDS, particularly, among depressed patients and be proactive in its management so as to reduce the burden of depressive disorder in the developing countries.

Declaration of Interest

No conflict of interest.

References

1. Rosenthal L, Roehrs TA, Rosen A, Roth T (1993) Level of sleepiness and total sleep time following various time in bed conditions. Sleep 16: 226-232.
2. Bonnet MH, Arand DL (1995) We are chronically sleep deprived. Sleep 18: 908-911.
3. Pagel JF (2009) Excessive daytime sleepiness. Am Fam Physician 79: 391-396.
4. Edd EM, Flores S (2009) Sleepiness or excessive daytime somnolence. Geriatr Nurs 30: 53-60.
5. Lessov-Schlaggar CN, Bliwise DL, Krasnow RE, Swan GE, Reed T (2008) Genetic association of daytime sleepiness and depressive symptoms in elderly men. Sleep 31: 1111-1117.
6. Bittencourt LR, Silva RS, Santos RF, Pires ML, Mello MT (2005) Excessive daytime sleepiness. Rev Bras Psiquiatr 27 Suppl 1: 16-21.
7. Ulfberg J, Carter N, Talbäck M, Edling C (1996) Excessive daytime sleepiness at work and subjective work performance in the general population and among heavy snorers and patients with obstructive sleep apnea. Chest 110: 659-663.
8. Lindberg E, Carter N, Gislason T, Janson C (2001) Role of snoring and daytime sleepiness in occupational accidents. Am J Respir Crit Care Med 164: 2031-2035.

9. Melamed S, Oksenberg A (2002) Excessive daytime sleepiness and risk of occupational injuries in non-shift daytime workers. Sleep 25: 315-322.

10. Garbarino S (2008) Sleep disorders and road accidents in truck drivers. G Ital Med Lav Ergon 30: 291-296.

11. Hublin C, Kaprio J, Partinen M, Heikkilä K, Koskenvuo M (1996) Daytime sleepiness in an adult, Finnish population. J Intern Med 239: 417-423.

12. Breslau N, Roth T, Rosenthal L, Andreski P (1996) Sleep disturbance and psychiatric disorders: a longitudinal epidemiological study of young adults. Biol Psychiatry 39: 411-418.

13. Silber MH (2001) Sleep disorders. Neurol Clin 19: 173-186.

14. Fava M (2004) Daytime sleepiness and insomnia as correlates of depression. J Clin Psychiatry 65 Suppl 16: 27-32.

15. Tylee A, Gastpar M, Lépine JP, Mendlewicz J (1999) DEPRES II (Depression Research in European Society II): a patient survey of the symptoms, disability and current management of depression in the community. DEPRES Steering Committee. Int Clin Psychopharmacol 14: 139-151.

16. Kroenke K, Spitzer RL, Williams JB (2003) The Patient Health Questionnaire-2: validity of a two-item depression screener. Med Care 41: 1284-1292.

17. Spitzer RL, Williams JB, Kroenke K, Linzer M, DeGruy FV 3rd, et al. (1997) Utility of a new procedure for diagnosing mental disorders in primary care. The PRIME-MD 1000 study. JAMA 272: 1749-1756.

18. Johns MW (1991) A new method for measuring daytime sleepiness: the Epworth sleepiness scale. Sleep 14: 540-545.

19. Kroenke K, Spitzer RL, Williams JB (2001) The PHQ-9: validity of a brief depression severity measure. J Gen Intern Med 16: 606-613.

20. Johns MW (1993) Daytime sleepiness, snoring, and obstructive sleep apnea. The Epworth Sleepiness Scale. Chest 103: 30-36.

21. Berry JM, Storandt M, Coyne A (1984) Age and sex differences in somatic complaints associated with depression. J Gerontol 39: 465-467.

22. Hara C, Lopes Rocha F, Lima-Costa MF (2004) Prevalence of excessive daytime sleepiness and associated factors in a Brazilian community: the Bambuí study. Sleep Med 5: 31-36.

23. Blazer DG (2000) Mood disorders: epidemiology. Comprehensive textbook of psychiatry, 7th ed, Philadelphia, Lippincott Williams & Wilkins, 1298-1308.

24. Eldevik MF, Flo E, Moen BE, Pallesen S, Bjorvatn B (2013) Insomnia, excessive sleepiness, excessive fatigue, anxiety, depression and shift work disorder in nurses having less than 11 hours in-between shifts. PLoS One 8: e70882.

25. Young TB (2004) Epidemiology of daytime sleepiness: definitions, symptomatology, and prevalence. J Clin Psychiatry 65 Suppl 16: 12-16.

26. Chellappa SL, Araújo JF (2006) Excessive daytime sleepiness in patients with depressive disorder. Rev Bras Psiquiatr 28: 126-129.

27. Mume CO (2010) Excessive daytime Sleepiness among depressed patients. Libyan J Med 5.

28. Hayley AC, Williams LJ, Berk M, Kennedy GA, Jacka FN, et al. (2013) The relationship between excessive daytime sleepiness and depressive and anxiety disorders in women. Aust N Z J Psychiatry. 47: 772-778.

29. Cano-Lozano MC, Espinosa-Fernández L, Miró E, Buela-Casas G (2003) A review of sleep disorders in depression. Rev Neurol 36: 366-375.

30. Johns M, Hocking B (1997) Daytime sleepiness and sleep habits of Australian workers. Sleep 20: 844-849.

31. Scott KM, McGee MA, Wells JE, Oakley Browne MA (2008) Obesity and mental disorders in the adult general population. J Psychosom Res 64: 97-105.

32. Guilleminault C, Brooks SN (2001) Excessive daytime sleepiness: a challenge for the practising neurologist. Brain 124: 1482-1491.

33. Stanton JM (1995) Weight gain associated with neuroleptic medication: a review. Schizophr Bull 21: 463-472.

34. Gallicchio L, Kalesan B (2009) Sleep duration and mortality: a systematic review and meta-analysis. J Sleep Res 18: 148-158.

35. Cui R, Tanigawa T, Sakurai S, Yamagishi K, Imano H, et al. (2008) Associations of sleep-disordered breathing with excessive daytime sleepiness and blood pressure in Japanese women. Hypertens Res 31: 501-506.

7

Exploring a Behavioural Therapy for Insomnia in Shift Workers

Annie Vallières[1,2,3,*], **Monica Roy**[1,2], **Emmanuelle Bastille-Denis**[1,2], **Sonia Claveau**[1,2] **and Tarek Simon**[1,2]

[1]*École de psychologie, Université Laval, Québec, Québec, Canada*

[2]*Laboratoire Psycho Socio Culturel du sommeil, Centre de recherche de l'Institut universitaire en santé mentale de Québec, Québec, Québec, Canada*

[3]*Centre de recherche du Centre hospitalier universitaire de Québec, Québec, Canada*

***Corresponding author:** Annie Vallières, 2325 rue des bibliothèques, École de psychologie, Pavillon Félix-Antoine-Savard, local 1044, Université Laval, Québec, G1V 0A6, Canada, E-mail: annie.vallieres@psy.ulaval.ca

Abstract

About 30% of Canadian workers are on shift work schedules, and 8% to 32% of them suffer from Shift Work Disorder (SWD). Only a few behavioural treatments exist to treat this population. This study explores the efficacy and feasibility of sleep restriction therapy for insomnia in a group of night shift workers. Six participants (3 women) meeting SWD criteria were recruited. Mean age was 45.7 years old (SD=8.2). A multiple baseline design was used. After baseline, each participant received six to eight weekly treatment sessions. They completed several self reported questionnaires and a daily sleep diary throughout the study. For each sleep period, sleep variables were calculated from the sleep diary. Two participants had a high treatment response and all others participants had a moderate response. Moreover, all participants presented at least two significant clinical improvements. Five participants presented a decreased in both sleepiness scores. The study suggests that sleep restriction therapy is effective, feasible, and reliable. Sleep restriction therapy for insomnia could improve sleep and diminish sleepiness in shift workers suffering from SWD. The present study opens new possibilities of treatment for shift workers that deserve greater attention in the future.

Keywords: Shift work; Insomnia; Behavioural therapy; Pilot study

Introduction

Shift work is a reality of our contemporary industrial world. Indeed, this work schedule involves approximately 28% of the Canadian work force [1]. Unfortunately, shift work can be accompanied by various problems such as sleep difficulties. When those sleep difficulties are insomnia or excessive sleepiness associated with the work schedule, they are called Shift Work Disorder (SWD) [2]. It is estimated that about 8% to 32% of shift workers [3-5] suffer from SWD. Specific negatives consequences are linked to SWD. For instance, it is associated with an increased risk of depression, morbidity and gastric ulcers [3], cardiovascular disease, cancer, reproductive troubles [6] and a decrease in quality of life [4,5,7]. Furthermore, it has a negative socio-economic impact as it is associated with increased absenteeism at work and to an increase in accidents caused by sleepiness [8] or insomnia [9]. Furthermore insomnia in the context of shift work seems to contribute to an aggravation of the overall clinical picture of shift workers [9]. Current interventions for SWD focus predominantly on alleviating sleepiness and increasing alertness in re-entraining the circadian rhythm. Most of the available treatments are pharmacological, such as hypnotics used to improve sleep [10,11], stimulants used to improve alertness [12,13], or luminotherapy used with or without dark sunglasses to shift the circadian rhythm at least partially to thereby improve sleep and alertness [14,15]. Other studies have evaluated the effect on the sleep of night workers, of a nap before [16-18] or during the night work [19,20]. Among all the interventions presently offered to shift workers, some provide improvement on either sleep or alertness but they fail to improve the whole symptomatology of SWD [21] and none of them, except hypnotics, specifically address insomnia in shift work. Furthermore, all pharmacological agents possess, the danger of developing physiological or psychological dependencies on medication, some provide insomnia rebound effects during withdrawal of the medication, and can also interfere with the sleep architecture [22]. Moreover, most of the studies evaluating intervention for SWD did not use specific diagnostic criteria [23] and only a few were conducted with a real shift worker population. Nonpharmacological treatments for insomnia such as CBT-I are recommended as a standard treatment for chronic insomnia [24].

CBT-I includes stimulus control therapy, sleep restriction therapy, relaxation training, sleep hygiene education and cognitive therapy [24-26]. Two studies have attempted to improve sleep in shift work with CBT-I [27-29]. In the first one, a nonrandomized group of 26 shift workers received seven sessions of CBT-I while 21 shift workers in the second one received a home-based cognitive-behavioral intervention for insomnia. Both studies show sleep improvement. More specifically, participants of the first study improved on sleep onset latency and sleep efficiency while participants of the second study improved on sleep quality. Perceived insomnia severity as well as sleep-related dysfunctional beliefs also improved in Jarnefelt et al. [27] whereas emotional distress decreased in the other study [29]. These two first studies [27,29] are a very promising step in addressing insomnia in shift work. However, several issues related to the methodology and to the intervention itself might limit the conclusions. The most important problem concerns the fact that no clinical interview was conducted to ascertain the diagnosis. CBT-I had been developed for chronic insomnia, which is a specific disorder. To know its efficacy in a shift work population, it should be evaluated within a shift worker population suffering from SWD with insomnia. Also, several aspects of the CBT-I assessed in the two studies may hide the real treatment effect. Indeed, numerous changes from the original content of CBT-I were made, the CBT-I was delivered as a package and in two different formats. Moreover, the designs used did not allow any control for spontaneous change. Therefore, it is impossible to know to what part of the treatment might have been responsible for improvements, and what would be the real effect of CBT-I on sleep in a clinical population.

The work schedule can lead to an insomnia different from that of people sleeping by night. These differences can be in terms of when insomnia occurs in a 24 h period, as well as why it occurs or is maintained. The etiology of insomnia in shift work has not yet been documented. Nothing is known regarding conditioning process, sleep habits, beliefs or cognitive processes involved in shift work insomnia. Consequently, in order to adapt a CBT-I to shift workers, each component of CBT-I should be evaluated separately to know the component of CBT-I that needs to be applied, when it should be applied, and which works best as a function of the work schedule. Among the behavioral therapies for insomnia, sleep restriction therapy should be useful for shift workers as it uses the process of sleep homeostasis to improve sleep. The objective of sleep restriction therapy is to facilitate and consolidate sleep, using and regulating homeostatic sleep pressure [30,31]. Indeed, the sleep homeostasis mechanism of shift workers is known to be deregulated and to contribute to their level of sleepiness. Therefore, a better management of this pressure through sleep restriction therapy should have a beneficial effect on sleep. This study aims at exploring the efficacy of sleep restriction therapy adapted for SWD including insomnia symptoms. More specifically, it is expected that sleep onset latency will decrease for sleep, and sleep efficiency will increase after treatment for all participants. The study also evaluates the feasibility and the treatment acceptability among shift workers.

Methods

Participants

Participants were recruited through press releases in local media, advertising in hospitals and through participation in another study at the Centre d'étude des troubles du sommeil (CETS) of the Institut universitaire en santé mental de Québec (IUSMQ). Inclusion criteria were: (a) being over 18 years old; (b) being a shift worker (work a minimum of eight nights per month); (c) working at least four hours between 24:00 and 8:00 and (d) reporting a sleep disorder related to the work schedule as defined by the ICSD-II [2]. The criterion of 8 nights per month was chosen to ensure that sleep difficulties were related to the work schedule. Exclusion criteria were: (a) being unable to answer questions during interviews or being unable to respond to questionnaires; (b) being unable to go to the sleep laboratory; (c) being blind; (d) travelling more than one hour to get home after work; (e) having traveled over three time zones in the last month; (f) presenting a severe psychological disorder such as major depression; (g) presenting alcohol or substance abuse; (h) presenting another possible sleep disorder such as sleep apnea or periodic limb movement; (i) using hypnotics on a regular basis in the last month and (j) drinking over 10 cups of coffee (or other stimulants) per day. The study was approved by the IUSMQ ethical committee (#185). Eight eligible participants responded to recruitment publicity and underwent telephone screening. Subsequently, they went through a multi-step screening evaluation, which includes two pre-treatment interviews. One participant was then excluded because sleep apnea was suspected and another one was no longer interested in the study. The final sample included six participants (3 men and 3 women). The mean age of participants was 45.7 years (ranging from 38 to 57 years old). The average duration of sleep difficulties was 15.3 years (ranging from 1 to 30 years) and the average duration of shift work was 11.4 years (ranging from 0.7 to 20 years). Participants 2, 3, 4 and 5 completed all the assessment phases. Participant 1 left shift work at week 5: at that moment, the treatment strategies concerned nocturnal sleep only. Participant 6 dropped out of the study at week 6 of the treatment without giving any reason. Participants' main characteristics are summarized in Table 1. Follow-up data are available for participant 2, 3, and 5 only.

Participant	Age/Gender	Duration of shift work (years)	Duration of sleep difficulties (years)	Nature of sleep complaint
1	38/M	1	1	Initiation, maintenance and premature termination
2	43/F	20	12	Premature termination
3	57/F	0.7	5	Maintenance and premature termination
4	42/F	20	20	Initiation and maintenance
5	39/M	10	24	Maintenance and premature termination
6	55/M	6	30	Maintenance

Table 1: Summary of participants' characteristics (Note. F: Female; M: Male).

Design

A single case design called multiple baseline across subjects design [32] was used to explore the efficacy of the sleep restriction therapy for shift workers with SWD. This particular single case design provides a controlled investigation of treatment mechanisms [33]. Baseline length has to be different for each participant to ensure that the introduction of the experimental treatment occurs at a different time for each participant. This particularity of the design provides a control for possible maturational or spontaneous changes. Maturation refers to natural changes over time of a participant's sleep that occurs without treatment. Figure 1 illustrates the design, showing a different baseline length for each participant.

Procedure

Before entering the study, participants were instructed to maintain their typical sleep habits. The study was conducted in French. At baseline and throughout the study, participants completed several self-report measures in French and continuous assessments of their sleep and sleepiness. Three months after the end of treatment, participants were as asked to complete the self-report measures about sleep, fatigue, depression, and anxiety.

Measures

Initial screening and evaluation: Initial screening consisted of a 20-minute telephone interview to determine participant eligibility. Subsequently, two pre-treatment interviews were conducted: a semi-structured psychological interview (SCID-IV evaluation) [34] and a sleep history interview adapted from the IIS (Insomnia Interview Schedule [35]) and the Standard Shift Work Index [36] to evaluate the presence of psychological disorders and sleep difficulties.

Sleep diary: Participants completed sleep diaries upon awakening after each sleep period. From these diaries Total Sleep Time (TST), Wake After Sleep Onset (WASO), Sleep Onset Latency (SOL), and Sleep Efficiency [SE; ratio of TST divided by Time in Bed (TIB)] were derived for each participant for diurnal and nocturnal sleep. Sleepiness according to the Stanford Sleepiness Scale [37] was also recorded in the sleep diary. Participants rated their level of sleepiness/alertness using a 7-point Likert scale (ranges from "1" to "7"). Higher scores represent a greater degree of sleepiness. This questionnaire is widely used in sleep and shift work population studies.

Questionnaires

Dysfunctional beliefs and attitudes about sleep-16: (DBAS-16 [38]) assesses with 16 items four domains of beliefs and attitudes regarding sleep: (a) misattribution or amplification of the causes of insomnia; (b) sleep concerns; (c) unrealistic sleep expectations and (d) faulty beliefs about insomnia consequences. Each item is scored on Likert-type scale ranging from "1" to "10". Higher scores indicate a high level of misconceptions and bad attitudes related to sleep. The psychometric properties of the French version are well documented in an insomnia population [38,39].

Glasgow content of thoughts inventory: (GCTI [40]) assesses with 25 items the nature and frequency of intrusive thoughts at bedtime. Each item is scored on Likert-type scale from "1" to "4" and the total score ranges between "25" to "100". Higher scores indicate a high degree of intrusive thoughts at bedtime. The psychometric qualities of the French version have not yet been evaluated.

The multidimensional fatigue inventory: (MFI [41]) assesses with 20 items global fatigue and five related domains: (a) general fatigue; (b) mental fatigue; (c) physical fatigue; (d) reduced motivation, and (e) decreased activity. Higher scores indicate a more severe fatigue. This French version of the questionnaire has good psychometric qualities [42] and is frequently used in an insomnia population.

Beck depression inventory: (BDI-II [43]) assesses with 21 items the presence and severity of depressive symptoms within the last two weeks. Each item is scored on scale from "0" to "3" and total score ranges between "0" and "63". Higher scores indicate a greater symptom severity. This questionnaire is widely used and the psychometric qualities of the French version are well established [43].

State-trait anxiety inventory: (STAI-Y [44]) assesses with 20 items state and trait anxiety. Each item is scored on a Likert-type scale ranging from "1" to "4". Higher scores indicate a high level of anxiety. The psychometric properties of the French version of the STAI-Y are excellent and well documented [45].

Compliance and acceptability measures: Compliance to behavioral procedure was computed from the sleep diaries. A weekly percentage of adherences to the prescribe time to go to bed as well as to arising time were computed separately for each participant and sleep episode. Nonadherence was considered as going to bed more than 15 minutes earlier and getting out of bed more than 15 minutes later than the prescribed nocturnal and diurnal sleep window. Moreover, more than 30 minutes of the prescribed TIB was also considered as nonadherance. There were then six criteria to be respected: three for nocturnal sleep and three for diurnal sleep. For each criterion, a score of 1 was assigned when it was respected and a score of 0 if not. For each day the maximum score was 3. Daily scores were computed, divided by the total expected score and multiplied by 100. The total expected score is based on the assumption that the participant had entirely respected the procedures.

Treatment acceptability scale: (TAS [46]) This 4-item scale assesses participants' perceptions of treatment acceptability. Each item is scored on Liker-type scale from "1" to "10". Higher scores indicate a high degree of acceptability of treatment. The psychometric qualities of the French version have not yet been evaluated.

Treatment

The sleep restriction therapy adapted to shift work and administered in this study is outlined in a treatment manual [47]. Use of the manual ensures treatment fidelity and facilitates treatment standardization and replication. The treatment includes five or six 50-minute individual consultation sessions. The first four sessions were administered weekly while the following two were at every two weeks. The content and aims of the sleep restriction therapy are summarized in Table 2. The treatment went from steps 1 to 3 where in step 1 sleep restriction was applied to night sleep, in step 2 to day sleep, and in step 3 to naps. At each step criterion SE level was reached before going to the next step. Therefore, the number of treatment session to reach criterion and pass to the next step could vary among participants. During the sleep restriction therapy, the first meeting with participants served to provide participants with information about sleep and its regulatory mechanisms, while the following meetings discussed the maintenance of therapeutic gains.

Sleep restriction therapy consists of curtailing the time spent in bed to conform to the reported amount of time asleep. A sleep window is determined using the average of TST reported by participants in their baseline weeks of sleep diaries. The sleep window is increased by 15-30 minutes, contingent upon reaching a SE of 85% or more. When SE is between 80% and 85%, the sleep window is kept stable and when SE is lower than 80%, the sleep window is shortened by 15-30 minutes. As suggested [14], bedtimes for daily sleep were set close to the time that participants arrived home after their work shift. The lower limit of the sleep window is five hours. Treatment sessions are conducted by a graduate student in psychology (EBD) and supervised by a clinical psychologist (AV).

Steps	Treatment guidelines
1: night sleep	Addressing insomnia symptoms occurring during night sleep
	• Applying sleep restriction therapy using a sleep window as for insomnia
	• Once average sleep efficiency for night sleep reaches 85% then go to step 2
2: day sleep	Addressing insomnia symptoms occurring during day sleep
	• Applying sleep restriction using a sleep window as for insomnia
	• Once average sleep efficiency for day sleep reaches 85% then go to step 3
3: naps	Addressing naps
	• Scheduled naps using sleep restriction therapy and a sleep window
	• Length and timing of naps should be adapted to lifestyle habits and without interfering with sleep homeostasis process
General recommendation with sleep restriction	• The sleep window for each sleep period should be adjusted after computing the sleep efficiency of each sleep period.
	• The time for going to bed, whether night sleep, day sleep or nap, should be determined regarding lifestyle habits and as a function of the sleep homeostatic drive.
Recall	Sleep restriction therapy for insomnia
	• Determined a sleep window length (time for going in and out bed) based on the total sleep time average
	• Modify the sleep window following these rules:
	• Increase of the sleep window if sleep efficiency is ≥ 85%
	• Decrease of the sleep window if sleep efficiency is < 80%
	• Otherwise maintain

Table 2: Summary of sleep restriction adapted for insomnia in shift work.

Data Analysis

The five dependent variables were derived from sleep diaries for nocturnal and diurnal sleep. Mean comparisons at each stage (baseline and post-treatment) were performed to determine the magnitude of change of nocturnal and diurnal sleep. Clinically significant change criteria, based on expected results obtained with CBT-I, were used to determine the clinical value of the change [48]. For WASO and SOL, the reduction at post-treatment must be between 50 and 60% compared to baseline. TST increases must be between 30 and 45 minutes at post-treatment, SE must be greater than 85% and sleepiness must decrease. Subsequently, treatment response was evaluated using the following criteria: (a) and (b) respectively, reduction of diurnal and nocturnal WASO or SOL greater than 50% at post-treatment; (c) and (d) respectively, increase of diurnal and nocturnal TST greater than 30 to 45 minutes at post-treatment; (e) and (f) respectively, diurnal and nocturnal SE greater than 85%; (g) and (h) respectively, diminution of nocturnal and diurnal sleepiness scores.

With CBT-I, one can reasonably expect a improvement of 75% of the problem for those with chronic insomnia [49]. Since there are eight criteria, an amelioration for at least six criteria would represent the expected 75% improvement. Treatment response is considered "high" when at least six criteria are met, "moderate" if three to five criteria are met and "low" if fewer than three criteria are met.

A nonparametric one-tailed test was used to assess the significance of responses after treatment. The questionnaire data were visually analyzed and described, confidence intervals were computed on the mean difference from post to baseline. Cronbach alpha consistency was measured for the two self-report questionnaires without French validation (GCTI and TAS) [50].

Results

Figures 1 and 2 illustrate daily changes in the percentage of nocturnal and diurnal sleep efficiency and total sleep time during each phase of the study (baseline, treatment and posttreatment) for each participant. The figures show night-to-night variability for nocturnal sleep and diurnal sleep, confirming the presence of insomnia.

Moreover, the figures show that no changes in sleep occurred before treatment introduction, for each participant and sleep variable, indicating an adequate control in this respect. The internal consistency of the GCTI at baseline and posttreatment is excellent, with Cronbach alphas of .95 and .92, respectively. For the TAS, internal consistency is excellent at baseline and good at post-treatment with Cronbach alphas of 0.94 and 0.88, respectively.

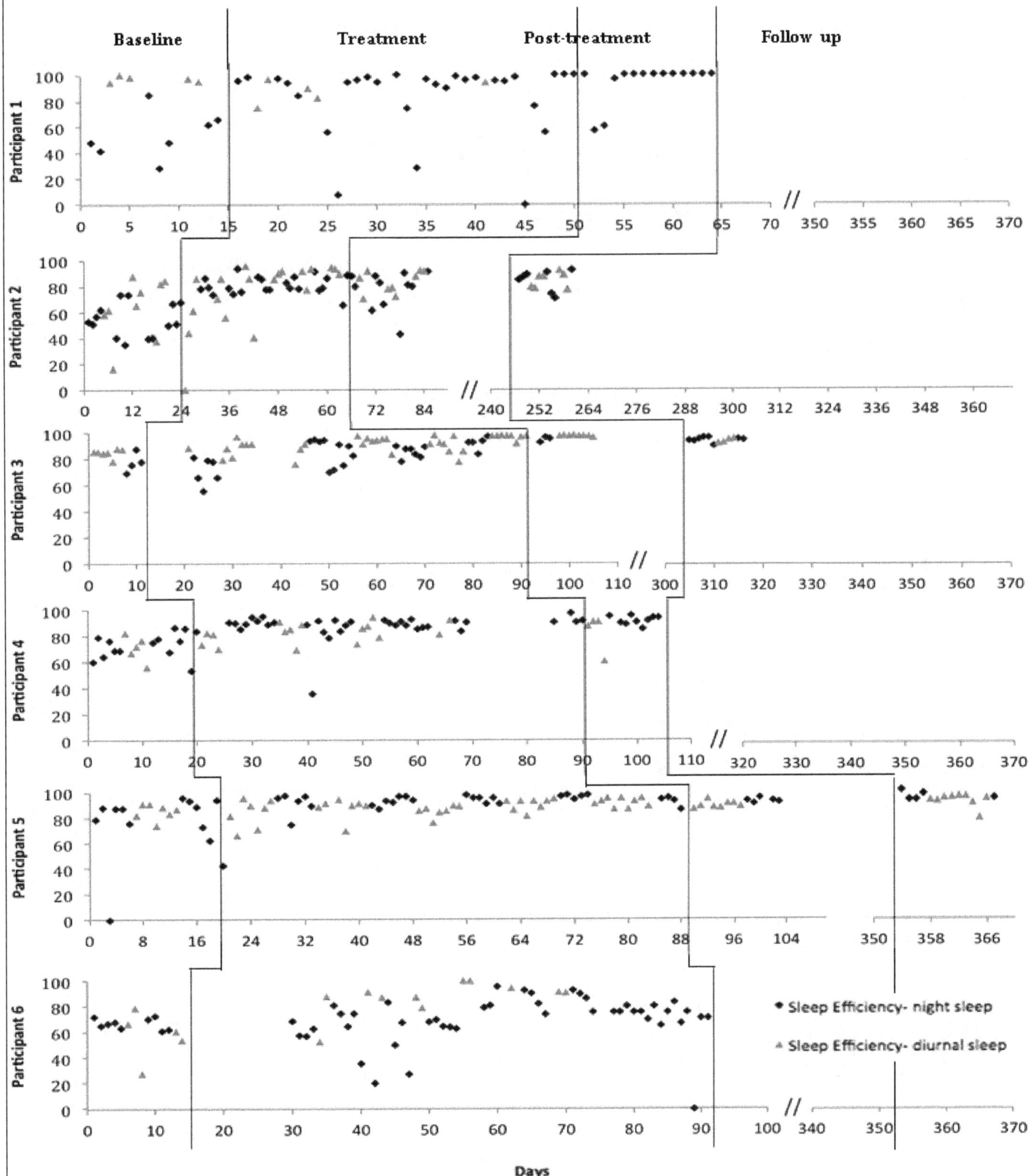

Figure 1: Sleep efficiency for each participant.

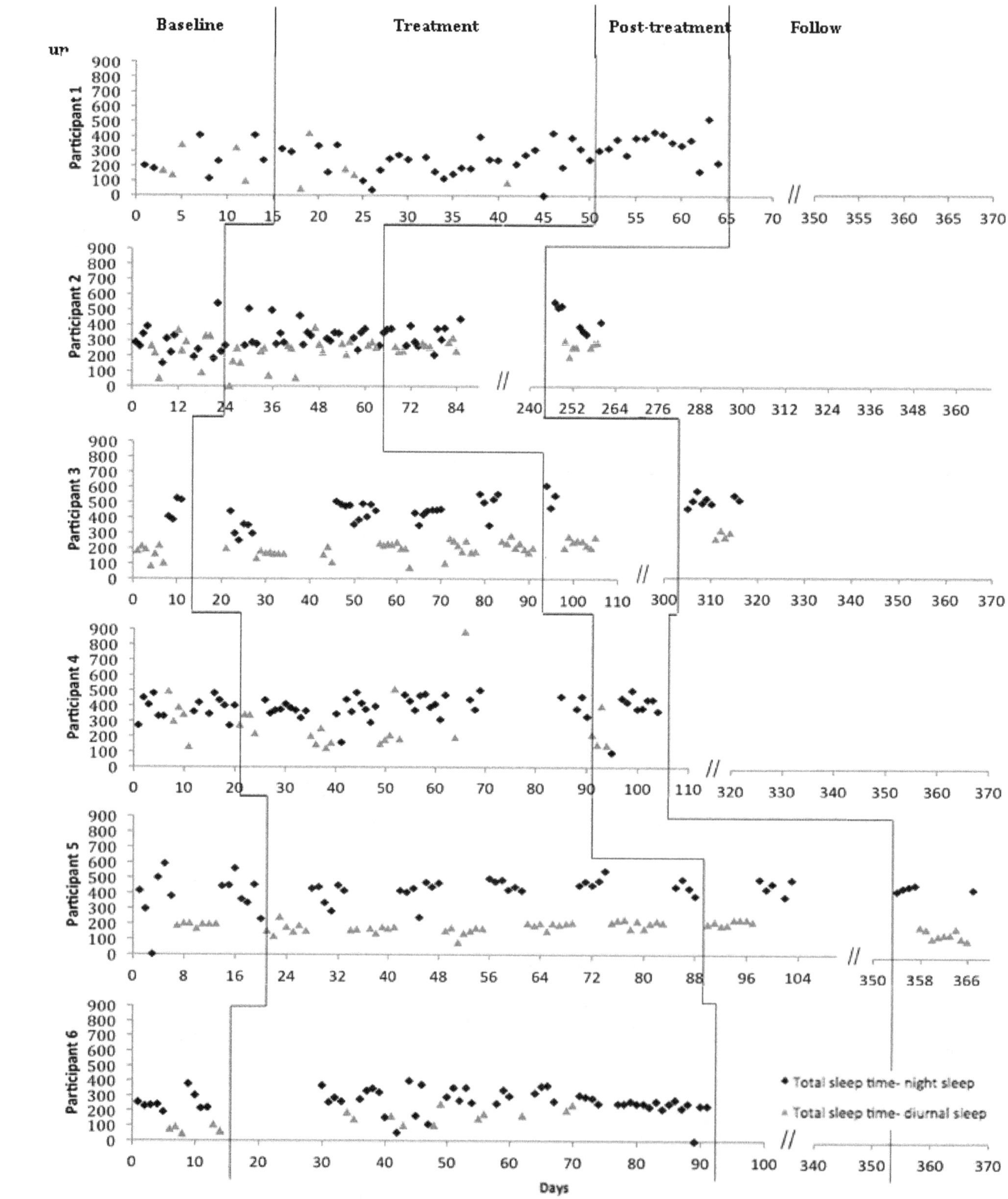

Figure 2: Total sleep time in minutes for each participant.

Participant 1

Participant 1 was a man of 38 years old with sleep difficulties since beginning night work a year previously (Table 1). Before treatment, diurnal SOL and WASO were low while nocturnal SOL and WASO were respectively 25.6 and 72.3 minutes. Diurnal and nocturnal TST were 214.2 and 247.5 minutes, respectively. Diurnal SE was high but nocturnal SE was 52.6%. Diurnal and nocturnal sleepiness scores were 1.7 and 2.1, respectively (Tables 3 and 4).

	Participant 1			Participant 2			Participant 3			Participant 4			Participant 5			Participant 6		
Sleep parameters	Pre	Post	F/U	Pre	Post	F/U	Pre	Post	F/U	Pre	Post	F/U	Pre	Post	F/U	Pre	Post	F/U
Sleep onset latency																		
Diurnal sleep	5	n/a	n/a	14.2	10.7	10.4	12.1	5	5	24	11.3	n/a	6.2	10.6	15.4	7.9	n/a	n/a
Nocturnal sleep	25.6	1.8	n/a	13.3	11	11.3	18.8	6.3	7.5	32.2	15.4	n/a	25.8	22.1	7.7	9.8	n/a	n/a
Number of awakenings																		
Diurnal sleep	0	n/a	n/a	0.7	0.2	0.3	1	0	0.7	3.4	3.5	n/a	1	0.4	0.3	1.5	n/a	n/a
Nocturnal sleep	0.9	0.1	n/a	2.2	0.6	1.6	2.3	1.5	0.4	4.6	2.3	n/a	0.8	0.8	1.3	3	n/a	n/a
Wake after sleep onset																		
Diurnal sleep	0	n/a	n/a	11.3	1.1	1.7	10.7	0	6.7	66	26.3	n/a	30.4	22.2	15.6	49.4	n/a	n/a
Nocturnal sleep	72.3	34.3	n/a	31.9	8	7.9	97.5	12.5	4.2	78.3	38.1	n/a	51.7	45	50.6	139.6	n/a	n/a
Total sleep time																		
Diurnal sleep	214.2	n/a	n/a	193.3	213.9	175	167.1	242.1	303.3	333	227.5	n/a	242.8	264.4	297.7	119	n/a	n/a
Nocturnal sleep	247.5	348.9	n/a	432.2	447	492.1	457.5	540	560.8	385.3	345.8	n/a	286.3	334.2	505.6	265.7	n/a	n/a
Time in bed																		
Diurnal sleep	220.4	n/a	n/a	229.6	237.9	192.1	196.4	247.5	315	456	272.5	n/a	367.2	318.9	352.5	188.7	n/a	n/a
Nocturnal sleep	470.6	385	n/a	511.7	479	526.9	588.8	570	575	521.7	429.6	n/a	533.8	427.9	598.8	415.1	n/a	n/a
Sleep efficiency (%)																		
Diurnal sleep	97.2	n/a	n/a	84.2	89.9	91.1	85.1	97	96	73	83.5	n/a	65.2	83.2	84.4	66.2	n/a	n/a
Nocturnal sleep	52.6	91.6	n/a	84.9	93.3	93.4	77.7	95	97.5	74	91.9	n/a	53.6	78	84.1	64.2	n/a	n/a

Table 3: Sleep measures across assessment phases for individual participants (Note. All times recorded are in minutes. Diurnal sleep refers to the sleep period after shift work. Nocturnal period refers to sleep periods when the participant has days off or working days. Pre= pre-treatment; Post=post-treatment; F/U= follow-up; n/a= not applicable).

	Participant 1			Participant 2			Participant 3			Participant 4			Participant 5			Participant 6		
Questionnaires	Pre	Post	F/U	Pre	Post	F/U	Pre	Post	F/U	Pre	Post	F/U	Pre	Post	F/U	Pre	Post	F/U
GCTI	38	47	n/a	42	33	29	60	44	43	48	29	n/a	82	60	68	75	n/a	n/a
DBAS	2.4	2.4	n/a	1.3	2.6	2	5.1	3	2.7	3.9	3.3	n/a	5.7	5.5	5	6.1	n/a	n/a

MFI	41	53	n/a	53	29	26	40	45	31	35	25	n/a	76	60	68	50	n/a	n/a
BDI	2	4	n/a	4	0	0	21	10	6	3	0	n/a	30	19	21	20	n/a	n/a
STAI-Y																		
State anxiety	31	27	n/a	35	32	21	34	29	28	33	21	n/a	43	56	-	40	n/a	n/a
Trait anxiety	24	33	n/a	31	36	23	36	31	29	31	24	n/a	59	49	-	49	n/a	n/a
Sleepiness																		
Diurnal sleep	1.7	n/a	n/a	2.5	4.2	3.5	3.3	2.4	2	3.4	1	n/a	3.2	2.4	2.4	3.2	n/a	n/a
Nocturnal sleep	2.1	1.6	n/a	2.9	3.4	2	1.5	1	1.3	3.3	1.2	n/a	3.5	1.4	1.6	3.1	n/a	n/a

Table 4: Total score on questionnaire across assessments phases (Note. GCTI: Glasgow Content of Thoughts Inventory; DBAS: Dysfunctional Beliefs and Attitudes about Sleep; MFI: Multidimensional Fatigue Inventory, BDI: Beck Depression Inventory; STAI-Y: State-Trait Anxiety Inventory; Pre: Pre-treatment; Post: Post-treatment, F/U: Follow-up; n/a: Not Applicable; (-): Missing Data).

After treatment, there was a clinical significant change for all criteria of nocturnal sleep. Indeed, nocturnal SOL and WASO decreased by 93.0% and of 52.6%, respectively while TST increased by 101.4 minutes, SE increased to 91.6%. Diurnal sleepiness decreased by 0.5 point. Participant 1 had an increased level of general fatigue. Intrusive thoughts at bedtime increased also, but the level of endorsement of dysfunctional beliefs and attitudes about sleep remained low. Depression and anxiety increased slightly (Table 4). Participant 1 did not complete the follow-up assessment. Finally, participant 1 had a moderate response to treatment, meeting all criteria for nocturnal sleep (criteria b, d, f, and h) but only one criterion for diurnal sleep (criterion g) (Tables 3 and 4). Participant 1 moderately accepted treatment and had diurnal and nocturnal sleep compliance of 55.6% and 58.7%, respectively (Table 5).

Statements	Participant 1		Participant 2		Participant 3		Participant 4		Participant 5		Participant 6	
	Pre	Post	Pre	Post	Pre	Post	Pre	Post	Pre	Post	Pre	Post
Acceptance of treatment	5	7	8	10	5	8	6	10	9	9	10	n/a
Expected short-term effect	5	8	7	10	6	9	7	10	9	8	10	n/a
Expected long-term effect	7	5	8	10	7	7	7	10	8	9	10	n/a
Treatment satisfaction	n/a	7	n/a	10	n/a	9	n/a	10	n/a	8	n/a	n/a
Mean total score	5.7/10	6.8/10	7.7/10	10/10	6/10	8.3/10	6.7/10	10/10	8/10	8.5/10	10/10	n/a

Table 5: Treatment acceptability (Note: Pre: Pre-treatment; Post: Post-treatment; n/a: Not Applicable).

Participant 2

Participant 2, a woman of 43 years old, had been a shift worker for 20 years and complained of sleep difficulties for 12 years (Table 2). Before treatment, the diurnal and nocturnal SOL and nocturnal WASO were less than 15 minutes while the nocturnal WASO were 31.9 minutes. Diurnal and nocturnal TST were 193.3 and 432.2 minutes and diurnal and nocturnal SE were 84.2% and 84.9% respectively. Nocturnal and diurnal sleepiness scores were 2.5 and 2.9 respectively (Tables 3 and 4). At post-treatment, diurnal WASO decreased by 90.3% and SE increased by 6.8%. TST increased by 20.6 minutes. Nocturnal sleepiness increased 1.7 points. Nocturnal WASO decreased by 74.9% and post-treatment SE increased by 9.9%. Diurnal TST increased by 14.8 minutes. Diurnal sleepiness increased by 0.5 points (score 3.4) (Table 3). Participant 2 had a decreased level of general fatigue at post-treatment. Intrusive thoughts at bedtime decreased, but level of endorsement of dysfunctional beliefs and attitudes about sleep increased. Depression and state anxiety decreased, but trait anxiety increased (Table 4). Most sleep improvement was maintained at the 3-month follow-up except for diurnal TST that decreased to baseline level (Table 3). Nocturnal TST increased while diurnal and nocturnal WASO remained low. Intrusive thoughts at bedtime, endorsement of dysfunctional beliefs about sleep, fatigue, depression, and anxiety remained at the post-treatment level (Table 4). Diurnal sleepiness decreased at follow-up but remained higher than baseline. Finally, participant 2 had a moderate treatment response, meeting four criteria (criteria a, b, e, and f) for diurnal sleep (a and e) and two for nocturnal sleep (b and f). Participant 2 readily accepted treatment but her compliance rate is missing (Table 5).

Participant 3

Participant 3, a woman of 57 years old, had been a night worker for 8.5 months, but had had sleep difficulties for 5 years (Table 2). Before treatment, diurnal SOL and WASO were less than 20 minutes while nocturnal SOL and WASO were of 18.8 and 97.5 minutes, respectively. Diurnal and nocturnal TST were 167.1 and 457.5 minutes, respectively, and diurnal and nocturnal SE were 85.1% and 77.7%. Nocturnal and diurnal sleepiness were of 3.3 and 1.5, respectively (Tables 3 and 4). After treatment, diurnal SOL and WASO decreased by 58.7% and 100%, respectively, while TST increased by 75 minutes. SE presented an increase of 14.0% and nocturnal sleepiness decreased by 0.9 point (Tables 3 and 4). For nocturnal sleep changes, SOL and WASO decreased by 66.5% and 87.2%, respectively, while TST increased by 82.5 minutes. SE increased by 22.3%. Diurnal sleepiness decreased by 0.5 point (Tables 3 and 4). Participant 3 presented an increase in general fatigue at post-treatment, while intrusive thoughts at bedtime, and level of endorsement of dysfunctional beliefs and attitudes about sleep decreased. The levels of depression and anxiety also decreased (Table 4). Finally, participant 3 had a high treatment response meeting all criteria for diurnal and nocturnal sleep. Participant 3 accepted treatment, having diurnal and nocturnal sleep compliances of 85.4% and 84.0%, respectively (Table 5). Most sleep improvement was maintained at the 3-month follow-up (Table 3). Diurnal and nocturnal TST further increased at the 3-month follow-up compared to post-treatment. Intrusive thoughts at bed time, endorsement of dysfunctional beliefs about sleep, depression, and anxiety remained at the post-treatment level (Table 4). Fatigue presents an additional decrease compare to post-treatment.

Participant 4

Participant 4, a woman of 42 years old, had been a shift worker for 20 years, with sleep difficulties during that whole time (Table 2). Before treatment, diurnal and nocturnal SOL were about 30 minutes, while diurnal and nocturnal WASO were 66.0 and 78.3 minutes, respectively. Diurnal and nocturnal TST were 333.0 and 385.3 minutes, respectively. Diurnal and nocturnal SE were of 73.0 and 74.0% and nocturnal and diurnal sleepiness of 3.4 and 3.3 (Tables 3 and 4). Participant 4 did not complete the follow-up assessment. After treatment, diurnal SOL and WASO decreased by 52.9% and of 60.2%, respectively, and sleepiness decreased by 2.4 points. Meanwhile, TST decreased of 105.5 minutes. Nocturnal SOL and WASO decreased respectively by 52.2% and 51.3%, and sleepiness decreased by 1.1 points. Post-treatment nocturnal SE increased by 24.2%. (Tables 3 and 4) and TST decreased by 39.5 minutes. Participant 4 had a decreased level of general fatigue at post-treatment: intrusive thoughts at bedtime, level of endorsement of dysfunctional beliefs and attitudes about sleep, and depression and anxiety levels also decreased (Table 4). Finally, participant 4 had a moderate response to treatment, meeting five criteria (criteria a, b, f, g, and h). Participant 4 accepted treatment, having diurnal and nocturnal sleep compliances of 45.0% and 66.4% respectively (Table 5).

Participant 5

Participant 5, a man of 39 years old, was a night worker for 10 years and had sleep difficulties for 24 years (Table 2). Before treatment, the diurnal and nocturnal SOL were 6.2 and 25.8 minutes while the diurnal and nocturnal WASO were 30.4 and 51.7 minutes. Diurnal and nocturnal TST were 242.8 and 286.3 minutes and diurnal and nocturnal SE were 65.2% and 53.6%. Nocturnal and diurnal sleepiness were 3.2 and 3.5, respectively (Tables 3 and 4). After treatment, there were clinically significant changes for two criteria of nocturnal sleep; nocturnal TST increased by 47.9 minutes and diurnal sleepiness decreased by 2.1 point. There was also a 0.8 point decrease in nocturnal sleepiness (Tables 3 and 4). Participant 5 had a decreased level of general fatigue. Intrusive thoughts at bedtime decreased also, as well as the level of dysfunctional beliefs and attitudes about sleep. The level of depression and trait anxiety decreased while state anxiety increased (Table 4). Most sleep improvement was maintained at the 3-month follow-up (Table 3). Diurnal and nocturnal TST further increased at the 3-month follow-up compared to post-treatment. Nocturnal WASO remained at baseline. Intrusive thoughts at bedtime, endorsement of dysfunctional beliefs about sleep, depression, and sleepiness remained at the post-treatment level (Table 4). Finally, participant 5 accepted treatment, having a diurnal and nocturnal sleep compliance of 80.0% and 78.3%, respectively (Table 5). This participant had a moderate treatment response, meeting three criteria (criterion d, g, and h).

Participant 6

Participant 6 was a man of 55 years old. He had been a rotated shift worker for 6 years and complained of sleep difficulties for 30 years (Table 2). Before treatment, the diurnal and nocturnal SOL were less than 10 minutes while the diurnal and nocturnal WASO were 49.4 and 139.6 minutes, respectively. Diurnal and nocturnal TST were 119.0 and 265.7 minutes and diurnal and nocturnal SE were 66.2% and 64.2% respectively. Nocturnal and diurnal sleepiness scores were 3.2 and 3.1, respectively (Tables 3 and 4). Participant 6 did not complete the follow-up assessment. Participant 6 dropped out of the study at the end of treatment and before post-treatment. When he dropped out of treatment his diurnal WASO decreased by 64.6%, TST increased by 106.0 minutes. SE increased by 37.4%, and diurnal sleepiness decreased by 0.2 points. Nocturnal WASO decreased by 52.5% and diurnal sleepiness decreased by 0.5 point. Nocturnal TST remained unchanged. At that time, participant 6 had a high treatment response, meeting six criteria (a, b, c, e, g, and h) (Tables 3 and 4). Finally, participant 6 readily accepted treatment (Table 5) but his compliance rate is missing.

Summary of treatment response

Two of the six participants (3 and 6) had a high treatment response, one of them meeting all criteria (Table 6). All others participants had a moderate response to treatment. Moreover, all participants presented at least two significant clinical improvements, one in diurnal and one in nocturnal sleep. Five participants presented a decrease in both sleepiness scores. Only one participant showed no WASO improvement. All participants, except one, presented at least one increase in SE. Four participants presented an increase in at least one TST. SOL is the sleep variable showing the least improvement. Given that all six participants had a moderate to high treatment response, the nonparametric sign test provided a significant one tailed p-value of 0.0156 (6 successes out of 6 trials).

Participant	Sleep parameters	Diurnal sleep Criterion met no/yes	Nocturnal sleep Criterion met no/yes	Treatment response
1	SOL/WASO (↓50-60%)	no (↑ 266.6%)/no(↑ +400%)	Yes (↓93.0%)/ Yes (↓52.6%)	5/8 : 62.5%; moderate
	TST (↑30-45 min)	no (↓ 74,87 min)	Yes (↑101.4 min)	

	SE (↑85%)	no (76.12%)	Yes (91.6%, ↑74.1%)	
	Sleepiness (↓)	Yes (↓0.7 pt)	Yes (↓0.5 pt)	
2	SOL/WASO (↓50-60%)	no (24.6%)/Yes (↓90.3%)	no (↓ 17.3%)/Yes (↓74.9%)	4/8 : 50%; moderate
	TST (↑30-45 min)	no (↑20.6 min)	no(↑14.8 min)	
	SE (↑85%)	Yes (89.9%, ↑ 6.8 %)	Yes (93.3%, ↑ 9.9%)	
	Sleepiness (↓)	no (↑ 1.7 pt)	no (↑ 0.5 pt)	
3	SOL/WASO (↓50-60%)	Yes (↓58.7%)/ Yes (↓100%)	Yes (↓66.5%)/ Yes (↓87.2%)	8/8 : 100%; high
	TST (↑30-45 min)	Yes (↑75.0 min)	Yes (↑82.5 min)	
	SE (↑85%)	Yes (97.0%, ↑14.0%)	Yes (95%, ↑22.3%)	
	Sleepiness (↓)	Yes (↓0.9 pt)	Yes (↓0.5 pt)	
4	SOL/WASO (↓50-60%)	Yes (↓52.9%)/ Yes (↓60.2%)	Yes (↓52.2%)/ Yes (↓51.3%)	5/8 : 62.5%; moderate
	TST (↑30-45 min)	no (↓ 105.5 min)	no (↓ 39.5 min)	
	SE (↑85%)	no (83.5%)	Yes (91.9%, ↑24.2%)	
	Sleepiness (↓)	Yes (↓2.4 pt)	Yes (↓1.1 pt)	
5	SOL/WASO (↓50-60%)	no (↑ 71%)/no (↓27%)	no (↓ 14.3%)/ no (↓13%)	3/8 : 37.5% moderate
	TST (↑30-45 min)	no (↑21.6 min)	Yes (↑47.9 min)	
	SE (↑85%)	no (83.2%)	no (78.0%))	
	Sleepiness (↓)	Yes (↓0.8 pt)	Yes (↓2.1 pt)	
6	SOL/WASO (↓50-60%)	no (↓ 36.7%)/Yes (↓64.6%)	no (↓ 29%)/ Yes (↓52.5%)	6/8 :75%; high
	TST (↑30-45 min)	Yes (↑106.0 min)	no (↑1.47 min)	
	SE (↑85%)	Yes (90.93%, ↑37.4%)	no (78.3%)	
	Sleepiness (↓)	Yes (↓0.2 pt)	Yes (↓0.5 pt)	

Table 6: Treatment response of each participant for diurnal and nocturnal sleep (Note: SOL: Sleep Onset Latency; WASO: Wake After Sleep Onset; TST: Total Sleep Time; SE: Sleep Efficiency; ↑: Increase of; ↓: Decrease of; pt: Point; min: Minute).

Questionnaires	n	Mean of difference	CI
GCTI	5	-11.4	[-26.77, 4.0]
DBAS	5	-0.35	[-1.86, 1.2]
MFI	5	-6.6	[-25.05, 11.9]
BDI-II	5	-5.2	[-11.85, 1.5]
STAI-Y			
State anxiety	5	-2.2	[-13.63, 9.2]
Trait anxiety	5	-1.6	[-11.75, 8.5]
TAS	3	45.33	[22.25, 68.4]

Table 7: Mean difference scores for self-reported questionnaires and confidence intervals (Note: GCTI: Glasgow content of thoughts inventory; DBAS: Dysfunctional beliefs and attitudes about sleep; MFI: Multidimensional Fatigue Inventory; BDI-II: Beck Depression Inventory; STAI-Y: State-Trait Anxiety Inventory; Mean of Difference: Mean of Difference Score between Post and Pre-treatment).

Mean of the difference scores from post-treatment to baseline for self-report questionnaires indicate negative change for all questionnaires except for TAS. These changes are in the expected direction, meaning that symptoms assessed improved with treatment and that treatment is more acceptable after treatment than before. Confidence intervals indicate non-significant changes except for TAS (Table 7).

Discussion

The findings of this study suggest that sleep restriction therapy adapted to treat SWD with insomnia symptoms is feasible and effective. All participants presented sleep improvement, the most frequently observed being a decrease in WASO. Moreover, either diurnal or nocturnal TST increased while subjective sleepiness decreased for five participants. Nocturnal and diurnal SE increased or remained over 85% for most of participants. The majority of participants reported a decrease in intrusive thoughts while falling asleep. Depression and anxiety levels were improved or remained low for five participants as shown by the difference scores between post and pre-treatment. Most of the improvement remained stable at follow-up; these measures were available for only half of the participants. Furthermore, the treatment was well accepted by participants while compliance rates were moderate.

Taken together, these preliminary results suggest that shift workers with SWD may benefit from a direct intervention targeting insomnia symptoms. They also underline the importance and relevance of addressing night and day sleep for shift workers. Overall, these results converge with those reported by Jarnefelt et al. [27] and Lee et al. [29] who use a CBT-I in a population of shift workers. The first study demonstrated some improvement on SOL and SE while sleep quality improved for participants of the second study. The present study seems to show even more sleep improvement regarding WASO and TST. These results are probably due to the fact that our participants received a diagnosis of SWD based on a clinical interview, which was not the case in the two previous studies. In other words, they were more likely to improve because they were more severely disrupted before treatment. Results for nocturnal sleep are very interesting, showing that the sleep improvement obtained compares with that seen in other studies using sleep restriction therapy for day workers [30,31].

Results on TST are highly promising and deserve attention. Indeed, several of our participants presented an increase in TST or a stable TST for nocturnal and diurnal sleep. The increase in TST obtained for diurnal sleep varies from 20.6 to 106 minutes while nocturnal TST varies from 1.5 to 101.4 minutes. These results are unexpected for several reasons. First, the range of increases obtained seems to be higher than that reported in other interventions for shift workers. For instance, wearing dark sunglasses has been shown to increase diurnal TST by an average of 25 minutes [15] while luminotherapy has been shown to produce an increase of about 30 minutes for shift workers [51]. Second, in the present study TST increased in a way comparable to what is expected for TST after sleep restriction therapy for day workers. In fact, with a population sleeping by night, TST is expected to diminish in the first weeks of treatment and increase again later after treatment [31,52]. Furthermore, although sleepiness is a known side effect of sleep restriction [30,31,52], nearly all our participants improved on sleepiness. Taken together, these results suggest that insomnia responds faster to sleep restriction therapy in SWD than in day workers. Also, these results suggest that at least part of the sleepiness in shift work seems to be related to TST. Finally, these results underline the importance of having a well diagnosed population to evaluate treatment efficacy.

Sleep restriction therapy used alone seem also to have an effect on psychological distress. Results on depression and anxiety levels show clearly that most participants benefit from treatment. Intrusive thoughts at bedtime seem highly present before treatment and their diminution constitutes another improvement observed for most participants following sleep restriction. Interestingly, our study shows that a specific insomnia treatment might produce mood relief even if the intervention does not specifically address depression. Again, these results are in line with Jarnefelt et al. [27] and Lee et al. [29].

The feasibility of sleep restriction for SWD is also demonstrated in the present study. First of all, sleep restriction therapy was well accepted by the participants as shown by the scores obtained on the treatment acceptability scale. Second, results on TST and sleepiness also support the feasibility of sleep restriction therapy, showing that there are no potential side-effects such as have been observed with day workers with insomnia. In addition, most of participants completed the treatment sessions. The greatest obstacle to sleep restriction therapy we faced were changes in the participants' work schedule, changes which are more related to workplace constraints than to the treatment itself. Subsequent assessments such as post-treatment and follow-up were more difficult to obtain. This situation could reflect the fact that, due to their work schedule, the workers have less time for meetings or participation in a demanding study. Finally, the compliance data showed that treatment procedures were moderately followed. This last result might negatively affect treatment efficacy and feasibility. The question of compliance in this population should be taken into account in other studies.

The present study suggests guidelines as well as some methodological issues. The first and most important is that this study shows the usefulness of assessing nocturnal and diurnal sleep for shift workers. It is clear that sleeping by both day and night is part of the reality of shift workers, and that they benefit from addressing both periods of sleep during treatment. In addition, it appears that several questionnaires assessing insomnia components need to be adapted to shift work in order to capture insomnia during diurnal sleep as well. Another methodological issue rising from the present study regards the use of semi-structured clinical interviews that ascertain the diagnosis of the population studied. This methodology presents two advantages. First, it ascertains the presence of the disorder to be studied in the population, decreasing interpretive biases. Second, sleep restriction therapy, as CBT-I, is a treatment developed and tested for a specific disorder, which is insomnia. Therefore, it is likely to be effective within other populations having a specific disorder with insomnia symptoms.

These preliminary results possess also some methodological limitations. First, the absence of a control group limits the interpretation of the results as nonspecific factors cannot be separated. Second, given the small sample size the study needs to be replicated in larger sample size. Doing so, a randomized design with a control group would be mandatory. Third, long-term effects of treatment were difficult to assess. Future studies should have reliable follow-up data to confirm the long term efficacy of sleep restriction therapy for shift workers. In addition, sleep diaries are subjective measures and, although important, the absence of more objective measures precludes definite conclusions about objective sleep changes. Finally, the lack of measure of the circadian rhythm markers precludes any conclusions about the circadian misalignment of shift workers and its possible realignement due to sleep restriction therapy.

In conclusion, the present study is one of the first evaluating a specific intervention for insomnia in a shift workers population diagnosed for SWD. The preliminary results obtained are promising, showing that sleep restriction therapy adapted for SWD produces sleep, sleepiness, and mood benefits. Further studies should investigate side-effects of sleep restriction therapy for shift workers to clarify the surprising results of an increase in TST and a decrease in sleepiness. Future studies could also consider adding stimulus control therapy for insomnia in shift workers as it is known for its efficacy and commonly used with sleep restriction therapy for insomnia. After a specific investigation of cognition for shift workers, cognitive interventions could be added to the treatment protocol and evaluated as well. In conclusion, the present study opens a new possibility of treatment for shift workers that deserves greater attention in the future.

Acknowledgements

This research was supported by a grant from the Faculté des sciences sociales of Université Laval and from the Research center of the Institut universitaire en santé mentale de Québec. The authors wish to thank Dr. James Everett for English revision.

References

1. Shields M (2002) Shift work and health. Health Rep 13: 11-33.
2. American Academy of Sleep Medicine (2005) The International Classification of Sleep Disorders II. (2ndedn). Westchester, IL: American Academy of Sleep Medicine.
3. Drake CL, Roehrs T, Richardson G, Walsh JK, Roth T (2004) Shift work sleep disorder: prevalence and consequences beyond that of symptomatic day workers. Sleep 27: 1453-1462.
4. Flo E, Pallesen S, Magerøy N, Moen BE, Grønli J, et al. (2012) Shift work disorder in nurses--assessment, prevalence and related health problems. PLoS One 7: e33981.
5. Di Milia L, Waage S, Pallesen S, Bjorvatn B (2013) Shift work disorder in a random population sample--prevalence and comorbidities. PLoS One 8: e55306.
6. Culpepper L (2010) The social and economic burden of shift-work disorder. J Fam Pract 59: S3-3S11.
7. Puca FM, Perrucci S, Prudenzano MP, Savarese M, Misceo S, et al. (1996) Quality of life in shift work syndrome. Funct Neurol 11: 261-268.
8. Ohayon MM, Lemoine P, Arnaud-Briant V, Dreyfus M (2002) Prevalence and consequences of sleep disorders in a shift worker population. J Psychosom Res 53: 577-583.
9. Vallières A, Azaiez A, Moreau V, LeBlanc M, Morin CM (2014) Insomnia in shift work. Sleep Med 15: 1440-1448.
10. Gigli GL, Maschio MC, Diomedi M, Moroni M (1993) Brotizolam and cognitive performance: A double-blind, crossover study versus placebo in a population of shift workers. Curr Ther Res 2: 129-136.
11. Hart CL, Ward AS, Haney M, Nasser J, Foltin RW (2003) Methamphetamine attenuates disruptions in performance and mood during simulated night-shift work. Psychopharmacology 1: 42-51.
12. Czeisler CA, Walsh JK, Roth T, Hughes RJ, Wright KP, et al. (2005) Modafinil for excessive sleepiness associated with shift-work sleep disorder. N Engl J Med 353: 476-486.
13. Neubauer DN (2006) Does modafinil safely and effectively treat shift-work sleep disorder? Nat Clin Pract Neurol 2: 134-135.
14. Boivin DB, James FO (2002) Circadian adaptation to night-shift work by judicious light and darkness exposure. J Biol Rhythms 17: 556-567.
15. Sasseville A, Benhaberou-Brun D, Fontaine C, Charon MC, Hebert M (2009) Wearing blue-blockers in the morning could improve sleep of workers on a permanent night schedule: a pilot study. Chronobiol Int 26: 913-925.
16. Bonnet MH, Arand DL (1994) Impact of naps and caffeine on extended nocturnal performance. Physiol Behav 56: 103-109.
17. Garbarino S, Mascialino B, Penco MA, Squarcia S, De Carli F, et al. (2004) Professional shift-work drivers who adopt prophylactic naps can reduce the risk of car accidents during night work. Sleep 27: 1295-1302.
18. Schweitzer PK, Randazzo AC, Stone K, Erman M, Walsh JK (2006) Laboratory and field studies of naps and caffeine as practical countermeasures for sleep-wake problems associated with night work. Sleep 29: 39-50.
19. Bonnefond A, Muzet A, Winter-Dill AS, Bailloeuil C, Bitouze F, et al. (2001) Innovative working schedule: introducing one short nap during the night shift. Ergonomics 44: 937-945.
20. Purnell MT, Feyer AM, Herbison GP (2002) The impact of a nap opportunity during the night shift on the performance and alertness of 12-h shift workers. J Sleep Res 11: 219-227.
21. Boivin DB, Tremblay GM, James FO (2007) Working on atypical schedules. Sleep Med 8: 578-589.
22. Bastien CH, LeBlanc M, Carrier J, Morin CM (2003) Sleep EEG power spectra, insomnia, and chronic use of benzodiazepines. Sleep 26: 313-317.
23. Schwartz JR, Roth T (2006) Shift work sleep disorder: burden of illness and approaches to management. Drugs 66: 2357-2370.
24. Morin CM, Bootzin RR, Buysse DJ, Edinger JD, Espie CA, et al. (2006) Psychological and behavioral treatment of insomnia:update of the recent evidence (1998-2004). Sleep 29: 1398-1414.
25. Passarella S, Duong MT (2008) Diagnosis and treatment of insomnia. Am J Health Syst Pharm 65: 927-934.
26. Smith MT, Perlis ML, Park A, Smith MS, Pennington J, et al. (2002) Comparative meta-analysis of pharmacotherapy and behavior therapy for persistent insomnia. Am J Psychiatry 159: 5-11.
27. Järnefelt H, Lagerstedt R, Kajaste S, Sallinen M, Savolainen A, et al. (2012) Cognitive behavioral therapy for shift workers with chronic insomnia. Sleep Med 13: 1238-1246.
28. Järnefelt H, Sallinen M, Luukkonen R, Kajaste S, Savolainen A, et al. (2014) Cognitive behavioral therapy for chronic insomnia in occupational health services: analyses of outcomes up to 24 months post-treatment. Behav Res Ther 56: 16-21.
29. Lee KA, Gay CL, Alsten CR (2014) Home-based behavioral sleep training for shift workers: a pilot study. Behav Sleep Med 12: 455-468.
30. Spielman AJ, Saskin P, Thorpy MJ (1987) Treatment of chronic insomnia by restriction of time in bed. Sleep 10: 45-56.
31. Vallières A, Ceklic T, Bastien CH, Espie CA (2013) A preliminary evaluation of the physiological mechanisms of action for sleep restriction therapy. Sleep Disord 2013: 726372.
32. Barlow DH, Hersen M (1984) Single-case experimental designs: Strategies for studying behavior change (2ndedn). New York, NY: Pergamon Press.
33. Kazdin AE (2003) Methodological issues and strategies in clinical research (3rdedn). Washington, DC: American Psychological Association.
34. First MB, Spitzer RL, Gibbon M, Williams JBW (1997) Structured Clinical Interview for DSM-IV Axis I Disorders, Clinical Version (SCID-IV). Washington, DC: American Psychiatric Association.
35. Morin CM, Insomnia: Psychological assessment and management. 1993, New York, NY: The Guilford Press.
36. Barton J, Spelten E, Totterdell P, Smith L, Folkard S, et al. (1995) The Standard Shiftwork Index - a Battery of Questionnaires for Assessing Shiftwork-Related Problems. Work and Stress 1: 4-30.
37. Hoddes E, Zarcone V, Smythe H, Phillips R, Dement WC (1973) Quantification of sleepiness: a new approach. Psychophysiology 10: 431-436.
38. Morin CM, Vallières A, Ivers H (2007) Dysfunctional beliefs and attitudes about sleep (DBAS): validation of a brief version (DBAS-16). Sleep 30: 1547-1554.
39. Blais FC, Gendron L, Mimeault V, Morin CM (1997) [Evaluation of insomnia: validity of 3 questionnaires]. Encephale 23: 447-453.
40. Harvey KJ, Espie CA (2004) Development and preliminary validation of the Glasgow Content of Thoughts Inventory (GCTI): a new measure for the assessment of pre-sleep cognitive activity. Br J Clin Psychol 43: 409-420.
41. Smets EM, Garssen B, Bonke B, De Haes JC (1995) The Multidimensional Fatigue Inventory (MFI) psychometric qualities of an instrument to assess fatigue. J Psychosom Res 39: 315-325.
42. Fillion L, Gélinas C, Simard S, Savard J, Gagnon P (2003) Validation evidence for the French Canadian adaptation of the Multidimensional Fatigue Inventory as a measure of cancer-related fatigue. Cancer Nurs 26: 143-154.
43. Beck AT, Steer RA, Brown GK (1996) Inventaire de Dépression de Beck (2ndedn). Toronto: The Psychological Corporation.
44. Spieldberger CD (1983) Manual for the State-Trait Anxiety Inventory: STAI (Form Y).
45. Gauthier J, Bouchard S (1993) A French-Canadian adaptation of the revised version of Spielberger's State-Trait Anxiety Inventory/Adaptation

canadienne-française de la forme révisée du State-Trait Anxiety Inventory de Spielberger. Canadian Journal of Behavioural Science 4: 559-578.

46. Morin CM, Gaulier B, Barry T, Kowatch RA (1992) Patients' acceptance of psychological and pharmacological therapies for insomnia. Sleep 15: 302-305.

47. Morin CM, Espie CA (2012) The oxford handbook of sleep and sleep disorders. Oxford University Press: New York.

48. Morin CM (2004) Cognitive-behavioral approaches to the treatment of insomnia. J Clin Psychiatry 65 Suppl 16: 33-40.

49. Morin CM, Culbert JP, Schwartz SM (1994) Nonpharmacological interventions for insomnia: a meta-analysis of treatment efficacy. Am J Psychiatry 151: 1172-1180.

50. Peterson RA (1994) A Meta-Analysis of Cronbach's Coefficient Alpha. Journal of Consumer Research 2: 381-391.

51. Boivin DB, Boudreau P, James FO, Kin NM (2012) Photic resetting in night-shift work: impact on nurses' sleep. Chronobiol Int 29: 619-628.

52. Kyle SD, Miller CB, Rogers Z, Siriwardena AN, Macmahon KM, et al. (2014) Sleep restriction therapy for insomnia is associated with reduced objective total sleep time, increased daytime somnolence, and objectively impaired vigilance: implications for the clinical management of insomnia disorder. Sleep 2: 229-37.

8

Functional Cognitive Disorders: Can Sleep Disturbance Contribute to a Positive Diagnosis?

Elhadd K[1], Bharambe V[1] and Larner AJ[2*]

[1] *Specialist Registrar in Neurology, Walton Centre for Neurology and Neurosurgery, United Kingdom*

[2] *Consultant Neurologist, Walton Centre for Neurology and Neurosurgery, United Kingdom*

[*] **Corresponding author:** AJ Larner, Cognitive Function Clinic, Walton Centre for Neurology and Neurosurgery, Lower Lane, Fazakerley, Liverpool, L9 7LJ, United Kingdom, E-mail: a.larner@thewaltoncentre.nhs.uk

Abstract

Study background: Sleep disturbance may contribute to subjective memory complaints which are frequently encountered in cognitive disorders clinics. Identification of sleep disturbance may contribute to a positive diagnosis of functional cognitive disorders (FCD) compared to dementia or mild cognitive impairment.

Methods: Jenkins Sleep Scale (JSS), a validated sleep scale, was administered to consecutive new patients attending a dedicated cognitive disorders clinic based in a regional neuroscience Centre.

Results: Sleep disturbance identified using JSS was more frequent in patients with functional cognitive disorders ($p<0.001$). Dichotomised JSS showed reasonable sensitivity (>0.8) for FCD when used as a diagnostic test.

Conclusion: Identifying sleep disturbance using a simple sleep screening scale may contribute to a positive diagnosis of functional cognitive disorders in a dedicated cognitive disorders clinic. This may have pragmatic implications for the treatment of subjective memory complaints.

Keywords: Diagnosis; Functional cognitive disorders; Memory clinic; Sleep screening

Introduction

Many patients referred to dedicated cognitive disorders clinics with complaints of cognitive impairment, chiefly of memory, are found on assessment and investigation not to harbour evidence of a neurodegenerative or cognitive neurological disorder. In our clinic such patients account for between 50-60% of referrals [1]. Whereas previously these individuals were variously labelled as being "Worried well" or "Memory complainers", or having subjective memory impairment, mild cognitive dysfunction, or functional memory disorder [2,3], more recently Stone, et al. have proposed the category of "Functional cognitive disorders"(FCD) [4].

Analogous to other functional disorders (e.g. movement, epilepsy), FCD should be a positive diagnosis, based on inconsistency or incongruence of symptoms, rather than a diagnosis of exclusion. Factors which may be more commonly observed in patients with FCD compared to patients with dementia/MCI have been suggested [1,4,5] which if confirmed may facilitate positive diagnosis of FCD. We have previously suggested that bringing a symptom list (handwritten or typed on an ipad), the phenomenon known as la maladie du petit papier, may be helpful in diagnosis of FCD [6].

Previously, it has been shown that impaired sleep quality, as measured using the Pittsburgh Sleep Quality Index (PSQI) [7], was worse in patients attending a dedicated cognitive disorders clinic whose eventual diagnosis was "Not dementia" [8]. It is possible that many of these non-demented patients may have qualified for a diagnosis of FCD.

The aim of the current study was to administer a simple sleep questionnaire to patients attending a dedicated cognitive disorders clinic to examine whether sleep impairment was more common in FCD patients and hence a possible marker for a positive diagnosis of FCD.

Methods

As part of an ongoing study of FCD in a dedicated cognitive disorders clinic, consecutive new patient referrals seen over a 6-month period (November 2017-April 2018) were assessed for sleep disturbance by administration of the Jenkins Sleep Scale (JSS) or Questionnaire which addresses four sleep-related symptoms over the previous four week period (Table 1) [9]. The scale was chosen for its brevity (administration time ca. 1 m), and because a dichotomous index may be easily computed based on the presence of any one of the four symptoms occurring on 15 or more nights during the four week period under consideration (JSS+, JSS-) [10]. JSS is considerably quicker and easier to administer, score and categorize than PSQI.

During the previous 4 weeks have you experienced:
Difficulty falling asleep?
Waking up several times per night?
Difficulty staying asleep (including waking up too early)?
Waking up feeling tired and worn out after usual amount of sleep?
If yes to any one of these, ask frequency question: 15 or more nights?
A dichotomous index was computed and coded as JSS+ if the respondents reported that any of the above sleep disturbances occurred 15 or more nights during the previous 4 weeks or as JSS-, if not.

Table 1: Jenkins Sleep Scale (JSS) or Questionnaire and its dichotomisation (after Jenkins et al.; Lallukka et al.).

Because inadequate sleep, even a mild insufficiency, may be linked to mood disturbance [11], both of which may impact on memory function, a two question screener for depression (M2Q) was also administered (Table 2) [12]. Again this scale was chosen for its brevity (administration time ca. 1 m), and because a dichotomous index may be easily computed based on the presence of either one of the two symptoms occurring ($M2Q^+$, $M2Q^-$) [12]. M2Q is considerably quicker and easier to administer, score and categorise than other mood screeners, such as the Patient Health Questionnaire 9 (PHQ^{-9}) which has previously been examined in a dedicated cognitive disorders clinic [13].

During the past month:
Have you often been bothered by feeling down, depressed, or hopeless?
Have you often been bothered by little interest or pleasure in doing things?
If yes to either one of these, coded as $M2Q^+$

Table 2: Mood 2 Question screener (M2Q) and its dichotomisation (after Arroll et al.).

Reference standard diagnosis of cognitive impairment (dementia, mild cognitive impairment) was by judgment of an experienced clinician based on standard diagnostic criteria (DSM-IV, Petersen, respectively) but did not use JSS or M2Q scores in order to avoid review bias. Reference standard diagnosis relied on clinical interview, informant interview (where possible), neuropsychological testing (bedside +/- formal as required) and structural neuroimaging (CT +/- MRI as required).

FCD was diagnosed on the basis of a typical profile of clinical features, including, but not limited to, the ability to describe in detail memory symptoms despite assertions of having a poor or terrible memory (often contrasted with a previously "Brilliant" memory); being more aware of the problems than others; variability of symptoms on a day to day basis and a relative lack of impact on social and/or occupational function [4].

Pragmatic diagnostic test accuracy study of both dichotomised instruments was undertaken. Results of the index tests and the reference standard diagnoses were cross-classified in a 2 × 2 contingency table, from which standard measures of discrimination with 95% confidence intervals were calculated, both paired (sensitivity and specificity; positive and negative predictive values [PPV, NPV], likelihood ratios [LR^+, LR^-] and clinical utility indexes [CUI^+, CUI^-]) and unitary measures (correct classification accuracy [CCA], Youden index [Y], predictive summary index [PSI], diagnostic odds ratio [DOR], area under the receiver operating characteristic curve [AUC ROC]) [14]. Dichotomised JSS and M2Q results were also combined either in series (both tests required to be positive before diagnosis of cognitive impairment is made: the "And" rule) or in parallel (either test positive sufficient for diagnosis to be made: "Or" rule) [15].

Results

Of 89 consecutive new referrals seen over the study period (F:M=43:46, 48% female; age range 22-88 years, median 62), 38 (=43%) were diagnosed with a cognitive disorder: 9 dementia (DSM-IV-TR criteria), 26 with MCI (Petersen criteria), and 3 with cognitive disorder without current cognitive impairment (e.g. transient global amnesia, transient epileptic amnesia). The remainder (51; =57%) were diagnosed with FCD.

Comparing JSS outcomes in the groups with cognitive disorders and with FCD, a higher percentage of FCD patients had markers of disturbed sleep on the dichotomised JSS (83% JSS+, *vs.* 50% of the cognitive disorders group) and this was statistically significant (chi square=11.2; $p<0.001$). JSS was negatively correlated with patient age ($r=-0.30$).

Comparing M2Q outcomes in the groups with cognitive disorders and with FCD, a higher percentage of FCD patients had markers of disturbed mood on the dichotomised M2Q (80% $M2Q^+$, *vs.* 47% of the cognitive disorders group) and this was statistically significant (chi square=10.9; $p<0.001$). M2Q was negatively correlated with patient age ($r=-0.38$).

Using either JSS or M2Q as a screening instrument for the diagnosis of FCD (Table 3), both showed a similar profile of reasonable sensitivity (≥ 0.8) but poor specificity (around 0.5) and positive predictive value (<0.7). Clinical utility indexes suggested both tests might be adequate to rule in a diagnosis of FCD, but very poor for ruling out the diagnosis.

Combining JSS and M2Q either in series or in parallel (Table 4) produced the anticipated changes [14], namely increased specificity, NPV, and LR- in series, and increased sensitivity, PPV, and LR+ in parallel. None of these changes was dramatic. JSS and M2Q were positively correlated ($r=0.33$).

Test	JSS+	M2Q+
Sens	0.83	0.8
	(0.73-0.94)	(0.68-0.92)
Spec	0.5	0.53
	(0.34-0.66)	(0.36-0.69)
Y	0.33	0.33
CCA	0.69	0.68
	(0.59-0.79)	(0.58-0.78)
PPV	0.69	0.68
	(0.57-0.81)	(0.55-0.80)
NPV	0.69	0.68
	(0.51-0.87)	(0.51-0.85)
PSI	0.38	0.36
LR+	1.67=unimportant	1.69=unimportant
	(1.17-2.37)	(1.16-2.46)
LR-	0.33=small	0.38=small
	(0.23-0.47)	(0.26-0.55)
DOR	5	4.47
	(3.52-7.10)	(3.07-6.50)
CUI+ (rule in)	0.57=adequate	0.54=adequate
CUI- (rule out)	0.35=very poor	0.358=very poor
AUC ROC	0.67 (0.62-0.72)	0.66 (0.61-0.72)

Table 3: Measures of discrimination for diagnosis of FCD using dichotomised JSS or M2Q (with 95% confidence intervals).

Test	JSS+/M2Q+ series	JSS+/M2Q+ parallel
Sens	0.69	0.93
	(0.55-0.82)	(0.86-1.00)
Spec	0.69	0.33
	(0.54-0.84)	(0.18-0.49)
Y	0.38	0.26
CCA	0.69	0.67
	(0.59-0.79)	(0.56-0.77)
PPV	0.74	0.64
	(0.61-0.87)	(0.52-0.75)
NPV	0.64	0.8
	(0.49-0.79)	(0.60-1.00)
PSI	0.38	0.44
LR+	2.25=small	1.40=unimportant
	(1.33-3.83)	(1.10-1.79)
LR-	0.45=small	0.20=small
	(0.26-0.76)	(0.16-0.26)
DOR	5.03	7
	(2.96-8.55)	(5.49-8.93)
CUI+ (rule in)	0.51=adequate	0.59=adequate
CUI- (rule out)	0.45=poor	0.27=very poor

Table 4: Measures of discrimination for diagnosis of FCD using dichotomised JSS or M2Q in series or parallel (with 95% confidence intervals).

Discussion

This study has shown that sleep disturbance and mood disturbance are associated with a diagnosis of functional cognitive disorders in a dedicated cognitive disorders clinic. The findings suggest that in clinical practice enquiries for sleep and mood disturbance may facilitate a positive diagnosis of FCD.

Study shortcomings include the small size of the cohort (lower than anticipated for the study period, due to local changes in clinic scheduling outside the authors' control). Other issues may relate to the index tests and the reference diagnosis.

The limitations of JSS are recognised: the four items cannot address the spectrum of sleep disorders and hence this can only be used as a preliminary screener [16]. Moreover, dichotomising any test results in loss of statistical power, although clinicians generally prefer tests which can be easily categorised in practice.

Reference diagnoses are hampered by the lack of diagnostic criteria for FCD, with the possibility of incorrect diagnoses (e.g. MCI might be mistaken for FCD, since neither impact on activities of daily living). Moreover this was a cross sectional study with potential for diagnostic errors in the absence of longitudinal patient follow up. However, the observed frequency of FCD was very similar to that recorded in a previous series from this clinic [1] suggesting consistency in diagnostic approach. FCD is a heterogeneous group, with various suggested typologies (e.g: mood disorder, other functional disorders, medication effects, dementia health anxiety, normal cognitive experience, dissociative amnesia, malingering, or combinations thereof). The cognitive disorders group is also heterogeneous, including dementia, MCI, and occasional patients without cognitive impairment (e.g. patients seen after an episode of transient global amnesia).

Enquiries about sleep should be a routine component of health assessment in patients with memory complaints since these may represent a pragmatic treatment target [8]. The study suggests that screening for sleep disturbance may contribute to a positive diagnosis of FCD, as may other demographic and clinical parameters [1,5,6]. This finding will need to be corroborated in larger, independent, patient cohorts and by using other, more comprehensive, sleep screeners.

Acknowledgements

No sources of funding received.

References

1. Bharambe V, Larner AJ (2018) Functional cognitive disorders: memory clinic study. Prog Neurol Psychiatry 22: in press.
2. Blackburn D, Wakefield S, Bell S, Harkness K, Venneri A, et al. (2014) Functional memory disorder: review from a memory clinic. J Neurol Neurosurg Psychiatry 85: e4.
3. Schmidtke K, Pohlmann S, Metternich B (2008) The syndrome of functional memory disorder: Definition, etiology, and natural course. Am J Geriatr Psychiatry 16: 981-988.
4. Stone J, Pal S, Blackburn D, Reuber M, Thekkumpurath P, et al. (2015) Functional (psychogenic) cognitive disorders: A perspective from the neurology clinic. J Alzheimers Dis 48: S5-S17.
5. Mirheidari B, Blackburn D, Harkness K, Walker T, Venneri A, et al. (2017) Toward the automation of diagnostic conversation analysis in patients with memory complaints. J Alzheimers Dis 58: 373-387.
6. Randall A, Larner AJ (2018) La maladie du petit papier: A sign of functional cognitive disorder? Int J Geriatr Psychiatry 33: 800.
7. Buysse DJ, Reynolds CF 3rd, Monk TH, Berman SR, Kupfer DJ (1989) The Pittsburgh Sleep Quality Index: A new instrument for psychiatric practice and research. Psychiatry Res 28: 193-213.
8. Hancock P, Larner AJ (2009) Diagnostic utility of the Pittsburgh Sleep Quality Index in memory clinics. Int J Geriatr Psychiatry 24: 1237-1241.
9. Jenkins CD, Stanton BA, Niemcryk SJ, Rose RM (1988) A scale for the estimation of sleep problems in clinical research. J Clin Epidemiol 41: 313-321.
10. Lallukka T, Dregan A, Armstrong D (2011) Comparison of a sleep item from the general health questionnaire-12 with the Jenkins sleep questionnaire as measures of sleep disturbance. J Epidemiol 21: 474-480.
11. Sullivan K, Ordiah C (2018) Association of mildly insufficient sleep with symptoms of anxiety and depression. Neurol Psychiatry Brain Res 30: 1-4.
12. Arroll B, Khin N, Kerse N (2003) Screening for depression in primary care with two verbally asked questions: Cross sectional study. BMJ 327: 1144-1146.
13. Hancock P, Larner AJ (2009) Clinical utility of patient health questionnaire-9 (PHQ-9) in memory clinics. Int J Psychiatry Clin Pract 13: 188-191.
14. Larner AJ (2015) Diagnostic test accuracy studies in dementia. A pragmatic approach. London: Springer.
15. Flicker L, Logiudice D, Carlin JB, Ames D (1997) The predictive value of dementia screening instruments in clinical populations. Int J Geriatr Psychiatry 12: 203-209.
16. Shahid A, Wilkinson K, Marcu S, Shapiro CM (2011) Jenkins sleep scale. In: Shahid A, Wilkinson K, Marcu S, Shapiro CM (eds). STOP, THAT and one hundred other sleep scales. New York: Springer, 203-204.

9

Infant Sleep Duration is Related to Externalizing Behavior at the Age of 18 Months

Ilona Quaak[1*], Marijke de Cock[1], Michiel de Boer[2] and Margot van de Bor[1]

[1]*Department of Health and Life Sciences, Faculty of Earth and Life Sciences, VU University, De Boelelaan 1085, 1081 HV Amsterdam, The Netherlands*

[2]*Department of Health Sciences, Faculty of Earth and Life Sciences, VU University, De Boelelaan 1085, 1081 HV Amsterdam, The Netherlands*

[*]**Corresponding author:** Ilona Quaak, Department of Health and Life Sciences, Faculty of Earth and Life Sciences, VU University, De Boelelaan 1085, 1081 HV Amsterdam, The Netherlands, E-mail: i.quaak@vu.nl

Abstract

Background: Sleep is essential for children's daytime functioning. Sleep problems have been related to several behavioral disorders. In the last few decades, growing attention has been given to externalizing problem behavior. Previous work has indicated that children and adolescents presenting externalizing problem behavior are at risk for an array of disorders in adulthood, including anxiety, disruptive behavior, mood problems and substance use. Several studies have shown that sleep problems may be related to externalizing problem behavior; research however is limited, especially among children younger than 18 months.

Methods: Data from the Dutch mother-child cohort LINC (Linking Maternal Nutrition to Child Health) were used. Sleep patterns were assessed by sleep diaries, which were filled out by the parents or caretaker when the child was three, six, nine, twelve and eighteen months old. Using the sleep diaries, sleep duration, nocturnal awakenings and early awakenings were calculated for each child at each time point.

Externalizing behavior was assessed by using the scale 'Externalizing behavior' of the Child Behavior Checklist 1.5-5. Mixed model analyses were conducted to determine whether random intercepts and/or slopes had to be included in analyses regarding the development of the sleep variables over time (0-18 months).

A random intercept and random slope was included for sleep duration and nocturnal awakenings, while for early awakenings only a random intercept was added. Subsequently, linear regression analyses were carried out to study the relationship between sleep characteristics over time with externalizing behavior as continuous, dependent variable. Family history, educational level, smoking, alcohol use and illicit drug use during pregnancy were checked for possible confounding effects. In total, data from 85 to 91 mother-child pairs were included, depending on the sleep variable.

Results: The intercept of sleep duration was found to be significantly related to externalizing scores on the CBCL (β=-2.35; CI=-4.31, -0.16; p=0.03). No other significant results were found.

Conclusion/discussion: We found that sleep duration was significantly related to externalizing behavior at 18 months. More specifically our results indicate that children who sleep less on average show more externalizing behavior. However, results should be interpreted with caution as the sample size was limited. Future studies should make use of longitudinal designs and larger sample sizes to confirm the relationship between sleep patterns and behavioral development over time.

Keywords: Infant sleep duration; Dutch cohort study; Sleep problems; Behavioral disorders; Externalizing behavior

Abbreviations:

ADHD: Attention Deficit Hyperactivity Disorder; CBCL 1.5-5: Child Behavior Checklist 1.5-5.

Introduction

During our lives, we spend almost one third of our time sleeping. Despite extensive research, there is no consensus on the function of sleep. It has been suggested that adequate sleep represents a restorative function which is crucial to control attention, emotion and behavior [1-5]. Deviant sleep patterns have been related to various adverse neurobehavioral effects in children, such as reduced cognitive functioning and poor school performance [6-10].

Therefore, it might not be a surprise that in literature sleep problems have been related to emotional as well as behavioral problems in both children and adolescents, although causal effects could not be demonstrated. In a study by Vriend et al. among 8 to 12 year old children, sleep duration was reduced or increased with one hour for four nights [11].

Children then completed the opposite condition. Depending on the group, significant associations were found with emotional functioning, memory, attention, and math fluency. The authors therefore state that even minor differences in sleep duration over a couple of nights can have significant consequences for children's emotional and cognitive functioning, emphasizing the importance of sleep duration for children's daytime functioning [11].

Furthermore, work from Sivertsen et al. has indicated that sleep problems, including short sleep duration, predict concurrent and later emotional as well as behavioral problems in children at the age of 18 months [12].

The sleep duration of children has steadily declined [13,14]. For example, in an Australian study Dollman et al. reported a decline in sleep duration between 1985 and 2004 of respectively 33 minutes in boys aged ten to fifteen years (from 9 hours 13 minutes to 8 hours and 40 minutes) [13]. For girls a decline of 28 minutes was reported: from 9 hours and 16 minutes to 8 hours and 48 minutes. In addition, in a Swiss study it was found that the sleep duration of 2-year old children decreased with 38 minutes between 1974 and 1986.

The authors suggest this trend is caused by an increasingly delayed bedtime, but unchanged wake time across decades [14]. Currently, 25% of the children is affected by sleep problems, including a disturbed sleep duration [15]. When left untreated, temporary sleep problems may persist to become chronic [16].

Simultaneously with increasing rates of sleep deprivation among children, prevalence rates of behavioral disorders among children are rising. Over the last 20 years, the number of children in contact with health care systems for the diagnosis and treatment of behavioral disorders has grown [17].

Increasing prevalence rates have been reported for obsessive-compulsive disorder, hyperkinetic disease, Tourette syndrome and Autism Spectrum Disorder [17]. With regard to Attention Deficit Hyperactivity Disorder (ADHD), prevalence rates in the United States were estimated at 7.8% in 2003, which increased to 9.5% in 2007 and 11.0% in 2011 [18]. Similar trends are also reported in other parts of the world, making it a global concern [19-21].

Several behavioral disorders have been related to sleep problems. In the last few decades, special attention has been given to externalizing problem behavior which is problem behavior directed toward the external environment.

In preschoolers externalizing problem behavior may include non-compliance, irritability, motor overactivity, aggressiveness or inattention [22]. Externalizing problem behavior has both concurrent and long-term consequences for the individual, family and friends, as well as the society in general [23].

Previous work has indicated that children and adolescents with externalizing problem behavior are at risk for an array of disorders in adulthood, including anxiety, disruptive behavior, mood problems and substance use [24-36]. Hence, externalizing problem behavior in childhood may predict behavioral problems later in life.

In a Canadian study parents had to rate sleep problems in their children on a 5-point Likert scale (1=almost never, 5=almost all the time). Problems included falling asleep, particular and long bedtime routine, nocturnal awakenings and restless sleep. An overall sleep problems score was calculated. The authors found that sleep problems accounted for a significant percentage of the variance in externalizing behavior, including inattentiveness, hyperactivity and physically aggressive behavior [37].

In another study, mothers had to indicate the presence and length of nocturnal awakenings of their 29-month old child. Three groups were created: no nocturnal awakenings, total nocturnal awakenings of less than 20 minutes and total nocturnal awakenings of more than 20 minutes. Using parental reports, children with nocturnal awakenings of more than 20 minutes scored higher on externalizing behavior [38].

Given the high prevalence rate of sleep problems among children and their possible impact on behavioral development in children, it seems essential to further investigate this relationship. Externalizing problem behavior in childhood may predict behavioral problems later in life; it therefore seems essential to further explore the role of this variable.

However, data on the relationship between sleep problems and externalizing behavior in preschool children are limited, especially with regard to preschool children. This is the first study to assess this relationship prospectively. We hypothesize that children with a shorter sleep duration, show more externalizing behavior. In addition, children presenting disrupted sleep patterns, are also expected to show more externalizing and problem behavior.

Methods

Study population

Data were used from the Dutch prospective mother-child cohort LINC (Linking EDCs in Maternal Nutrition to Child Health). The cohort was set up in the region of Zwolle, both a rural and urban setting in the Netherlands. Women were recruited from 2011 to 2013 during their first antenatal visit to the midwifery clinic. Women who were not able to fill out Dutch questionnaires were excluded from participation. Other exclusion criteria were pre-eclampsia, twin pregnancies and major congenital anomalies at birth.

After inclusion, participants were followed during pregnancy and after birth, until the child was 18 months old. During this period, the parents filled out questionnaires every three months on, amongst others, life style, mental wellness and environment. The LINC-study has been approved by the Medical Ethical Committee of the VU University Medical Centre (VUmc).

Sleep diaries

Sleep patterns were assessed by sleep diaries (appendix I), which were filled out by the parents or caretaker when the child was three, six, nine, twelve and eighteen months old. Parents could indicate for every hour of the day if the child was sleeping, was awake, was crying, or was being fed. Parents reported this for seven consecutive days in total. Using the sleep diaries, sleep duration, nocturnal awakenings and early awakenings were calculated for each child at each time point.

Daily sleep duration was calculated by summing up the total amount of time spent sleeping in one week, and dividing this number by seven. A child was defined as having nocturnal awakenings (yes: 1 or no: 0) if it woke up between 11pm and 5am, at least two times a week. A child was defined as having early awakenings (yes: 1 or no: 0) if it woke up between 5am and 6am, at least two times a week. Parents could make notes for each day separately in an additional table. If a child was ill, data from that day were excluded from further analysis.

Externalizing behavior

When children were 18 months of age, parents filled out the Child Behavior Checklist 1.5-5 to assess the behavioral development of the child [39]. The questionnaire consists of 99 items. Parents had to indicate on a 3-point Likert scale whether an item was very true (2), somewhat true (1) or not true (0) for the child. Scores were calculated according to the algorithm of the manual [39].

The subscale 'Externalizing' was used for the analysis. The scale 'Externalizing' consists of two other sub scales: 'Attention Problems' and 'Aggressive Behavior'.The scale consists of twenty-four items. A raw sum score (range 0-48) was used for the analyses. The software program Assessment Data Manager was developed by Achenbach for data management purposes of the CBCL and was used for the calculation of these raw scores.

According to Achenbach and Rescorla, for statistical analyses raw scores are usually preferable, as they directly reflect all differences among scores [39]. In addition, there are no effects of transformations and differences at the low end of the normal range are maintained.

Covariates

Covariates were selected based on literature [40-45]. Family history, educational level, smoking, alcohol use and illicit drug use during pregnancy were checked for possible confounding effects.

Questionnaires were used for the collection of these data. For family history, parents were asked if the child had family members with ADHD (yes or no). With regard to educational level, parents were asked to indicate the highest educational level they had completed, using eight different categories. The educational level was labeled as 'high' if at least one of either parent(s) had obtained a Bachelor's or a Master's Degree, and 'low' otherwise.

For the assessment of alcohol use the mother was asked if she had used alcohol during pregnancy (yes or no). Smoking and illicit drug uses during pregnancy were assessed similarly. Under 'Analysis', information if provided on the covariate selection for the statistical models.

Analysis

First, selective non-response was studied by comparing included and excluded mother-child pairs on a number of demographic variables (means of gestational age, maternal BMI, age of the mother at birth and level of maternal education).

Stata 12.1 was used to conduct mixed model analyses in order to analyze the development of the three sleep variables (sleep duration, early awakening and nocturnal awakenings) over the first 1.5 years of life. In these analyses we included random intercepts and/or slopes at the individual level based on the Akaike information criterion (AIC) of the models.

Linear mixed models were estimated for sleep duration and logistic mixed models were estimated for early awakenings and nocturnal awakenings. A continuous time variable was added to the models as a fixed effect. For nocturnal awakenings we assumed a quadratic development over time by adding time squared to the model, based on an improved fit of the model.

A random intercept and random slope was included for sleep duration and nocturnal awakenings, while for early awakenings only a random intercept was added. For example, with regard to sleep duration a random intercept of 1 would mean the child sleeps 1 hour more on average in comparison to the estimated mean sleep duration in the population.

The random slope ld refers to the degree to which the sleep duration of a child decreases or increases more rapidly over time than that of others. The individual intercepts and slopes based on these models were saved and used in the subsequent analyses.

Linear regression analyses were carried out to study the relationship of sleep characteristics over time with externalizing behavior as continuous, dependent variable. In these analyses the random intercepts and slopes from the analyses on sleep patterns (sleep duration, nocturnal and early awakenings) were added to the models as central independent variables. Bootstrap methods were applied, based on 1000 bootstrap samples, in order to estimate the confidence intervals. When bootstrapping, pseudo-samples (named bootstraps) are drawn from the original sample.

The method is convenient for nonlinear statistics or when the sample size is small as there are no distributional assumptions. Bootstrapping may provide more accurate confidence intervals than the standard methods in these cases. It should be noted that, although we believe that for the current study this was the most valid approach, null-hypothesis tests based on p-values did not resemble those based on the bootstrapping confidence intervals.

A confidence interval that did not cross the null was considered to be statistically significant. Adjusted analyses included covariates that changed the regression coefficients of the central determinants with 10% or more after adding them to the statistical models. All analyses were carried out in SPSS 21.

Results

Sample characteristics

A flow chart of the number of participants is presented in Figure 1. A total of 144 mother-child pairs was included in the study. Twenty-six pairs dropped out of the study.

In addition, one participant had a miscarriage, and from 18 mother-child pairs no CBCL or sleep data was available. Therefore, the total number of included mother-child pairs was 99.

The included mother-child pairs were compared to the 45 excluded pairs on a number of demographic variables, which were available for most pairs.

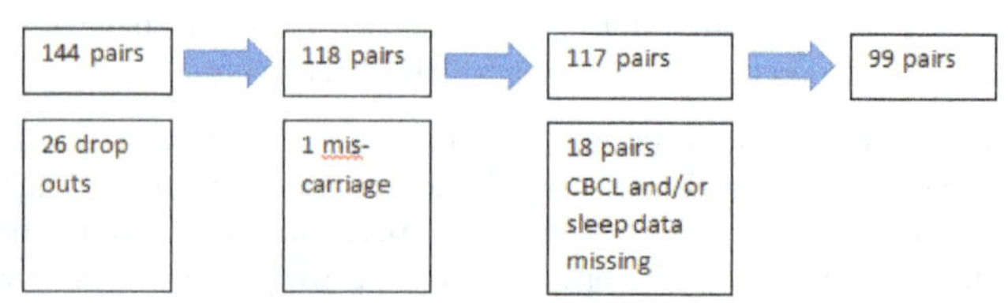

Figure 1: Flow chart of the number of participants.

No significant mean differences were found for gestational age, maternal BMI and the age of the mother at birth. The median level of maternal education was at least a Bachelor's degree in both groups.

Characteristic	N		Range
Gestational age in weeks (mean, SD)	92	39.9 (1.2)	36.4-42.1
Age mother in years (mean, SD)	97	30.5 (3.7)	21-40
Educational level (high, %)	85	74 (76.3)	-
Smoking pregnancy (yes, %)	97	5 (5.2)	-
Alcohol use pregnancy (yes, %)	97	11 (11.3)	-
Illicit drug use pregnancy (yes, %)	97	0 (0)	-
Family history ADHD (yes, %)	96	13 (13.5)	-
Externalizing behavior score (mean, SD)	99	10.4 (6.2)	0-27

Table 1: Maternal characteristics and externalizing behavior scores in 18 months old children. ADHD=Attention Deficit Hyperactivity Disorder; CBCL=Child Behavior Checklist; N=sample size; SD=standard deviation.

In Tables 1 and 2, an overview is provided of the characteristics of the study population. The mean score on the Externalizing Behavior scale was 10.4. More than 13 percent of the children had a family member affected by ADHD.

In Table 2, study characteristics are provided with regard to the sleep patterns. The number of included mother-child pairs varies over time, limiting comparability of the data.

When looking at the percentages, the data seems to indicate a slow decline over time for sleep duration, nocturnal and early awakenings.

However, when taking only the numbers into account, for nocturnal and early awakenings, the data does not seem consistent as the number of children with either nocturnal or early awakenings at 18 months seems to increase compared to the time point of 12 months.

	Sleep duration (hrs)		Early awakenings		Nocturnal awakenings	
	N	Mean (SD)	N	Yes (%)	N	Yes (%)
3 months	64	14.1 (1.6)	64	26 (40.6)	64	41 (64.1)
6 months	53	14.1 (1.3)	53	14 (26.4)	52	22 (42.3)
9 months	48	13.9 (1.4)	48	8 (16.7)	48	17 (35.4)
12 months	53	13.9 (1.1)	53	5 (9.4)	53	18 (34.0)
18 months	90	13.5 (1.1)	89	6 (6.7)	89	24 (27.0)

Table 2: Sleep behavior during the first 18 months of life. SD=standard deviation

Associations between sleep patterns and externalizing problems at 18 months

Mixed models were used to study the associations between sleep patterns and externalizing problems at 18 months, using random intercepts and random slopes. With regard to sleep duration, the random intercepts ranged from -2.47 to 1.85. This means that the variation in sleep duration ranged from 2.47 hours below, to 1.85 hours above the average sleep duration. The random slopes for sleep duration varied between 0.08 to 0.11. The range of the random intercepts for nocturnal awakenings varied from -37.10 to 2.83, while the random slope varied between -1.08 to 0.51. For early awakening, only a random intercept was added to a model, ranging from -1.07 to 2.46. In Table 3, the results of the crude and adjusted analyses for the relation between the random coefficients of the sleep variables and externalizing problems are presented. In the crude analysis, the intercept of sleep duration was found to be significantly related to externalizing scores on the CBCL (β=-2.35; CI=-4.31, -0.16; p=0.03). This means, that with every hour of increase in average sleep duration, a child scored 2.35 points lower on the externalizing scale of the CBCL (Table 3). As none of the covariates caused at least a 10% change in the regression coefficient after adding the variable to the model, no adjusted analysis was performed with regard to sleep duration. No other significant results were found.

Variable	Crude analysis				Adjusted analysis			
	N	β	95% CI	p-value	N	β	95% CI	p-value
Sleep duration[1]								
Random intercept	99	-2.35	-4.31, -0.16	0.03	-	-	-	-
Random slope	99	-32.31	-70.49, 6.19	0.09	-	-	-	-
Nocturnal awakenings[2]								
Random intercept	92	0.01	-0.17, 0.28	0.87	92	0	-0.19, 0.28	0.99
Random slope	92	3.4	-0.27, 6.97	0.05	92	3.51	-0.66, 7.19	0.06
Early awakenings[3]								

Random intercept	95	0.67	-0.93, 2.25	0.39	95	0.57	-1.13, 2.18	0.51

Table 3: Regression coefficients, confidence intervals and p-values for sleep and score on the scale 'Externalizing problems' of the CBCL 1.5-5. Significant at an alpha of 0.05, β=regression coefficient; CI: Confidence Interval; N: Sample Size; [1]No confounders caused a ≥10% change in the regression coefficient, [2]Adjusted for smoking pregnancy, Family history of ADHD, Alcohol use pregnancy, [3]Adjusted for smoking pregnancy, Alcohol use pregnancy.

Discussion

To our knowledge, this is the first study to prospectively examine the relationship between sleep patterns in the first 18 months of life and their relation with externalizing behavior at the age of 18 months. Sleep characteristics were assessed at different time points using sleep diaries, while for the assessment of behavioral development the CBCL 1.5-5 was used. We found that sleep duration was significantly related to externalizing behavior. More specifically our results indicate that children who sleep less on average show more externalizing behavior. As the sample size was small, results should be interpreted with caution.

We found a significant association between the intercept of sleep duration and externalizing behavior. Children who slept an hour more scored 2.60 points lower on the externalizing scale of the CBCL. The effect is moderate, as the maximum score on the scale is equal to 48. However, our findings are in line with previous studies conducted in somewhat older children. In a recent study from the United States in children of four years old, parents reported their children's bed and wake times on weekdays in order to assess sleep duration [5]. Parents also rated their child on six different types of externalizing behavior. Children sleeping <9.44 hours (1 standard deviation below the mean of 10.47 hours) presented a significantly higher odds of all aspects of externalizing behavior, including over activity, anger, aggression, impulsivity, tantrums and annoying behavior [5]. In a different study, a short sleep duration in eight year old children was related to an increased risk for externalizing behavior (2.9 to 3.9-fold increased risk) [46]. In addition, in a meta-analysis of 86 studies conducted in 2012, a shorter sleep duration was significantly related to more behavioral problems in children aged five to twelve years (r=0.09; CI: 0.07, 0.11). Subsequent analysis showed that both internalizing (r=0.09; CI: 0.06, 0.12) and externalizing behavior (r=0.08; CI: 0.06, 0.11) were positively associated to a shorter sleep duration [47]. Finally, in a longitudinal study, a reduced sleep duration and sleep quality in school-aged children (6-17 years old) predicted symptoms of externalizing behavior over time, as well as depression and anxiety [48]. To a lesser extent, behavioral problems predicted changes in sleep characteristics as well, indicating a potential reciprocal relationship.

Although research in especially preschool children is limited, studies conducted so far have reported similar results, with a shorter sleep duration being related to more externalizing behavior. In only one study, using teacher and parent reports, a shorter sleep duration was not significantly related to externalizing problems in children aged five to six [49]. However, the direction of the results was the same, with a shorter sleep duration being related to more externalizing problems.

Recent research indicates that emotional disruption might be the mechanism at work in the association between sleep patterns and externalizing behavior. In a review, Kouros and El-Sheikh suggest that emotional regulation may present a pathway linking sleep patterns and behavioral outcomes [1]. In a study by Yoo and colleagues, participants deprived from sleep for approximately 35 hours showed an increase of 60% in the response of the amygdala to negative stimuli, compared to the control group [3]. In addition, participants deprived from sleep showed a decrease in functional connectivity between the amygdala and the medial-prefrontal cortex, which has been related to affective processing.

Findings from the above studies should be interpreted with caution as a reduction in sleep duration is not equal to sleep deprivation. However, it has been suggested that a lack of sleep may modulate the response of the human brain to negative stimuli and that sleep deprivation may lead to a reduction in top-down, prefrontal control [3]. Sleep may provide a framework in which the neuronal systems that are involved in emotion regulation and the processing of recent emotional experiences are 'reset' [2,3]. Therefore, it is speculated that sleep deprivation could be implied in the etiology of behavioral disorders, especially mood disorders [1,3].

Strengths of the current study include the homogeneity of the study population in educational level and ethnicity, which decreases the likelihood of confounding by demographic factors. To assess externalizing behavior, the CBCL 1.5-5 was used. The CBCL is a well-known and widely used screening instrument in clinical practice for behavioral problems as it is considered both a reliable and valid instrument [50]. When examining the psychometric properties of the CBCL 1.5-5, with regard to the (test-retest) reliability of the scales, a mean correlation was found of 0.85 across all scales, with most correlations falling in the 0.80s or 0.90s [39]. Across all scales, a mean correlation of 0.61 was found with regard to both cross-informant agreement and the stability of the scale scores (using an interval of 12 months). The content and criterion-related validity were positively evaluated, as the questionnaire was found to significantly discriminate between referred and nonreferred children (p<0.01). Although the CBCL should be combined with observational techniques for diagnostical purposes, it is a useful screening method for behavioral problems [50]. Furthermore, data with regard to sleep patterns was collected over several days (one week) which may increase the reliability of the parameters assessed. Moreover, as data was collected at five different time points, individual sleep patterns could be analyzed. However, we did not assess information on daytime napping, which has been related to behavioral outcomes in preschool children in previous work [51,52]. In addition, the sleep diaries used in this study have not been validated previously, which is a possible weakness. Up to our knowledge, this is the first study using this sleeping diary, limiting comparability with other studies (hiscock & Jordan, 2004). As the sleep diaries depend on parental observation, information might be less accurate when compared to more objective measurements such as a sleep actigraphy or polysomnography.

Previous work has indicated that the sleep diary is cost-effective and useful when administered to larger samples, but is also characterized by lower response rates and a higher risk of missing or incomplete data [53-56]. In addition, only externalizing behavior was included in the current study, while sleep patterns may also be related to other behavioral outcomes. Unfortunately, the other subscales of the CBCL

1.5-5 were not normally distributed in our sample. Only the Attention Deficit Hyperactivity subscale was normally distributed. However, we did not find any significant results for this subscale (supplemental materials) in our cohort. This does not seem surprising, as most children do not receive a diagnosis of ADHD before the age of 7 (Visser et al.). Hence, the age of 18 months may be too young to successfully differentiate age appropriate from disturbed behavior. Finally, the sample size in this study was small, which reduced the power of our study. Therefore, the results should be interpreted with caution.

A healthy sleep duration is critical for the emotional well-being of children [5]. At this moment, sleep disturbances are often considered to be symptoms of other disorders [57]. Despite an overlap in symptoms, there are strong arguments not to regard sleep disturbances only as secondary to other disorders [58]. Sleep disturbances may already exist before other problems develop. In the current study, differences in sleep patterns were already observed in children from three to 18 months. Moreover, these differences were shown to be related to externalizing problem behavior. These results may be an indication to start interventions in children with sleep problems at a younger age. In addition, the treatment of sleep problems may lead to a reduction in symptoms of other disorders [57,58].

Conclusions and Recommendations

The objective of the current study was to explore the relationship between sleep patterns and externalizing behavior at the age of 18 months. In the current study, differences in sleep patterns were already observed in children from three to 18 months. Moreover, differences in sleep duration over time were negatively related to externalizing behavior. Although the results from the current study should be seen as exploratory, health care professionals are encouraged to advocate for a healthy sleep hygiene as well as regular sleep habits and bedtime routines for children. Future studies should make use of longitudinal designs and higher sample sizes to confirm the relationship between sleep patterns and behavioral development over time, while exploring the role of daytime napping.

References

1. Kouros CD, El-Sheikh M (2015) Daily mood and sleep: reciprocal relations and links with adjustment problems. J Sleep Res 24: 24-31.
2. van der Helm E, Walker MP (2011) Sleep and Emotional Memory Processing. Sleep Med Clin 6: 31-43.
3. Yoo SS, Gujar N, Hu P, Jolesz FA, Walker MP (2007) The human emotional brain without sleep--a prefrontal amygdala disconnect. Curr Biol 17: R877-878.
4. Fallone G, Acebo C, Arnedt JT, Seifer R, Carskadon MA (2001) Effects of acute sleep restriction on behavior, sustained attention, and response inhibition in children. Percept Mot Skills 93: 213-229.
5. Scharf RJ, Demmer RT, Silver EJ, Stein RE (2013) Nighttime sleep duration and externalizing behaviors of preschool children. J Dev Behav Pediatr 34: 384-391.
6. Vaughn BE, Elmore-Staton L, Shin N, El-Sheikh M (2015) Sleep as a support for social competence, peer relations, and cognitive functioning in preschool children. Behav Sleep Med 13: 92-106.
7. Gruber R, Laviolette R, Deluca P, Monson E, Cornish K, et al. (2010) Short sleep duration is associated with poor performance on IQ measures in healthy school-age children. Sleep Med 11: 289-294.
8. Dewald JF, Meijer AM, Oort FJ, Kerkhof GA, Bögels SM (2010) The influence of sleep quality, sleep duration and sleepiness on school performance in children and adolescents: A meta-analytic review. Sleep Med Rev 14: 179-189.
9. Steenari MR, Vuontela V, Paavonen EJ, Carlson S, Fjallberg M, et al. (2003) Working memory and sleep in 6- to 13-year-old schoolchildren. J Am Acad Child Adolesc Psychiatry 42: 85-92.
10. El-Sheikh M, Buckhalt JA, Mark Cummings E, Keller P (2007) Sleep disruptions and emotional insecurity are pathways of risk for children. J Child Psychol Psychiatry 48: 88-96.
11. Vriend JL, Davidson FD, Corkum PV, Rusak B, Chambers CT, et al. (2013) Manipulating sleep duration alters emotional functioning and cognitive performance in children. J Pediatr Psychol 38: 1058-1069.
12. Sivertsen B, Harvey AG, Reichborn-Kjennerud T, Torgersen L, Ystrom E, et al. (2015) Later emotional and behavioral problems associated with sleep problems in toddlers: a longitudinal study. JAMA Pediatr 169: 575-582.
13. Dollman J, Ridley K, Olds T, Lowe E (2007) Trends in the duration of school-day sleep among 10- to 15-year-old South Australians between 1985 and 2004. Acta Paediatr 96: 1011-1014.
14. Iglowstein I, Jenni OG, Molinari L, Largo RH (2003) Sleep duration from infancy to adolescence: reference values and generational trends. Pediatrics 111: 302-307.
15. Owens J (2008) Classification and epidemiology of childhood sleep disorders. Prim Care 35: 533-546, vii.
16. Mindell JA (2006) Behavioral treatment of bedtime problems and night wakings in infants and young children. Sleep 29: 1263-1276.
17. Atladottir HO (2015) The increasing prevalence of reported diagnoses of childhood psychiatric disorders: a descriptive multinational comparison. Eur Child Adolesc Psychiatry 24: 173-183.
18. Division of Human Development, N.C.o.B.D.a.D.D, (2015) Centers for Disease Control and Prevention, Attention-Deficit/Hyperactivity Disorder (ADHD) - Data & Statistics.
19. Brugha TS, McManus S, Bankart J, Scott F, Purdon S, et al. (2011) Epidemiology of autism spectrum disorders in adults in the community in England. Arch Gen Psychiatry 68: 459-465.
20. Baron-Cohen S, Scott FJ, Allison C, Williams J, Bolton P, et al. (2009) Prevalence of autism-spectrum conditions: UK school-based population study. Br J Psychiatry 194: 500-509.
21. Nygren G, Cederlund M, Sandberg E, Gillstedt F, Arvidsson T, et al. (2012) The prevalence of autism spectrum disorders in toddlers: a population study of 2-year-old Swedish children. J Autism Dev Disord 42: 1491-1497.
22. Roskam I (2015) Stimulating parents' self-efficacy beliefs or verbal responsiveness: Which is the best way to decrease children's externalizing behaviors? Behav Res Ther 72: 38-48.
23. Janssens A, Van Den Noortgate W, Goossens L, Verschueren K, Colpin H, et al. (2015) Externalizing Problem Behavior in Adolescence: Dopaminergic Genes in Interaction with Peer Acceptance and Rejection. J Youth Adolesc 44: 1441-1456.
24. Reef J (2011) Developmental trajectories of child to adolescent externalizing behavior and adult DSM-IV disorder: results of a 24-year longitudinal study. Soc Psychiatry Psychiatr Epidemiol 46: 1233-41.
25. Broidy LM, Nagin DS, Tremblay RE, Bates JE, Brame B, et al. (2003) Developmental trajectories of childhood disruptive behaviors and adolescent delinquency: a six-site, cross-national study. Dev Psychol 39: 222-245.
26. Copeland WE, Miller-Johnson S, Keeler G, Angold A, Costello EJ (2007) Childhood psychiatric disorders and young adult crime: a prospective, population-based study. Am J Psychiatry 164: 1668-1675.
27. Mannuzza S, Klein RG, Moulton JL (2008) 3rd, Lifetime criminality among boys with attention deficit hyperactivity disorder: a prospective follow-up study into adulthood using official arrest records. Psychiatry Res 160: 237-246.
28. Odgers CL, Moffitt TE, Broadbent JM, Dickson N, Hancox RJ, et al. (2008) Female and male antisocial trajectories: from childhood origins to adult outcomes. Dev Psychopathol 20: 673-716.

29. Simonoff E, Elander J, Holmshaw J, Pickles A, Murray R, et al. (2004) Predictors of antisocial personality. Continuities from childhood to adult life. Br J Psychiatry 184: 118-127.
30. Sourander A, Jensen P, Davies M, Niemelä S, Elonheimo H, et al. (2007) Who is at greatest risk of adverse long-term outcomes? The Finnish From a Boy to a Man study. J Am Acad Child Adolesc Psychiatry 46: 1148-1161.
31. Sourander A (2006) Early predictors of parent- and self-reported perceived global psychological difficulties among adolescents: a prospective cohort study from age 3 to age 15. Soc Psychiatry Psychiatr Epidemiol 41: 173-82.
32. Moffitt TE, Caspi A, Harrington H, Milne BJ (2002) Males on the life-course-persistent and adolescence-limited antisocial pathways: follow-up at age 26 years. Dev Psychopathol 14: 179-207.
33. Nock MK (2007) Lifetime prevalence, correlates, and persistence of oppositional defiant disorder: results from the National Comorbidity Survey Replication. J Child Psychol Psychiatry 48: 703-713.
34. Zoccolillo M (1992) Co-occurrence of conduct disorder and its adult outcomes with depressive and anxiety disorders: a review. J Am Acad Child Adolesc Psychiatry 31: 547-556.
35. Fergusson DM, Horwood LJ, Ridder EM (2007) Conduct and attentional problems in childhood and adolescence and later substance use, abuse and dependence: results of a 25-year longitudinal study. Drug Alcohol Depend 1: S14-26.
36. Huesmann LR, Dubow EF, Boxer P (2009) Continuity of aggression from childhood to early adulthood as a predictor of life outcomes: implications for the adolescent-limited and life-course-persistent models. Aggress Behav 35: 136-149.
37. Reid GJ, Hong RY, Wade TJ (2009) The relation between common sleep problems and emotional and behavioral problems among 2- and 3-year-olds in the context of known risk factors for psychopathology. J Sleep Res 18: 49-59.
38. Zaidman-Zait A, Hall WA (2015) Children's night waking among toddlers: relationships with mothers' and fathers' parenting approaches and children's behavioural difficulties. J Adv Nurs.
39. Achenbach TMR (2000)Manual for the ASEBA Preschool forms and Profiles. Burlington, Vermont: University of Vermont Department of Psychiatry.
40. Linnet KM (2003) Maternal lifestyle factors in pregnancy risk of attention deficit hyperactivity disorder and associated behaviors: review of the current evidence. Am J Psychiatry 160: 1028-1040.
41. Mick E, Biederman J, Faraone SV, Sayer J, Kleinman S (2002) Case-control study of attention-deficit hyperactivity disorder and maternal smoking, alcohol use, and drug use during pregnancy. J Am Acad Child Adolesc Psychiatry 41: 378-385.
42. Silva D, Colvin L, Hagemann E, Bower C (2014) Environmental risk factors by gender associated with attention-deficit/hyperactivity disorder. Pediatrics 133: e14-22.
43. Piper BJ, Corbett SM (2012) Executive function profile in the offspring of women that smoked during pregnancy. Nicotine Tob Res 14: 191-199.
44. Bada HS, Bann CM, Whitaker TM, Bauer CR, Shankaran S, et al. (2012) Protective factors can mitigate behavior problems after prenatal cocaine and other drug exposures. Pediatrics 130: e1479-1488.
45. Han JY, Kwon HJ, Ha M, Paik KC, Lim MH, et al. (2015) The effects of prenatal exposure to alcohol and environmental tobacco smoke on risk for ADHD: a large population-based study. Psychiatry Res 225: 164-168.
46. Pesonen AK, Räikkönen K, Paavonen EJ, Heinonen K, Komsi N, et al. (2010) Sleep duration and regularity are associated with behavioral problems in 8-year-old children. Int J Behav Med 17: 298-305.
47. Astill RG, Van der Heijden KB, Van Ijzendoorn MH, Van Someren EJ (2012) Sleep, cognition, and behavioral problems in school-age children: a century of research meta-analyzed. Psychol Bull 138: 1109-1138.
48. Kelly RJ, El-Sheikh M (2014) Reciprocal relations between children's sleep and their adjustment over time. Dev Psychol 50: 1137-1147.
49. Paavonen EJ, Porkka-Heiskanen T, Lahikainen AR (2009) Sleep quality, duration and behavioral symptoms among 5-6-year-old children. Eur Child Adolesc Psychiatry 18: 747-754.
50. Skovgaard AM, Houmann T, Landorph SL, Christiansen E (2004) Assessment and classification of psychopathology in epidemiological research of children 0-3 years of age: a review of the literature. Eur Child Adolesc Psychiatry 13: 337-346.
51. Miller AL, Seifer R, Crossin R, Lebourgeois MK (2015) Toddler's self-regulation strategies in a challenge context are nap-dependent. J Sleep Res 24: 279-287.
52. Hall WA, Scher A, Zaidman-Zait A, Espezel H, Warnock F (2012) A community-based study of sleep and behaviour problems in 12- to 36-month-old children. Child Care Health Dev 38: 379-389.
53. Arora T, Broglia E, Pushpakumar D, Lodhi T, Taheri S (2013) An investigation into the strength of the association and agreement levels between subjective and objective sleep duration in adolescents. PLoS One 8: e72406.
54. Werner H, Molinari L, Guyer C, Jenni OG (2008) Agreement rates between actigraphy, diary, and questionnaire for children's sleep patterns. Arch Pediatr Adolesc Med 162: 350-358.
55. Gregory AM, Cousins JC, Forbes EE, Trubnick L, Ryan ND, et al. (2011) Sleep items in the child behavior checklist: a comparison with sleep diaries, actigraphy, and polysomnography. J Am Acad Child Adolesc Psychiatry 50: 499-507.
56. Kaplan KA, Talbot LS, Gruber J, Harvey AG (2012) Evaluating sleep in bipolar disorder: comparison between actigraphy, polysomnography, and sleep diary. Bipolar Disord 14: 870-879.
57. Gregory AM, Sadeh A (2012) Sleep, emotional and behavioral difficulties in children and adolescents. Sleep Med Rev 16: 129-136.
58. Harvey AG (2001) Insomnia: symptom or diagnosis? Clin Psychol Rev 21: 1037-1059.

Appendix 1:

Characteristic	Mean	SD	Range	N and % of children subclinical or clinical
Emotionally reactive	1.5	1.6	0-7	3 (3%)
Anxious/depressed	0.9	1	0-5	0 (0%)
Somatic complaints	1	1.2	0-5	2 (2%)
Withdrawn	0.6	1	0-5	1 (1%)
Sleep problems	1.4	2.2	0-12	2 (2%)
Attention problems	2.3	1.7	0-6	3 (3%)

Aggressive behavior	8.1	5.1	0-22	2 (2%)
Affective problems	1.3	1.7	0-8	4 (4%)
Anxiety problems	1.6	1.7	0-10	2 (2%)
Pervasive developmental problems	1.5	1.6	0-8	1 (1%)
Attention deficit hyperactivity problems	3.7	2	0-8	0 (0%)
Oppositional defiant problems	3.3	2.3	0-10	5 (5%)
Internalizing behavior	4	3.5	0-17	3 (3%)
Externalizing behavior	10.4	6.2	0-27	7 (7%)
Total problems score	21	12.7	Feb-55	-2%

Table 1: CBCL scores in 18 months old children (n=99). CBCL = Child Behavior Checklist; N = sample size; SD = standard deviation.

Appendix 2:

Variable	Crude analysis				Adjusted analysis			
	N	β	95% CI	p-value	N	β	95% CI	p-value
				Sleep duration[1]				
Random intercept	88	-0.45	-1.22, 0.01	0.15	88	-0.37	-1.00, 0.37	0.27
Random slope	88	-6.68	-19.21, 5.59	0.25	88	-5.37	-17.28, 6.37	0.35
				Nocturnal awakenings[2]				
Random intercept	85	0.02	-0.06, 0.12	0.56	85	0.02	-0.05, 0.12	0.68
Random slope	85	0.36	-0.80, 1.38	0.51	85	0.45	-0.92, 1.53	0.46
				Early awakenings[3]				
Random slope	85	0.2	-0.28, 0.69	0.42	85	0.13	-0.37, 0.67	0.6

Table 2: Regression coefficients, confidence intervals and p-values for sleep and ADHD score on the CBCL 1.5-5.β = regression coefficient; CI = confidence interval; N = sample size; [1] Adjusted for: Alcohol use pregnancy, Smoking pregnancy, [2] Adjusted for: Smoking pregnancy, Alcohol use pregnancy, Family history of ADHD, [3] Adjusted for: Smoking pregnancy, Alcohol use pregnancy, Family history of ADHD.

10

Modification of a Motor-Response Dependent Measure of Daytime Sleepiness (OSLER-2)

Jayne Roberts[1], **David J Berlowitz**[1,2*] **and Jo Spong**[2]

[1]*Department of Medicine, Austin Health and Northern Health, University of Melbourne, Parkville, Victoria, Australia*

[2]*Institute for Breathing and Sleep, Austin Hospital, Heidelberg, Victoria, Australia*

[*]**Corresponding author**: David J Berlowitz, Institute for Breathing and Sleep, Bowen Centre, Austin Health, Heidelberg, Victoria, 3084, Australia, E-mail: david.berlowitz@austin.org.au

Abstract

Background: A simple, portable measure of daytime sleepiness is the Oxford Sleep Resistance (OSLER-2) test; however its use is limited to those with good hand function. This study modified the OSLER-2 test to assess the measurement of daytime sleepiness using two alternative, non-hand-held response switches.

Methods: The unit was modified to accept the standard hand-held switch, a head-tap switch ("Jelly-bean") and chin-tap switch ("Wand"). Participants were required to respond to a central LED light presented for one second every three seconds. It terminated following either seven consecutive missed responses (participant asleep) or forty minutes (maximum test length, "performance time"). Twenty-two able-bodied participants with no diagnosed sleep disorders were sleep restricted prior to three testing days where switch order was randomized. The test was performed four times over each day. Sleep latency, performance times and errors were recorded along with video of the switch use.

Results: Sleep latency was longer with the Wand (M=1265 sec (546)) than the Jelly-bean (M=1102 (544)) and hand-held switch (M=1037 sec (557), $p<0.05$). Performance times were longer with the Wand (M=1788 sec (695)) than the Jelly-bean (M=1530 sec (758); $p<0.05$) and hand-held switch (M=1459 sec (784); $p<0.01$). Sleep latency, performance times and errors did not differ significantly between the Jelly-bean and hand-held switches. Video suggested the Wand was occasionally activated erroneously by forward (drowsy) head-drops.

Conclusion: The Jelly-bean provides a possible alternative response switch to measure daytime sleepiness in those with limited hand function.

Keywords: Hand function; Performance; Sleep latency; Switches; Vigilance

Introduction

Daytime sleepiness is a common, debilitating symptom for those suffering with a sleep disorder. It decreases work productivity [1], and impairs both mental health status [2] and the ability to perform daily activities [3]. Tests used to measure daytime sleepiness include the Multiple Sleep Latency Test (MSLT) and the Maintenance of Wakefulness Test (MWT) [4-6]. Both the MSLT and MWT are multi-nap approaches in which the ability to fall asleep and the ability to remain awake are tested respectively in the absence of alerting factors. Though simple tests, the use of Electro-encephalogram (EEG) monitoring to determine time of sleep onset makes these tests costly, labor intensive and typically confines their performance to specialized sleep units.

A behavioral equivalent called the Oxford Sleep Resistance (OSLER) test [7] was developed to reproduce many of the characteristics of the MWT [7,8]. Without the need for EEG monitoring or a trained technician, the OSLER test is a simple to use, less expensive and more portable method of measuring sleep latency than both the MSLT and MWT. The OSLER test requires a simple button response to a light flashed at pseudo-random intervals for one second every three seconds. Failure to respond to seven flashes is interpreted as sleep having occurred, otherwise the test continues for its complete duration of forty minutes. The test is limited in its present form however; it requires the participant to have adequate hand function to operate a response switch. Given that daytime sleepiness is a particularly common symptom amongst people with a spinal cord injury (SCI) [9,10], who have limited or no hand function, the inability to apply the portable, inexpensive benefits of the OSLER test to this population, in which travel to a sleep unit can be burdensome, is complexing. This study aimed to take the first steps in modifying the OSLER-2 test to incorporate switches that do not rely on hand function. This study performed an OSLER-2 switch comparison; it examined sleep latency measured on the OSLER-2 test using the modified switches compared to the standard hand-held one.

Methods

Study participants

Healthy, able-bodied people aged between 18 and 70 years, with no previous diagnosis of a sleep disorder were recruited from the community. Exclusion criteria included: visual problems not corrected by glasses or contact lenses; psychiatric or neurological disorders;

addiction to nicotine; use of benzodiazepines; recent travel or planned travel across time zones during the study or shift work. Participants provided written informed consent and the study was approved by the Austin Health Human Research Ethics Committee. Participants who completed the study were remunerated for their time. The study is registered at www.anzctr.org.au (335819).

Procedure

Participants attended three days of testing at the Austin hospital sleep laboratory, each on the same weekday and separated by one week. One participant was unable to attend a day of testing due to illness and so completed the testing sessions over a four week period.

The night prior to each testing day, participants restricted their sleep to between 02:00 and 05:00. Sleep restriction was confirmed by a Sense Wear Pro3 armband (BodyMedia, Pittsburgh, USA) which records movements and sleep habits. Participants wore the armband for the 14 hours prior to each testing day.

The OSLER-2 test was conducted four times on each testing day, at 09:30, 11:30, 13:30 and 15:30 hours. The test records participant responses made via response switch to a light-emitting diode (LED) illuminated for one second every three seconds. The OLSER-2 test lasts for forty minutes unless the participant fails to respond to seven consecutive LED illuminations (21 sec) which is interpreted as the participant falling asleep and the test subsequently stops. The OSLER-2 records the times at which the test terminates, which is considered the sleep latency (minutes and seconds), along with the number of missed responses ("errors"). If a participant does not fall asleep, then the total time of forty minutes is displayed.

Three different response switches were used in this study, the standard OSLER-2 hand-held switch and two modified, non-hand-held switches not currently used in the OSLER-2 test, but commonly used by people with disabilities. The modified switches are: the "Jelly-bean" and "Magic Wand-Pad" ("Wand") switches which are activated using a single, light touch head tap and a chin tap respectively which can be audible (Figures 1 and 2; note written consent to publish these photographic images was obtained by the person presented in these images). A different switch was used on each of the three days of testing, the order of which was blocked and randomized.

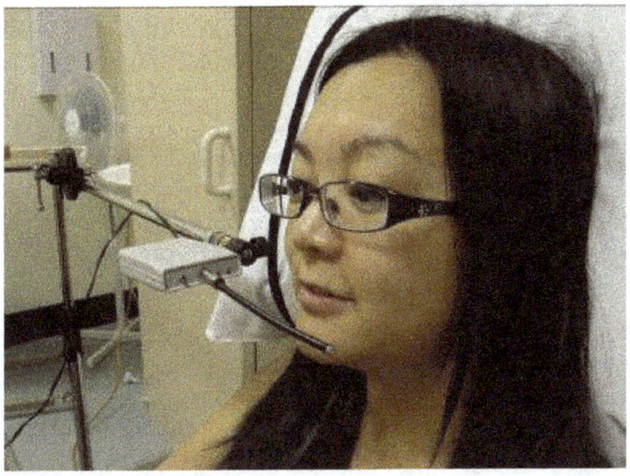

Figure 1: The Jelly-bean switch (button on pillow) with illustration of its placement for a head tap.

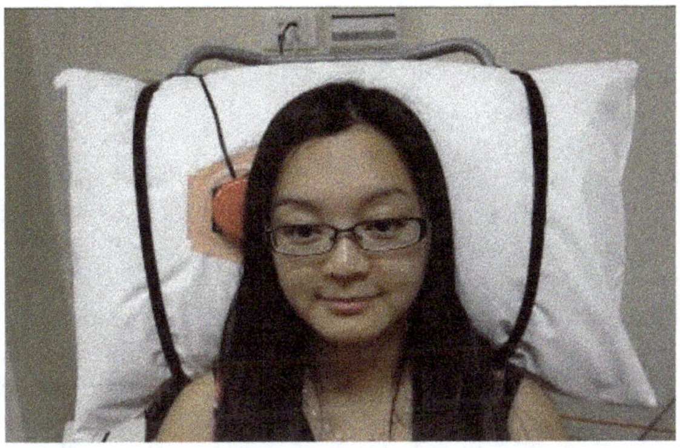

Figure 2: The Magic Wand-Pad switch with illustration of its placement for a chin tap.

During the OSLER-2 tests, participants sat in an isolated, noise proof room, darkened to approximately 0.1 Lux, with temperature between 21 and 24 degrees Celsius. The LED was placed at eye-level, two meters in front of the participant. The participant sat slightly reclined in a wheelchair to mimic the posture in which people with a motor disability, such as quadriplegia, would be expected to perform the test. Participants were asked to remain awake without using extraordinary measures to do so and to trigger the switch every time the LED illuminated. To help prevent the occurrence of deliberately terminated tests, participants were informed that test times may vary, but were not told that a failure to trigger the switch seven times consecutively would result in test termination. A video feed of the room was monitored during all tests to assess compliance to instructions.

To measure trait and state sleepiness and circadian rhythm type, participants completed the Epworth Sleepiness Scale (ESS) [11] and the Morningness-Eveningness Questionnaire (MEQ) [12] the morning of their first testing day and the Karolinska Sleepiness Scale (KSS) [13] immediately prior to and following each of the four testing sessions. The ESS asks participants to rate on a scale of 0-3 (0 being "would never doze", 3 being "high chance of dozing") how likely they would doze off or fall asleep in eight different situations and the scores are then totaled. The MEQ is a seven item questionnaire which measures the circadian rhythm type of a person, such as whether they are a "morning" person or an "evening" person. Three to four possible answers are given for each question, with each answer corresponding scores ranging from 0-6. These scores are totaled at the end of the questionnaire with results falling into one of six categories. The possible categories include "definitely morning type", "moderately morning type", "neither type", "moderately evening type" and "definitely evening type". The KSS is a nine-point Likert-type scale ranging in score from 1 ("very alert") to 9 ("extremely sleepy, fighting sleep"). The KSS asks participants to indicate on the scale how sleepy they are feeling at that current time.

Between OSLER-2 tests, participants were encouraged to engage in sedentary activities such as reading and watching TV and were monitored to avoid falling asleep. A light lunch was provided following the 11:30 testing session and participants were not exposed to bright sunlight during their stay.

Participants completed a sleep diary for the duration of their involvement of the study to identify their typical sleep behavior. The diary recorded nightly sleep behaviour and caffeine and alcohol intake. Participants were asked not to smoke or consume alcohol, caffeine or energy drinks from the day before testing until the completion of their testing day.

Data analysis

Summary statistics are presented to describe the sample. Data collected from the OSLER-2 on each of the three testing days, which comprised four OSLER-2 test per day, was examined. Analyses were performed on two sets of data. The first was on the portion of the sample who fell asleep during the testing session and thus obtained a "sleep latency". The second was on the entire sample, thus including those who did not fall asleep during the test, in order to examine switch "performance" times. Missed responses ("errors") were also examined for the sleep latency and performance portions of the sample.

OSLER-2 Sleep latency and performance times

The proportion of the sample that fell asleep, thus obtaining a sleep latency across switch type and testing time of day was tabulated. Linear Mixed Model (LMM) analysis was used to examine fixed effects of switch type (Jelly-bean, Wand and hand-held), testing time over the day (09:30, 11:30, 13:30, and 15:30), and study week/switch order (week 1, 2, and 3) for both sleep latency and performance times. The participant was included in the model as a random intercept to allow for repeated test results, with a compound symmetric covariance structure to adjust for serial correlation across time within any given day (SPSS software, version 21.0; SPSS, Chicago, Illinois). Significant fixed effects from the LMM analyses were explored using pairwise comparisons. The reported effect size and confidence intervals from the significant fixed effects are from the LMM. This LMM approach was also used to compare state sleepiness (KSS) at the beginning of each testing time.

Error analyses

The LMM approach described was also used to examine the percentage of time corresponding to the appearance of errors during the OSLER-2 test. The calculation used to determine the percentage of time spent by each participant in making errors was: (3 seconds x number of errors/sleep latency duration in seconds) x100 [14].

For all LMM analyses made in this study, the initial model included a switch*time interaction in order to assess whether the effect of switch differed by testing time of day however as this was not statistically significant in any analysis, it was subsequently removed and the model re-analyzed without the interaction term. P values less than 0.05 were considered significant.

Results

Participants

22 participants (15 female) were recruited into the study. Two failed to complete their third day of testing and one completed just one day of testing (three Wand and one hand-held switch testing days missed). The median (25th, 75th percentile ranges) age of the sample was 21 years (19.8, 26), BMI 22 kg/m^2 (20.5, 24.0), abdominal circumference 75.5 cm (71.0, 86.0) and neck circumference 32.5 cm (30.0, 36.3).

Sleep diary

On the nights prior to sleep restriction, participants reported having a median (25th, 75th percentile ranges) of 7.5 (7.0, 8.0) hours sleep per night and generally feeling refreshed most mornings. Ten participants reported alcohol intake during their participation in the study with 8.5 (2.7, 25.3) standard drinks over the three week study period. Fifteen participants reported caffeine intake during this time, with 9 (4.0, 20.0) cups during the study period.

Data from the BodyMedia SenseWear Pro3 Armband confirmed that participants had restricted their sleep on the night before testing with a median sleep time of 2.4 hours (1.9 hrs, 2.7 hrs).

Trait and state sleepiness and circadian type

The mean (SD) ESS was 6.3 (3.4) indicating that participants did not experience excessive daytime sleepiness. The Morningness-Eveningness Scale (MEQ) indicated that of the sample, there were two "moderate morning types", six "moderate evening types", three "definite evening types" and eleven being classified as "neither morning or evening types". The mean KSS score was 5.8 (1.6), which is interpreted as between "neither alert nor sleepy" and "sleepy-but no difficulty remaining awake". KSS scores did not differ significantly before each of the four testing times on each of the three testing days.

OSLER-2 sleep latency and performance times

The proportion of participants who fell asleep overall and at each testing time of the day for each switch type is presented in Table 1.

Overall Time points	Hand-held Switch		Jelly-bean Switch		Wand switch	
	(n=21)	%	(n=22)	%	(n=19)	%
	18	85.7	19	86.4	16	84.2
09:30	15	71.4	13	59.1	11	57.9
11:30	15	71.4	15	68.2	8	42.1
13:30	16	76.2	18	81.8	13	68.4
15:30	12	57.1	13	59.1	9	47.4

Table 1: Count of participants who demonstrated a sleep latency (7-missed responses) overall and at each testing time of day for each switch type.

The mean sleep latency and performance times for each switch type at each testing time of day are shown in Figures 3 and 4 respectively. The mean (SD) sleep latency and performance times for each switch are presented in Table 2.

The LMM showed a statistically significant effect for switch type ($p<0.05$) for both sleep latency and performance times and a significant effect for switch order ($p<0.05$) for performance times. Participants fell asleep significantly faster when using the hand-held than the Wand switch ($p<0.05$; mean difference: 301.3; CI: -59.9, -542.7). Sleep latency times did not differ significantly between the Wand and Jelly-bean switches or between the Jelly-bean and hand-held switches.

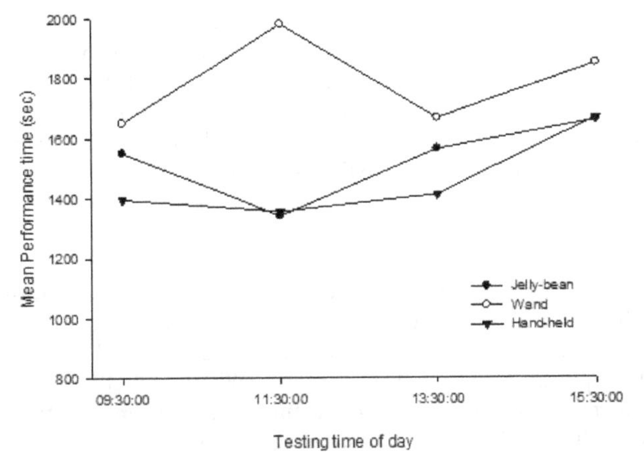

Figure 3: Mean sleep latency (sec) for each testing time of the day and for each switch type.

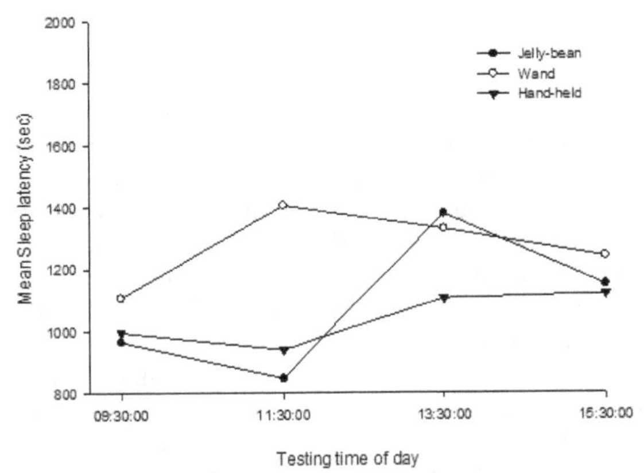

Figure 4: Mean performance times (sec) for each testing time of the day and for each switch type.

	Hand-held Switch		Jelly-bean Switch		Wand Switch	
	M (SD)	**N**	**M (SD)**	**N**	**M (SD)**	**N**
Sleep latency (sec)	1037 (557)	58	1102 (544)	59	1265 (546)	41
Performance time (sec)	1459 (784)	84	1530 (758)	88	1788 (695)	76
Time spent making errors (SL) (%)	15.1 (7.9)	58	16.0 (9.2)	59	13.5 (8.2)	41
Time spent making errors (Perf) (%)	11.4 (9.1)	84	11.6 (10.2)	88	9.9 (8.9)	76

Table 2: The mean (SD) sleep latency, performance times and time spent making errors for each switch type. (sec: second; Time spent making errors (SL): portion of sample who fell asleep as indicated by seven consecutive missed responses to the LED stimuli; Time spent making errors (Perf) is for the whole sample).

Performance times were significantly longer when using the Wand compared to the Jelly-bean ($p<0.05$; mean difference: 330.5; CI: 71.6, 589.3) and hand-held switch ($p<0.01$; mean difference: 359.7; CI: 100.7, 618.8). There was no significant difference in performance time between the Jelly-bean and hand-held switches.

Mean performance times were significantly longer for the first (1778 sec (707)) presented switch compared to both the second (1509 sec (766)) presented switch ($p<0.05$; mean difference: -284.4: CI: 35.2, 533.6) and the third (1445 sec (770)) presented switch ($p<0.05$; mean difference: 282.1; CI: 25.2, 539.0). There was no significant difference in performance times between the second and third presented switches.

Error analysis

The mean (SD) percent of time spent making errors on each switch are presented in Table 2 for the portion of the sample who obtained sleep latency and also for performance times (whole sample).

The LMM examining the percent of time spent making errors showed that there was a significant effect for the time of day the test was conducted for both the sleep latency ($p<0.01$) and performance ($p<0.01$) portions of the group. For the sleep latency group, a higher mean (SD) percentage of time making errors was observed during the 11:30 testing session (18.7% (9.8)) than the 09:30 (14.5% (7.6); $p<0.01$; mean difference: 4.0; CI: 1.2, 6.7), 13:30 (12.4% (7.1); $p<0.001$; mean difference: 5.3; CI: 2.6, 8.0) and 15:30 (15.2% (8.3); $p<0.05$; mean difference: 3.5; CI: 0.6, 6.3) testing sessions.

Similarly, for the performance time portion of the sample, the mean percentage of time making errors was also significantly higher during the 11:30 testing session (13.2% (11.2)) than the 09:30 (10.0% (9.2); $p<0.01$; mean difference: 3.2; CI: 1.2, 5.2), 13:30 (10.7%, (8.0); $p<0.05$; mean difference: 2.5; CI: 0.48, 4.45) and the 15:30 (10.2% (9.1); $p<0.01$; mean difference: 3.0; CI: 1.0, 5.0) testing sessions. There was no significant difference between switch type in the time spent making errors for both the sleep latency and performance time groups.

Discussion

This is the first study to examine the use of non-hand-held response switches to perform the OSLER-2 test as a measure of daytime sleepiness. The aim of this study was to examine sleep latency measured on the OSLER-2 test using modified non hand-held switches compared to the standard hand-held one. Comparable findings were observed between the Jelly-bean and hand-held switches. In contrast, the modified Wand switch presented longer sleep latency and performance times, and fewer errors.

The differences in response requirements along with design characteristics may account for the varying findings observed between the non-hand-held and hand-held switches. These include: the presence of audible feedback noise, the required muscle response ("button push") movement and the varying placement of the switch for response. Both modified switches provide an audible feedback noise when pushed and require a larger movement to respond to the LED light than the hand-held switch. The larger bodily movements with the head and chin taps were observed via the video link during the testing sessions, however not so for the simple finger response of the hand-held switch. The larger movements require slightly more response time and may heighten attention. The presence of audible feedback may have increased alertness and may also have increased participant's motivation which has been shown to effect sleep latency in similar tests [15]. Our results suggest that auditory feedback and greater bodily movement may have contributed to the poorer overall performance of the Wand.

The video feed also highlighted that the placement of the modified switches for response to the LED possibly contributed to the different results between the switches. When becoming drowsy during the test, the participants' head tended to move away from the Jelly-bean, and their finger away from the hand-held switch. In contrast, when using the Wand, drowsiness resulted in the head slumping forward and into the switch. Subsequently, participants who appeared to be close to falling asleep whilst using the Wand ultimately activated the switch and prevented the occurrence of a missed response. Fewer participants were then registered as having fallen asleep and less errors overall observed whilst using the Wand due to the switch being erroneously activated.

A significant effect of switch presentation order was observed when examining the performance times of the switches. Performance times were significantly longer for the switch which was first used by participants than the performance times of the second or third presented switches. This finding is likely reflective of the participants becoming familiar with the task requirements, experimental environment and protocol. Once becoming familiar after the first testing day, participants may have become more comfortable and less cautious about what was required and thus faster at completing the tests for the second and third testing days. As the switch order was randomised and counterbalanced, this effect of switch presentation order would be expected to have equalled out across switches.

It was also observed that there was an increase in errors during the 11:30 testing session which could be reflective of a "post-lunch dip" in performance which has been observed regardless of an individual having had lunch or not [16]. The dip in performance is believed to be related to an increased propensity towards sleep at this time of the day, driven by the homeostatic sleep drive and the circadian rhythm [16]. The longer a person remains awake, the greater the desire to sleep. Naturally this sleep drive peaks prior to night sleep, however it is also higher in the afternoon than the morning. Whilst the post-lunch dip is more often observed in the midafternoon hours, the fact that the participants in this study were sleep deprived the night before testing, may have potentially pushed this dip in performance to occur earlier.

Future research

The present study sought to compare the performance of the different switch types on the OSLER test. The logical proceeding research would administer the OSLER-2 test with modified non hand-held switches to a population with limited hand function. This would allow the determination of whether such modified switches, in particular the Jelly-bean, could in fact be used by people with inadequate hand function who may be exhibiting symptoms of a sleep disorder. Future research could also apply EEG whilst the OSLER test with modified switches was being performed to provide normative values for this modified test in order to understand what length of sleep latency is indicative of daytime sleepiness.

Conclusion

The findings from this study suggest that sleep latency as measured by the Jelly-bean switch is more comparable to sleep latency as measured with the standard hand-held OSLER-2 switch. The Wand switch appears to be unreliable for use with the OSLER-2 test. The Wand may result in misleading daytime sleepiness information and potentially contribute to a missed diagnosis of a sleep disorder. The alternative Jelly-bean switch, may provide a simple, inexpensive, portable means for people with limited or no hand function to have their daytime sleepiness examined in the assessment of an underlying sleep disorder.

Acknowledgements

We acknowledge the generous support of the participants and Steven Vander Hoorn for his statistical advice. This project is proudly supported by the Transport Accident Commission (TAC). This funding source had no involvement in the conduct or publication of this study.

Funding

This project is proudly supported by the Transport Accident Commission (TAC). This funding source had no involvement in the conduct or publication of this study.

References

1. Mulgrew AT, Ryan CF, Fleetham JA, Cheema R, Fox N, et al. (2007) The impact of obstructive sleep apnea and daytime sleepiness on work limitation. Sleep Med 9: 42-53.
2. Habukawa M, Uchimura N, Kakuma T, Yamamoto K, Ogi K, et al. (2010) Effect of CPAP treatment on residual depressive symptoms in patients with major depression and coexisting sleep apnea: Contribution of daytime sleepiness to residual depressive symptoms. Sleep Med 11: 552-557.
3. Dean B, Aguilar D, Shapiro C, Orr WC, Isserman JA, et al. (2010) Impaired health status, daily functioning, and work productivity in adults with excessive sleepiness. J Occup Environ Med 52: 144-149.
4. Carskadon MA, Dement WC, Mitler MM, Roth T, Westbrook PR, et al. (1986) Guidelines for the multiple sleep latency test (MSLT): a standard measure of sleepiness. Sleep 9: 519-524.
5. Mitler MM, Gujavarty KS, Browman CP (1982) Maintenance of wakefulness test: a polysomnographic technique for evaluation treatment efficacy in patients with excessive somnolence. Electroencephalogr Clin Neurophysiol 53: 658-661
6. Littner MR, Kushida C, Wise M, Davila DG, Morgenthaler T, et al. (2005) Practice parameters for clinical use of the multiple sleep latency test and the maintenance of wakefulness test. Sleep 28: 113-121.
7. Bennett LS, Stradling JR, Davies RJ (1997) A behavioural test to assess daytime sleepiness in obstructive sleep apnoea. J Sleep Res 6: 142-145.
8. Krieger AC, Ayappa I, Norman RG, Rapoport DM, Walsleben J (2004)

Comparison of the maintenance of wakefulness test (MWT) to a modified behavioral test (OSLER) in the evaluation of daytime sleepiness. J Sleep Res 13: 407-411.

9. McEvoy RD, Mykytyn I, Sajkov D, Flavell H, Marshall R, et al. (1995) Sleep apnoea in patients with quadriplegia. Thorax 50: 613-619.

10. Berlowitz DJ, Spong J, Gordon I, Howard ME, Brown DJ (2012) Relationships between objective sleep indices and symptoms in a community sample of people with tetraplegia. Arch Phys Med Rehabil 93: 1246-1252.

11. Johns MW (1991) A new method for measuring daytime sleepiness: the Epworth sleepiness scale. Sleep 14: 540-545.

12. Horne JA, Ostberg O (1976) A self-assessment questionnaire to determine morningness-eveningness in human circadian rhythms. Int J Chronobiol 4: 97-110.

13. Gillberg M, Kecklund G, Akerstedt T (1994) Relations between performance and subjective ratings of sleepiness during a night awake. Sleep 17: 236-241.

14. Mazza S, Pepin JL, Deschaux C, Naegele B, Levy P (2002) Analysis of error profiles occurring during the OSLER test - A sensitive mean of detecting fluctuations in vigilance in patients with obstructive sleep apnea syndrome. Am J Respir Crit Care Med 166: 474-78.

15. Shreter R, Peled R, Pillar G (2006) The 20-min trial of the maintenance of wakefulness test is profoundly affected by motivation. Sleep Breath 10: 173-179.

16. Monk TH (2005) The post-lunch dip in performance. Clin Sports Med 24: e15-23, xi-xii.

11

New Mandibular Advancement Device (BestMAD) in the Treatment of Obstructive Sleep Apnea

Enzo Iacomino[1*], Martina Pagliarella[2], Franco Pestilli[3], Giovanni Falisi[4] and Vittorio Bisogni[5]

[1]*ENT Department, Hospital "San Salvatore", L'Aquila, Italy*

[2]*Department of Biotechnological and Applied Clinical Sciences, University of L'Aquila, Italy*

[3]*Expert in Orthodontic Technique, freelancer, Italy*

[4]*Department of Life, Health and Environmental Sciences, University of L'Aquila, Italy*

[5]*Department of Pneumology, Hospital "San Pietro Fatebenefratelli", Rome, Italy*

[*]**Corresponding author:** Dr. Enzo Iacomino, ENT Department, Hospital "San Salvatore", Via Vetoio, 1-67100 Loc. Coppito, L'Aquila, Italy, E-mail: enzoiacomino74@hotmail.com

Abstract

Background: Oral appliances have emerged as an important alternative in treating patients with mild-moderate obstructive sleep apnea (OSA). They are effective, simple to use and well tolerated by the patient compared to other therapeutic solutions, such as continuous positive airway pressure (CPAP) or surgery of the upper airways. Aim: The aim of this preliminary study was to assess the effectiveness of a new mandibular advancement device, the BestMAD, in the treatment of OSA patients.

Materials and methods: We selected 10 patients, 9 males and 1 female, with an average age of 51.5 years, affected by OSA, with a BMI (Body Mass Index) value ≤25 kg/m2. All patients used the BestMAD for at least 6 months. A control polysomnography was repeated after 6 months and a questionnaire was administered to assess the side effects eventually felt by the patient.

Results: After treatment with BestMAD, a statistically significant improvement was found in AHI (p=0.0051), RDI (p=0.0051) and ESS (p=0.0049). With regard to adherence to the treatment, 8 patients claimed to have used the BestMAD for the entire duration of nocturnal rest, while the remaining 2 only for a few hours at night.

Conclusions: BestMAD is a comfortable device which has proved effective in improving the polysomnographic parameters.

Keywords: Obstructive sleep apnea; Oral appliance; Mandibular advancement device

Introduction

Obstructive sleep apnea (OSA) is a common clinical condition affecting 2-26% of the general population [1,2]. It is characterized by partial or complete obstruction of the upper airways during sleep, resulting in repetitive events of apnea and hypopnea with a consequent negative impact on the health and the behavior of patients [3,4]. Furthermore, OSAS is considered today a cardio-metabolic disease with a great impact on public health, related to increased risk of hypertension, cardiovascular disease and mortality, methabolic imbalance and cerebrovascular accidents [5-7]. The treatment with continuous positive airway pressure (CPAP) is considered the gold standard, but some patients find it intolerable [8]. A study assessing compliance with CPAP, found that only 46% of patients used the device for more than 4 hours per night for more than 70% of the nights [9]. For patients with mild or moderate OSA, oral appliances may be appropriate therapy as suggested by the Standards of Practice Committee of the American Academy of Sleep Medicine and the Deutshe Gesellschaft fur Zahnarztliche Schlafmedizin [10,11]. In recent years, several clinical randomized trials compared the effectiveness of treatment with CPAP and oral devices [12,13]. Although CPAP demonstrated superior efficacy in terms of apnea-hypopnea index (AHI) reduction, self-reported compliance with oral appliance was higher. The resulting effects on clinical outcomes in patients with mild, moderate or severe OSA were equivalent or better in the oral appliance. These devices are designed to increase the pharyngeal airway space (PAS) by three fundamental mechanisms: 1) the protrusion of the jaw and the tongue away from the back wall of the pharynx; 2) the stabilization of the jaw and the inhibition of the opening of the mouth, allowing the anterior positioning of the hyoid bone and the tongue; 3) the implementing of the vertical dimension to induce a reflex at the level of the TMJ, which activates the genioglossus muscle and tends to extend the tongue [13-16]. On the basis of scientific assessments and international guidelines, the use of the protrusion guides is recommended for the treatment of sleep-related breathing disorders as an alternative choice after a previous attempt treatment with CPAP, or as initial therapy in the presence of primary snoring, upper airway resistance syndrome (UARS), mild-moderate OSA with little symptoms in conditions of sufficient intraoral anchorage [17]. More than 60 different oral appliances are in use, with considerable variations in design [18-21]. Mandibular advancement devices (MAD) have been the most intensely researched, and their effectiveness documented by the Cochrane Collaboration as the highest level of scientific evidence [22,23]. In 2007, Dr. Enzo Iacomino, Dr. Vittorio Bisogni and the expert in orthodontic technique Mr. Franco Pestilli developed the BestMAD, a device for mandibular and tongue base advancement for the treatment of OSA in patients intolerant to CPAP, alone or in combination with other therapeutic options. The device was clinically applicable since 2008. The purpose of this study was to evaluate the effectiveness of BestMAD in the treatment of patients with OSA.

Materials and Methods

BestMAD

The BestMAD is a tailor-made patient device, structured in two arches that run on each other (Figure 1).

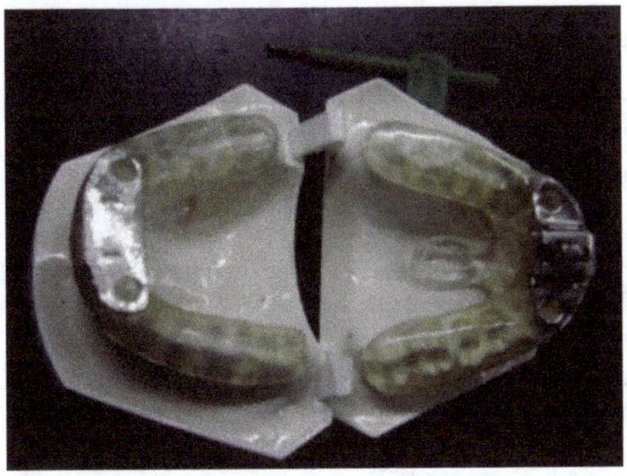

Figure 1: BestMAD determins a mandibular and tongue base advancement associated with the activation of the genioglossus muscle. It reduces the resistance of the upper airways, expanding the size of the oropharyngeal lumen and is therefore indicated for the symptomatic treatment of sleep apnea and snoring.

The part in contact with the teeth and the gingival mucosa (1 mm) is soft and made of vacuum-polyurethane, while the outside part is rigid and made of copolyester completed with acrylate (1 mm). An adjustable screw (MDSA® Pty Ltd, Australia) joins the two arches, and the protrusion is adjustable from a minimum of 4 mm to a maximum of 10 mm (2 mm in crackdown) (Figure 2).

The screw provides lateral movements (compatible with any physiological movements during the REM stage of sleep) (Figure 3) the initial adjustment of the protrusion is established on clinical and radiological data and is generally of 6 mm.

It is not advisable to exceed 10-12 mm in protrusion. A proprioceptive indicator or oral tongue stimulator (Figure 4) was included in the device as reference point for the anterior positioning of the tongue.

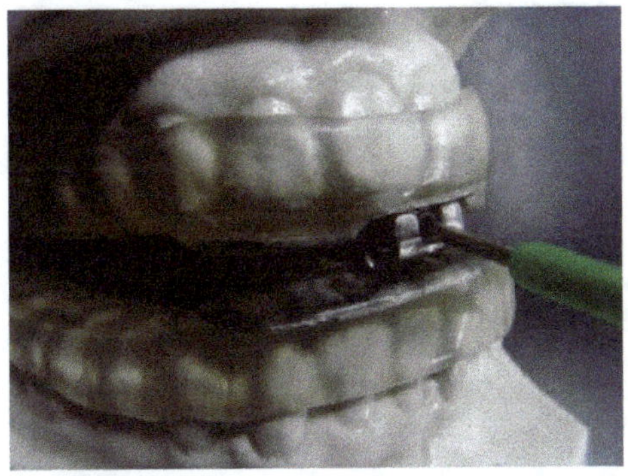

Figure 2: The screw connecting the two arches adjusts the protrusion (2 mm per revolution of the screw) and allows the physiological movements of laterality during REM sleep.

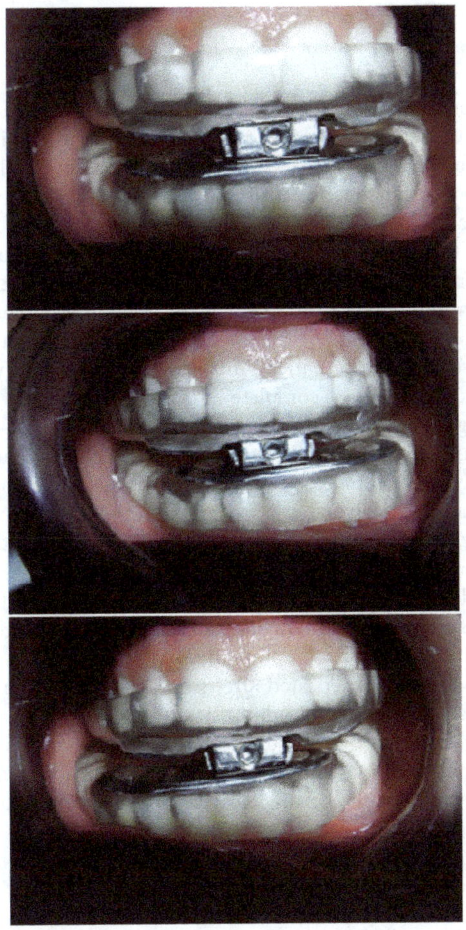

Figure 3: Lateral movements with BestMAD.

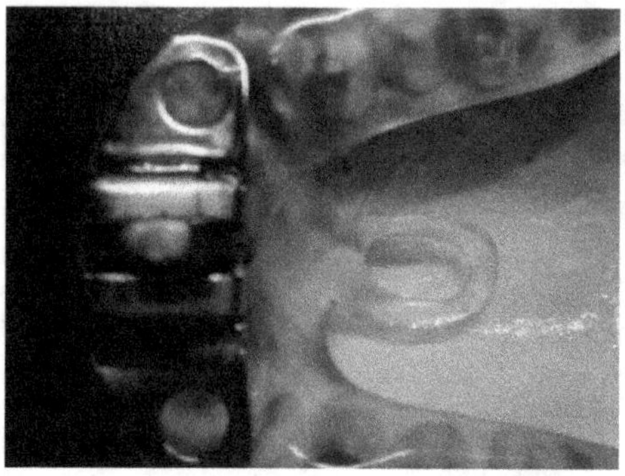

Figure 4: The proprioceptive indicator of the BestMAD is a tongue perforated platform, with holes of increasing diameter, which starts from the top of the superior arch of the device and reaches the anterior part of the hard palate to induces a continuous stimulation of the tongue.

Patients

A total of 10 patients (9 males and 1 female, mean age 51.5 years, range 20-70) selected from those relating to the service for the diagnosis and treatment of sleep-disordered breathing of the Hospital "San Pietro Fatebenefratelli" in Rome and to the ENT department of the Hospital "San Salvatore" in L'Aquila from 2008 to 2013, were enrolled in the study. The inclusion criteria were: a diagnosis of OSA with no compliance to the CPAP, BMI (Body Mass Index) ≤ 25 kg/m^2, hypopharyngeal collapse observed in the fiberoptic endoscopy with Muller maneuver and a positive mandibular advancement test at the sleep endoscopy. All the patients underwent a preliminary ENT and dental examination, complete overnight cardio-respiratory polysomnography, medical questionnaire on the sleep-disordered breathing and related conditions, Epworth Sleepiness Scale (ESS) to measure daytime sleepiness, nasolaryngeal fiberoptic endoscopy with Muller maneuver, sleep endoscopy with mandibular advancement test, Computerized Tomography (CT) of the facial bones. All the selected patients were treated with the BestMAD. Patients no. 4, 6, 7, 8, 9 and 10 also underwent oropharyngeal surgery before starting the therapy with the BestMAD. All of them had an uvulopalatopharyngoplasy, and one of them also had a septoplasty (patient no. 10). A control polysomnography was repeated after six months and a questionnaire we specifically created was administered to assess the side effects eventually felt by the patient (difficulty in chewing and/or breathing, drooling, xerostomia, dental, lingual, gingival and/or mandibular discomfort, headache, changes in occlusal, masseter and/or temporomandibular joint pain, spinal pain, dizziness).

Results

Clinical data collected before and after 6 month of treatment with BestMAD are shown in Tables 1 and 2.

Statistical analysis was performed using the Wilcoxon test for all the parameters. This entails the need to bring the threshold of statistical significance by α=0.05 to α^*=0.008.

The improvement of the values of AHI (Apnea-Hypopnea Index), RDI (Respiratory Disturbance Index) and ESS after treatment with BestMAD was statistically significant (p=0.0051, p=0.0051, and p=0.0049 respectively). The ODI (Oxygen Desaturation Index) and the index of arrhythmia were reduced drastically, even if the values were not statistically significant (p=0.0107 and p=0.0363 respectively). The snore index remained almost unchanged (p=0.0743).

Patients no.	AHI	RDI	Snore ind (/h)	ODI (/h)	ESS
1	32	44	330.7	18.8	5
2	28.5	52.1	359.7	23	12
3	20	24.8	435.3	5.8	9
4	3	41.4	145	0	7
5	2.3	4.2	32.5	0.4	8
6	46.4	38.8	294	67	8
7	10.2	92	389	1.2	11
8	34.8	63.8	224	21.1	7
9	36.7	30	250	5.3	6
10	27	49	327	19	8
Mean Values	24.09	44.01	278.72	16.16	8.1

Table 1: Clinical data before starting the therapy with Best-MAD. AHI: Apnea-Hypopnea Index. RDI: Respiratory Disturbance Index. ODI: Oxygen Desaturation Index. ESS: Epworth Sleepiness Scale.

Patients no.	AHI (/h)	RDI (/h)	Snore ind (/h)	ODI (/h)	ESS
1	0.1	25	184.3	0	3
2	14.1	28.7	408.5	12.8	4
3	1.1	2.9	488.1	0.1	3
4	2.5	35.5	198.6	0.7	4
5	0.7	0.7	56.7	0.4	3
6	16.6	20.3	194	15	3
7	4.6	33	33	0.3	2
8	7.8	22.8	120	1.1	2
9	12.7	10	150	1.3	3
10	2.6	5	128	1.9	2
Mean Values	6.28	18.39	196.12	3.36	2.9

Table 2: Clinical data after 6 months of therapy with Best-MAD. AHI: Apnea-Hypopnea Index. RDI: Respiratory Disturbance Index. ODI: Oxygen Desaturation Index. ESS: Epworth Sleepiness Scale.

With regard to adherence to the treatment and side effects, 8 patients claimed to have used the BestMAD for the entire duration of nocturnal rest, while the remaining 2 only for a few hours at night. Six of 10 patients complained of xerostomia, 6 of drooling, 4 of temporomandibular joint pain, 2 of dental discomfort, 2 of mandibular discomfort, 2 of respiratory irritation and 2 of masseter pain.

Discussion

Data emerging from this study suggested the efficacy of the therapy with BestMAD in patients with OSA, alone or in combination with surgery. In our clinical practice, the use of BestMAD in selected patients has proved of high clinical efficacy, especially in patients with sleep apnea that occur mainly in the supine position, with a positive mandibular advancement test detected during the sleep endoscopy and hypopharyngeal collapse observed in the fiberoptic endoscopy with Muller maneuver.

In our opinion, one of the greatest strengths of the BestMAD consists in the oral tongue stimulator. The neurological control of tongue posture is surely determined by many factors, but the current state of our knowledge does not yet allow us to know their mode of action. The central nervous system processes sensory information, in particular the tactile and proprioceptive, which come from the dorsal surface of the tongue. The ability to recognize the position of the tongue and the surrounding anatomical structures depends largely on these sensory afferents, determining stereognosic and tactile discriminative ability. In most cases, atypical swallowing, abnormal tongue rest position, decreased sensitivity and OSA are associated [24-26]. Sensory impulses necessary for the maintenance of a proper tongue posture come from mutual stimulation of the dorsum of the tongue with the teeth and the mucosa of the hard palate. In orthodontic practice, some devices are commonly used to change the neuromuscular behavior of the stomatognathic apparatus through automatic acts committed unintentionally. These are described in the literature as "oral stimulators" or "reminders". The function of these devices is to normalize the muscle behavior in the dynamic (mastication, deglutition, phonation and mimicry) and in the static phases. From these neurophysiological considerations was born the idea of applying a tongue proprioceptive stimulus to the BestMAD. For its realization, we started from the classic oral stimulators known in the orthodontic practice, such as perforated plates or Tucat palatine pearl. The oral tongue stimulator placed on the BestMAD consists in a perforated platform (Figure 4) which reaches the anterior part of the hard palate and induces a continuous anterior stimulation of the tongue, expanding the pharyngeal airway space (PAS) during sleep.

Another strength of BestMad is the screw that connects the two arches of the device. In the first equipment we use, and in most of those commercially available, the structure is represented by a single block that is anchored on the maxilla and holds the lower jaw in a forward position. An adjustment screw regulates its advancement. We noticed that, in some patients (especially those with obesity, hypertrophy of the masseter and bruxism), the device was often detached from the maxilla during sleep, probably under the pressure of the unconscious movements of the jaw, resulting in a fall back of the jaw and tongue. From this evidence the idea to replace the old screw with a new connection between the two arches of the device that allows the movements of laterality keeping the jaw protrusion. In this way the kinetic energy of the mandibular movements can dissipate, avoiding the detachment of the device during the night.

Conclusions

In conclusion, the BestMad has proved to be a good choice among the many oral devices available on the market, either alone or in combination with other procedures, for the treatment of selected patients with OSA.

Considering that the BestMad should be used mainly at night and for the whole life, we have tried to make it as comfortable as possible, trying to prevent, at the same time, any kind of unwanted tooth movement. However, there is the need for further studies involving a greater number of patients and with a long-term control of the results.

References

1. Tishler PV, Larkin EK, Schluchter MD, Redline S (2003) Incidence of sleep-disordered breathing in an urban adult population: the relative importance of risk factors in the development of sleep-disordered breathing. JAMA 289: 2230-2237.
2. Jordan AS, McEvoy RD (2003) Gender differences in sleep apnea: epidemiology, clinical presentation and pathogenic mechanisms. Sleep Med Rev 7: 377-389.
3. Bonsignore MR, Zito A (2008) Metabolic effects of the obstructive sleep apnea syndrome and cardiovascular risk. Arch Physiol Biochem 114: 255-260.
4. Kawada T (2013) Screening for obstructive sleep apnea syndrome in hypertensive outpatients: clinical characteristics of hypertension are important for their analysis. J Clin Hypertens 15: 856.
5. Fusetti M, Fioretti AB, Valenti M, Masedu F, Lauriello M, et al. (2012) Cardiovascular and metabolic comorbidities in patients with obstructive sleep apnoea syndrome. Acta Otorhinolaryngol Ital 32: 320-325.
6. Vgontzas AN, Bixler EO, Chrousos GP (2005) Sleep apnea is a manifestation of the metabolic syndrome. Sleep Med Rev 9: 211-224.
7. Macey PM, Kumar R, Woo MA, Yan-Go FL, Harper RM (2013) Heart rate responses to autonomic challenges in obstructive sleep apnea. PLoS One 23: e76631.
8. Queiroz DL, Yui MS, Braga AA, Coelho ML, Küpper DS, et al. (2014) Adherence of obstructive sleep apnea syndrome patients to continuous positive airway pressure in a public service. Braz J Otorhinolaryngol 80: 126-130.
9. Kribbs NB, Pack A, Kline LR, Smith PL, Schwartz AR, et al. (1993) Objective measurement of patterns of nasal CPAP use by patients with obstructive sleep apnea. Am Rev Respir Dis 147: 887-895.
10. Morgenthaler T, Kapen S, Lee-Chiong T, Alessi C, Boehlecke B, et al. (2006) Practice parameters for the medical therapy of obstructive sleep apnea. Standards of Practice Committee; American Academy of Sleep Medicine. Sleep 29: 1031-1035.
11. Schwarting S, Huebers U, Heise M, Schlieper J, Hauschild A (2007) Position paper on the use of mandibular advancement devices in adults with sleep-related breathing disorders. A position paper of the German Society of Dental Sleep Medicine (Deutsche Gesellschaft Zahnaerztliche Schlafmedizin, DGZS). Sleep Breath 11: 125-126.
12. Doff MH, Hoekema A, Wijkstra PJ, van der Hoeven JH, Huddleston Slater JJ, et al. (2013) Oral appliance versus continuous positive airway pressure in obstructive sleep apnea syndrome: a 2-year follow-up. Sleep 36: 1289-1296.
13. Phillips CL, Grunstein RR, Darendeliler MA, Mihailidou AS, Srinivasan VK, et al. (2013) Health outcomes of continuous positive airway pressure versus oral appliance treatment for obstructive sleep apnea: a randomized controlled trial. Am J Respir Crit Care Med 15;187: 879-887.
14. Johal A, Battagel JM, Kotecha BT (2005) Sleep nasendoscopy: a diagnostic tool for predicting treatment success with mandibular advancement splints in obstructive sleep apnoea. Eur J Orthod 27: 607-614.
15. Victores AJ, Hamblin J, Gilbert J, Switzer C, Takashima M (2014) Usefulness of sleep endoscopy in predicting positional obstructive sleep apnea. Otolaryngol Head Neck Surg 150: 487-493.
16. Sears CR, Miller AJ, Chang MK, Huang JC, Lee JS (2011) Comparison of pharyngeal airway changes on plain radiography and cone-beam computed tomography after orthognathic surgery. J Oral Maxillofac Surg 69: e385-e394.

17. Cohen-Levy J, Pételle B, Pinguet J, Limerat E, Fleury B (2013) Forces created by mandibular advancement devices in OSA patients: a pilot study during sleep. Sleep Breath 17: 781-789.

18. Canadian Agency for Drugs and Technologies in Health (CADTH) (2010) Oral appliances for treatment of snoring and obstructive sleep apnea: a review of clinical effectiveness. CADTH Technol Overv 1: e0107.

19. Gasparini G, Azzuni C, Rinaldo FM, Cervelli D, Marianetti TM, et al. (2013) OSAS treatment with oral appliance: assessment of our experience through the use of a new device. Eur Rev Med Pharmacol Sci 17: 385-391.

20. Lawton HM, Battagel JM, Kotecha B (2005) A comparison of the Twin Block and Herbst mandibular advancement splints in the treatment of patients with obstructive sleep apnoea: a prospective study. Eur J Orthod 27: 82-90.

21. Health Quality Ontario (2009) Oral appliances for obstructive sleep apnea: an evidence-based analysis. Ont Health Technol Assess Ser 9: 1-51.

22. Lim J, Lasserson TJ, Fleetham J, Wright J (2006) Oral appliances for obstructive sleep apnoea. Cochrane Database Syst Rev 25: CD004435.

23. Okuno K, Sato K, Arisaka T, Hosohama K, Gotoh M et al. (2014) The effect of oral appliances that advanced the mandible forward and limited mouth opening in patients with obstructive sleep apnea: a systematic review and meta-analysis of randomised controlled trials. J Oral Rehabil 41: 542-554.

24. Weiss TM, Atanasov S, Calhoun KH (2005) The association of tongue scalloping with obstructive sleep apnea and related sleep pathology. Otolaryngol Head Neck Surg 133: 966-971.

25. Coste A, Lofaso F, d'Ortho MP, Louis B, Dahan E, et al. (1999) Protruding the tongue improves posterior rhinomanometry in obstructive sleep apnoea syndrome. Eur Respir J 14: 1278-1282.

26. Ohkubo C, Morokuma M, Yoneyama Y, Matsuda R, Lee JS (2013) Interactions between occlusion and human brain function activities. J Oral Rehabil 40: 119-129.

12

Obesity, Cardiovascular Disease and Sleep Disorders: Insights into the Rising Epidemic

Navneet Sharma, Justin Lee, Irini Youssef, Moro O Salifu and Samy I McFarlane*

Department of Medicine, Divisions of Endocrinology and Nephrology, New York, USA

***Corresponding author:** Samy I McFarlane, Department of Medicine, Divisions of Endocrinology, State University of New York, Downstate Medical Center, Brooklyn District President, American College of Physicians, 450 Clarkson Avenue, Brooklyn, New York, 11203, USA; E-mail: Samy.McFarlane@downstate.edu

Abstract

Cardiovascular disease (CVD) is the main cause of death among adult men and women in the USA and impacts millions around the globe. Traditional risk factors for CVD include obesity, diabetes, hypertension and dyslipidemia. The modern-day epidemic of obesity not only increased the rate of CVD but also ushered in an additional CVD risk factor to be added to the list; that is obstructive sleep apnea (OSA). In this review, we discuss the growing epidemic of obesity and OSA, highlighting the common pathogenic hypotheses linking these risk factors to CVD. We will also highlight the therapeutic rationale of OSA as a way to reduce CVD risk.

Keywords: Obesity; Cardiovascular disease; Sleep disorders

Introduction

Obesity is a major public health problem in the United States; with more than 2 out of 3 adults considered to be either overweight or obese [1]. The rise in obesity has caused increase in the incidence of obesity-related diseases, such as diabetes mellitus type 2 (DM2), hypertension (HTN), chronic kidney disease (CKD) and cardiovascular diseases (CVD). This epidemic has in turn placed a significant amount of burden on healthcare expenditure in the management of these chronic diseases. Diabetes alone costs more than $245 billion every year in America, with one in three Medicare dollars being spent on care for people with diabetes [2]. Costs for other obesity-related diseases are astronomical as well, with the figures only expected to rise in the future. It is imperative to understand the cause of obesity and its pathophysiology with other chronic conditions that are becoming increasingly expensive.

Obesity is generally understood as a condition of energy imbalance, where there is a surplus of energy consumption compared to its expenditure. Increased caloric intake with modern American diet that is high in simple carbohydrates and saturated fatty acids, combined with sedentary lifestyle are thought to be the main culprits in the obesity pandemic in America.

Obstructive sleep apnea (OSA) has been studied closely as one of the major associated illness in obese patients. Not only is obesity one of the main causes of OSA, affecting 70% of the patients with OSA, also shares some of the underlying pathophysiologic mechanisms with obesity-related diseases, such as DM2, HTN and CVD [3,4]. Furthermore, OSA increases risk of end-organ damage in critically ill patients. In a propensity matched study, OSA patients were at statistically significant risk of Acute Kidney Injury compared to non-OSA patients [5]. Similarly, CPAP treatment has shown to improve glucose control in type 2 diabetics with blood sugars not controlled with medications. This effect is achieved by increasing insulin secretion and reduced counter-regulatory hormone production [6]. Therefore, development and treatment of OSA carries wide ranging systemic implications and prognosis for patients.

CVD is the number one causes of death in the United States with 1 in every 4 death are attributed to CVD [7]. Modifiable risk factors, such as being overweight and obese account for more than 70% of the risk for CVD and mortality caused by CVD. [8] Pathophysiology and prevention of CVD is also very complex as there are multiple risk factors besides obesity that could increase the risk. These risk factors include but are not limited to, smoking, alcohol and drug abuse along with HTN, DM2 and/or hyperlipidemia, which are all modifiable [9].

It has been shown that low socioeconomic status is positively correlated with obesity and its complications, such as DM2 [10]. It must be noted that obesity, associated with OSA and CVD, is also disproportionately high in black population, as 63% of men and 77% of women in this ethnic group is either overweight or obese [11]. Per the Multi-ethnic study of atherosclerosis (MESA), black population demonstrated the highest levels of sleep disturbance, shorter sleep duration, worse sleep quality and daytime sleepiness compared to Caucasians, Hispanics and Asians [12]. Higher poverty rate is also associated with higher apnea-hypopnea index (AHI) with relatively lower continuous positive airway pressure (CPAP) therapy acceptance rate [13,14].

A similar pattern is observed in CVD and its many risk factors, as the prevalence is disproportionately higher in black population compared to other ethnic groups. [15] People of low income (<$35,000 per year) are at increased risk of developing CVD, compared to individuals with higher income (HR 1.48, 95% CI 1.21-1.81) [16]. With recent studies showing evidence of correlation between socioeconomic status and risk of developing OSA and CVD, there seems to be more than just biological pathophysiology in the development of these diseases.

There are many proposed hypotheses as to why these discrepancies may exist, including poor access to health care services, non-adherence to treatment recommendations, inadequate training and environmental and genetic variations [12,15]. Although the existence of association in these conditions are widely acknowledged, the understanding of the roles in how these diseases influence each other is not well investigated. Summary of prevalence and risk factors of Obesity, OSA and CVD are illustrated in Table 1.

	Obesity	OSA	CVD
Prevalence	35.70%	3% to 7% (male)	28.90%
(In U.S.)	68.8% (either overweight or obese)	2% to 5% (female)	
	Higher amongst Blacks		
	(48.1%; 63% males, 77% females either overweight or obese)	Higher amongst Blacks	Higher amongst Blacks (46% males, 48% females)
		(OR=1.78, compared with Whites)	
	Sedentary lifestyle	Obesity (70%)	Obesity (>70%)
Risk factors	Increased caloric intake	DM2	DM2
	Diet high in simple carbohydrates and saturated fatty acids	HTN	HTN
		CVD	Smoking
			Poor diet
			Physical inactivity

Table 1: Summary of prevalence and risk factors of obesity, obstructive sleep apnea, and cardiovascular disease.

In this review article, we aim to better understand the relationship between OSA and CVD, by analyzing their underlying pathophysiology from molecular level to non-medical factors that have not been investigated from previous studies, which can significantly influence the clinical outcome. This information will be helpful in guiding future treatment strategies, especially in communities that have high representation of vulnerable ethnic groups. Figure 1 summarizes the interrelationship between Obesity, OSA, and CVD.

Pathophysiologic Mechanisms

Intermittent hypoxia

While in sleep, OSA causes intermittent periods of hypoxia followed by reoxygenation. Recurrent episodes of hypoxia stimulate the carotid chemoreceptors and results in secondary rise in blood pressure from sympathetic activation [17,18]. These episodes of intermittent hypoxia can range anywhere from 5 to more than 100 events per hour [18]. Although acute hypoxia is capable of activating responses that can lead to acute nocturnal cardiac event [19], the chronicity in recurrent sympathetic activation and its consequent vasoconstriction over many year, can cause unique profile of biological consequences in OSA patients [20]. For this reason, intermittent hypoxia is thought to be a major culprit in patients with OSA that can lead to CVD. It is also interesting to note that intermittent hypoxia can increase the risk of CVD at the molecular level. Intermittent hypoxia has shown to increase the levels of angiopoietin-like 4 (Angptl4), a potent inhibitor of lipoprotein lipase. This change decreases the body's clearance of lipoprotein and increases fasting serum levels of triglycerides and very low density lipoprotein cholesterol [21]. In addition, hypoxia-inducible factor-1 (HIF-1), a transcription factor that modulates the body's response to ischemic injuries has been shown to be up regulated in hypoxia, further demonstrating the evidence of molecular genetic association between hypoxia and ischemic CVD, secondary to impaired lipoprotein turnover (Figure 1) [22].

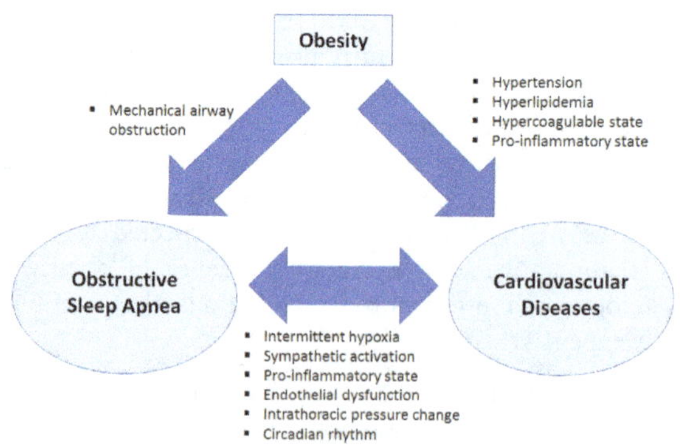

Figure 1: Interrelation between obesity, obstructive sleep apnea, and cardiovascular disease.

Sympathetic activation

It is known that sympathetic activations are caused by nocturnal intermittent hypoxia in OSA patients. However, it is interesting to note that, the sympathetic activations in these patients persist during daytime wakefulness in normoxic conditions [20,23]. This persistent sympathetic drive promotes systemic hypertension and increased cardiac sympathetic tone [24]. It also augments subsequent response to sympathetic stimuli [25]. In addition, sympathetic influence on renin-angiotensin system is another critical factor in the pathogenesis of systemic hypertension in OSA patients [19]. This change in autonomic regulation of blood pressure due to impaired baroreflex and renin-angiotensin system in these patients puts them at a higher risk of developing systemic HTN, persistent tachycardia and ultimately CVD.

Pro-inflammatory state

Chronic hypoxic stress can activate systemic inflammatory pathways, as OSA patients have increased level of plasma cytokines, serum amyloid-A and C-reactive protein (CRP) [20,26]. Obesity has also been shown to increase the level of pro-inflammatory cytokines and may cause hypercoagulable state in the bloodstream along with OSA [27]. Adipocyte hypertrophy results in altered expression of adipokines. Adipokines play crucial role in vascular function by influencing glucose and lipid metabolism. In fact, dysregulation of adipocytes leads to altered levels in pro- and anti-inflammatory adipokine expression. While altered adipokine expression has been demonstrated to be a predicative marker and associate with CVD in experimental in vitro and in vivo models, this impact of is less clear in humans [28]. Along with the buildup and the rupture of atherosclerotic plaques, these phenomena of pro-inflammatory and hypercoagulable state can be fatal in the development of CVDs, such as acute myocardial infarction (MI).

Endothelial dysfunction

OSA patients suffer from endothelial dysfunction due to decreased availability of nitric oxide (NO) and cell apoptosis, secondary to increased oxidative stress and systemic inflammation [20]. It is also thought that chronic hypoxic stress causes release of endothelin-1, a potent vasoconstrictor, in human endothelium [29]. Impaired NO production compounded with increase in endothelin-1 release in the vasculature can predispose OSA patients into systemic HTN and consequent CVD. Accumulation of reactive oxygen species also likely contributes to the pathogenesis of endothelial dysfunction in OSA patients by directly forming vascular lesions and CAD [19].

Intrathoracic pressure change

Repetitive inspiratory effort against closed upper airway generates intrathoracic pressure change that subsequently causes an increase in transmural gradients across the atria, ventricles and aorta [20,30]. Severe OSA can compromise left and right ventricular function, diastolic filling, and increase the afterload. These all impose risk of developing CVD, arrhythmias, and heart failure (HF) [20,31,32].

Circadian rhythm

Disruption in circadian rhythm and sleep homeostat has also shown its association with CVD. In OSA patients, insufficient duration, quality and timing of sleep, in addition to intermittent hypoxia can promote the development of CVD [33]. It is also interesting to note that people of African descent, who have a higher prevalence of CVD than others also have more disrupted sleep pattern, including period length and phase shifting, compared to the people from European heritage [33]. Figure 2 Sumarizes the pathophysiologic mechanisms linking OSA to CVD.

Clinical Association between CVD and OSA

Ischemic cardiovascular alterations

Coronary artery disease (CAD): Chronic intermittent hypoxia induced atherosclerosis with endothelial dysfunction are the thought to be the main causes of CAD in OSA patients. Many clinical studies have shown significant evidence to support the association between the two diseases. Severe OSA patients with AHI>30 showed significantly higher risk of cardiovascular events, including acute coronary syndrome (ACS), myocardial infarction (MI) and stroke [34]. AHI was also found to have strong correlation with atherosclerotic volume when measured by imaging through intravascular ultrasound. [20,35] An interesting finding to note is that MI's occurring in patients with OSA have a different timing pattern compared to others, as one study has shown that almost half of OSA patients had their MI's during sleeping hours (22:00 to 06:00) whereas in the general population, the most likely time for the onset of MI is between 06:00 and 11:00 [20,36]. This is likely explained by the fact that nocturnal hypoxia caused by OSA is predisposing this group of patients to nocturnal MI. Treating severe OSA patient has also shown significant reduction in the risk of CAD as patients who received successful CPAP therapy had lower incidence of fatal and nonfatal cardiovascular events [34,37].

Cerebrovascular accidents (CVA): Ischemic strokes or cerebrovascular accidents were found to be higher in patients with OSA from multiple cross-sectional and prospective cohort studies [38-40]. It is important to note that this higher risk of CVA in OSA patients are independent of other CVD risk factors whose incidence may have also been influenced by the presence of OSA, such as HTN, HF, Atrial Fibrillation(AF) and DM2 [19]. Association was also found between OSA and CVA, as higher AHI was correlated with higher risk of CVA (HR 2.85, 95% CI 1.10-7.39) and greater extent of metabolic impairment of cerebral white matter [40,41]. Proposed mechanisms of pathogenesis include altered cerebral autoregulation, endothelial dysfunction and pro-thrombotic/inflammatory state that place these patients at a higher risk of reduced cerebral blood flow, leading to ischemic stroke [20]. Potential therapeutic benefit from the treatment of OSA is unclear at the moment as limitations in maintaining chronic CPAP treatment with CVA patients have been identified [38]. Nevertheless, it may be beneficial to offer CPAP treatment initially to CVA patients as it would reduce the influence and recurrence of other cardiovascular risk factors as outlined previously (Figure 2).

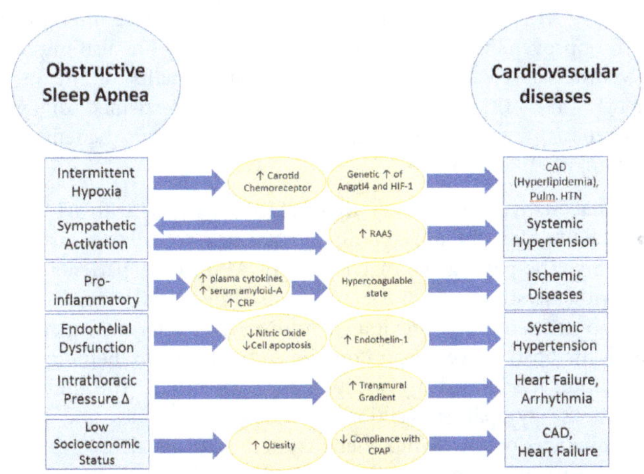

Figure 2: Pathophysiology of Obstructive sleep apnea leading to cardiovascular disease.

Nonischemic cardiovascular alterations

Systemic hypertension: From the Wisconsin cohort study, there was a dose-dependent relationship between the OSA status of an individual and the risk of developing HTN, as AHI of 15 events/hour or more showed 3-fold increase in the incidence of HTN [42]. Evidence of positive linear relationship between the severity of OSA and the incidence of CVD was also shown in the Sleep Heart Health Study, a large multi-center cross-sectional study [43]. As mentioned previously, the combination of sympathetic activation and renin-angiotensin system are thought to be possible mechanisms of OSA leading to HTN. One particularly important variant to consider is resistant HTN, defined as BP>140/90 mmHg despite being on combination of 3 or more anti-hypertensive medications titrated to their maximal doses OSA was found more frequently in the resistant HTN population, compared to controlled HTN (71% *vs.* 38%) [19,44]. This relationship was further strengthened by the evidence of decrease in daytime BP with the treatment of OSA in patients with resistant HTN [20,45].

Heart failure (HF): HF is also commonly associated with OSA. Sleep-disordered breathing (SDB), which encompasses OSA with central sleep apnea (CSA) are often found with HF patients up to 50% to 70% [19,46]. HF patient's exhibit mixed sleep apnea, characterized by initial CSA event followed by an obstructive component [47]. The initial CSA causes sympathetic activation, followed by elevated blood pressure and heart rate, which in turn causes left ventricular remodeling. When this remodeling process is combined with fluid retention from renin-angiotensin system activation, these phenomena can together drive patients into HF [48]. It is important to note that OSA can cause HF via same mechanism as well, via same mechanism responsible for sympathetic activation and HTN, namely intermittent hypoxia leading to alteration of carotid chemoreceptors. Respiration against occluded nasopharynx can also cause increased intrathoracic pressure and left ventricular transmural gradient, which can lead to an increase in cardiac afterload and decrease in cardiac output [19]. Symptomatic HF with peripheral edema can cause rostral fluid shift at night with supine position, which when occurs simultaneously with decreased pharyngeal muscle tone from Cheyne-Stokes respiration can cause airway collapse with subsequent worsening of OSA [47]. Treating primary symptoms of HF, including diuretics, angiotensin-converting enzyme inhibitors and implantable device therapy has shown improvement in SDB [19,48]. CPAP therapy has also improved left ventricular ejection fraction (LVEF) and quality of life in HF patients [49]. OSA and HF are closely intertwined in their pathogenesis and patients with both diseases can benefit from treatment of HF and/or OSA.

Cardiac arrhythmia: Prevalence of SDB in patients with AF is 40% to 50% [50]. AF is the most common sustained arrhythmia associated with OSA. The pathogenic mechanism of AF in OSA patients largely deals with the stretching of the atria caused by intrathoracic pressure variation as mentioned previously. Additionally, intermittent hypoxia caused by obstructive respiratory episodes leads to hemodynamic fluctuation, modulated by sympathetic activation. The imbalance between the sympathetic action from apneic episodes and natural predominance of parasympathetic system during sleep, results in sympatho-vagal imbalance, a mechanism widely thought to be responsible for initiation and maintenance of AF in humans [50,51]. Long term OSA is associated with extensive atrial remodeling that disturbs local conduction pathway and causes longer sinus node recovery period [50]. A recent meta-analysis has also shown the effectiveness of CPAP therapy in patients with AF, as patients treated with CPAP had 42% decreased risk of AF compared to ones who were not treated [52]. Recurrence of AF after radiofrequency ablation was also 25% higher amongst patients with OSA [53]. CPAP therapy was associated with lower rate of recurrent AF compared to untreated patients (HR 0.41, 95% CI, 0.22-0.76) [54]. Overall, the data supports a strong relationship between OSA and AF in their pathophysiology and reflects a potential benefit of CPAP therapy in improving cardiovascular outcomes in patients with AF.

Pulmonary hypertension: Several studies have shown association between OSA and pulmonary HTN, where prevalence of pulmonary HTN in OSA is estimated to be up to 20% [19]. Several risk factors for pulmonary HTN can be commonly found in OSA patients, such as high BMI, obesity-hypoventilation syndrome, left heart disease and nocturnal as well as daytime hypoxemia. Clinical significance in the coexistence of these two conditions was outlined from an observational study with 83 patients, as it was found that those with pulmonary HTN at the time of diagnosis of OSA had poorer outcomes at 1, 4, 8-year survival rate than those who did not [55]. Primary mechanisms of pulmonary HTN in OSA patients are thought to be hypoxic vasoconstriction in pulmonary vasculature and vascular remodeling after chronic stress [20]. CPAP treatment can effectively lower the pulmonary artery pressure and vascular reactivity to hypoxia, leading to treatment benefit of OSA in patients with Pulmonary HTN [56,57].

Treatment of OSA as a therapeutic guide to CVDs

CPAP is the treatment of choice in OSA patients that has been shown to be efficacious in the reduction of CVD. Of the cardiovascular comorbidities discussed, systemic HTN has shown the strongest evidence for benefit [19]. It is recommended that OSA patients with HTN, especially for those with moderate to severe symptoms, and those with resistant HTN be treated with CPAP [19].

Much of the existing literature supporting the use of CPAP as an augment therapy are single-center or smaller randomized trials. A larger, recent randomized controlled trial with 2,717 patients, where the treatment group received CPAP and the control group received usual care, showed no significant effect of CPAP therapy on the composite cardiovascular endpoint (HR 1.10, 95% CI 0.91-1.32), despite lowering the AHI. [58] Based on current literature, it seems unclear if there is a definitive treatment benefit from CPAP beyond symptomatic relief.

Other therapies besides CPAP may also be beneficial to OSA patients in reducing cardiovascular risks, as simple as lifestyle modifications such as weight loss, avoidance of alcohol and sedative medications before bedtime. These lifestyle modifications can all reduce symptoms in patients with mild OSA [19, 59].

Bi-level positive airway pressure (BiPAP) is also an option of treatment for patients who cannot tolerate CPAP treatment and for those with OSA associated with chronic obstructive pulmonary disease (COPD) [20]. At the moment, there is no definitive evidence of benefit from the use of BiPAP in lowering CVD risk.

Positional therapy with avoidance of supine position during sleep and mandibular advancement devices have also shown to reduce the AHI and symptoms of OSA, such as snoring. Currently these therapeutic modalities have not shown consistent therapeutic benefit in reducing CVD directly. (Table 2) [19].

CVD	Association with OSA	Literature
Systemic Hypertension	Positive, dose-dependent relationship with AHI	Wisconsin cohort (2000)
	Sympathetic activation	Sleep Heart Health (2000)
	RAAS activation	
	More frequent in resistant hypertension	
Ischemic Heart Disease	Higher risk of myocardial infarction (AHI>30)	Lancet (2005)
Coronary Artery Disease (CAD)	Positive relationship between atherosclerotic volume and AHI	American College of Cardiology (2008)
	Increased nocturnal MIs	International Journal of Cardiology (2009)
	Nocturnal hypoxia	
Heart Failure	High degree of association (50-70%)	European Journal of Heart Failure (2007)
	Initial central apnea causing sympathetic stimulation	Nature Reviews: Cardiology (2016)
	HTN, tachycardia causing cardiac remodeling	
	RAAS activation	
Arrhythmias	Moderate degree of association (40-50%)	American College of Cardiology (2014)
	Intrathoracic pressure change causing stretching of atria	Sleep Medicine (2016)
	Atrial remodeling disturbing conduction pathways	
	Sympatho-vagal imbalance from apneic episodes	
Strokes (CVA)	Risk independent of other CVD risk factors	Lancet (2004)
	Dose-dependent relationship with AHI	American Thoracic Society (2010)
	Altered cerebral autoregulation	
	Endothelial dysfunction	
	Pro-thrombic/inflammatory state	
Pulmonary Hypertension	Evidence of association (20%)	American Journal of Cardiology (2009)
	Obesity-hypoventilation syndrome	

Table 2: Association between OSA and its impact on known CVDs with available data.

Conclusion

Obesity in the United States has reached its epidemic state and the prevalence of its related diseases, such as OSA and CVD are also rising. Table 1 summarizes the pathophysiologic and clinical implications of OSA. With the trend expected to rise in the future, it is important to understand the association between these two obesity-related diseases, in efforts to reduce the burden on the rising healthcare expenditure that is increasing.

It is also important to understand that many of the patients with such conditions are minorities with considerable portion that remain undiagnosed. Current hypotheses suggest low socioeconomic status and lack of education on proper nutrition may have contributed to predisposition of this population into more risk factors.

In addition to environmental factors, variations in molecular genetics of different ethnicities are likely associated with differences in risk of progression to OSA and CVD As the number one cause of death in the United States, it is essential to recognize the pathophysiology of CVD and factors potentially contributing to its onset. In this article, we recognize OSA as an emerging risk factor for CVD and pathophysiologic relationship between OSA and CVD; these are summarized in Figure 3.

Figure 3 also provides possible interventions available currently to possibly halt the progression from OSA to CVD. It is not yet clear if the treatment of OSA would reduce the risk of CVD, due to conflicting results in current literature. Larger, multi-center trials are needed. Despite the lack of well-defined evidence based guidelines, clinicians should always keep prevention of obesity as one of their priorities, especially if practicing in an at-risk population (Figure 3).

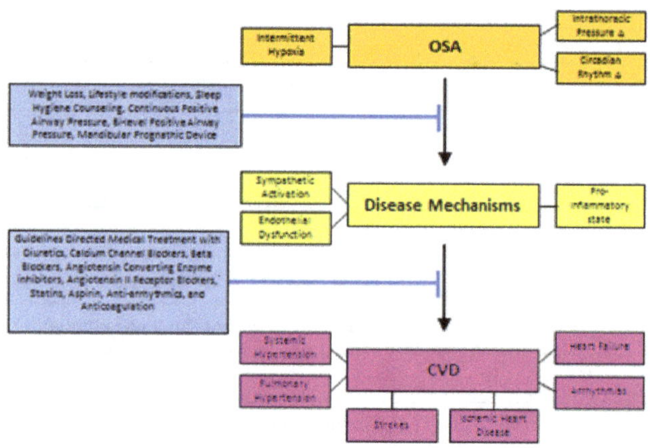

Figure 3: Progression of Obstructive Sleep Apnea to Cardiovascular Disease with potential treatments to inhibit or slow the progression from Obstructive Sleep Apnea to Cardiovascular Disease.

Acknowledgement

This work is sponsored in part by the Brooklyn Health Disparities Center NIH grant #P20 MD006875.

References

1. National Center for Health Statistics (2015) Obesity and Overweight. United States.
2. American Diabetes Association. The Staggering Costs of Diabetes in America.
3. Fritscher LG, Mottin CC, Canani S, Chatkin JM (2007) Obesity and obstructive sleep apnea-hypopnea syndrome: the impact of bariatric surgery. Obes Surg 17: 95-99.
4. Giunta J, Salifu M, McFarlane S (2016) Sleep Disorders and Cardio-Renal Disease: Implications for minority populations. Epidemiology 6: e120.
5. Dou L, Lan H, Reynolds DJ, Gunderson TM, Kashyap R, et al. (2017) Association between obstructive sleep apnea and acute kidney injury in critically Ill patients: A propensity-matched study. Nephron 135: 137-146.
6. Mokhlesi B, Grimaldi D, Beccuti G, Van Cauter E (2015) Effect of one week of CPAP treatment of obstructive sleep apnoea on 24-hour profiles of glucose, insulin and counter-regulatory hormones in type 2 diabetes. 19: 452-456.
7. Sardarinia M, Akbarpour S, Lotfaliany M, Farideh BK,Mohammadreza B,et al. (2016) Risk Factors for Incidence of Cardiovascular Diseases and All-Cause Mortality in a Middle Eastern Population over a Decade Follow-up: Tehran Lipid and Glucose Study. PLoS One 11: e0167623.
8. McFarlane SI, Sica DA, Sowers JR (2005) Stroke in patients with diabetes and hypertension. J Clin Hypertens 7: 286-292.
9. Myers CA, Slack T, Broyles ST, Heymsfield SM, Church TS, et al. (2016) Diabetes prevalence is associated with different community factors in the diabetes belt versus the rest of the United States. Obesity (Silver Spring).
10. American Heart Association. African-Americans and Heart Disease, Stroke. 2015 July.
11. Chen X, Wang R, Zee P, Lutsey PL, Javaheri S, et al. (2015) Racial/Ethnic Differences in Sleep Disturbances: The Multi-Ethnic Study of Atherosclerosis (MESA). Sleep 38: 877-888.
12. Wang R, Dong Y, Weng J, Kontos EZ, Chervin RD, et al. (2016) Associations among neighborhood, race and sleep apnea severity in children: a six city analysis. Ann Am Thorac Soc 14: 76-84.
13. Kendzerska T, Gershon AS, Tomlinson G, Leung RS (2016) The Effect of patient neighborhood income level on the purchase of continuous positive airway pressure treatment among patients with sleep apnea. Ann Am Thorac SocJan 13: 93-100.
14. Jones KM, Carter MM, Schulkin J (2015) Racial and Ethnic Disparities in Cardiovascular Disease: An Assessment of Obstetrician-Gynecologists' Knowledge, Attitudes, and Practice Patterns. J Racial Ethn Health Disparities 2: 256-266.
15. Sumner JA, Khodneva Y, Muntner P, Redmond N, Lewis MW, et al. (2016) Effects of concurrent depressive symptoms and perceived stress on cardiovascular risk in low- and high-income participants: findings from the reasons for geographical and racial differences in stroke (REGARDS) study. J Am Heart Assoc 5: e003930.
16. Fletcher EC, Lesske J, Behm R, Miller CC, Stauss H, et al. (1992) Carotid chemoreceptors, systemic blood pressure, and chronic episodic hypoxia mimicking sleep apnea. J Appl Physiol 72: 1978-1984.
17. Lesske J, Fletcher EC, Bao G, Unger T (1997) Hypertension caused by chronic intermittent hypoxia–influence of chemoreceptors and sympathetic nervous system. J Hypertens 15: 1593-1603.
18. Khayat R, Pleister A (2016) Consequences ofObstructive Sleep Apnea; Cardiovascular Risk of Obstructive Sleep Apnea and Whether Continuous Positive Airway Pressure Reduces that Risk. Sleep Med Clin 11: 273-286.
19. Sert Kuniyoshi FH, Pusalavidyasagar S, Singh P, Somers VK (2010) Cardiovascular consequences of obstructive sleep apnoea. Indian J Med Res 131: 196-205.
20. Drager LF, Yao Q, Hernandez KL, Shin MK, Bevans-Fonti S, Gay J, et al. (2013) Chronic intermittent hypoxia induces atherosclerosis via activation of adipose angiopoietin-like 4. Am J Respir Crit Care Med 188: 240-248.
21. Kasivisvanathan V, Shalhoub J, Lim CS, Shepherd AC, Thapar A, et al. (2011) Hypoxia-inducible factor-1 in arterial disease: a putative therapeutic target. Curr Vasc Pharmacol 9: 333-349.
22. Somers VK, Dyken ME, Clary MP, Abboud FM (1995) Sympathetic neural mechanisms in obstructive sleep apnea. J Clin Invest 96: 1897-1904.
23. Oparil S, Zaman MA, Calhoun DA (2003) Pathogenesis of hypertension. Ann Intern Med 139: 761-776.
24. Guo GB, Abboud FM (1984) Angiotensin II attenuates baroreflex control of heart rate and sympathetic activity. Am J Physiol 246: H80-H89.
25. Hartmann G, Tschop M, Fischer R, Bidlingmaier C, Riepl R, et al. (2000) High altitude increases circulating interleukin- 6, interleukin-1 receptor antagonist and C-reactive protein. Cytokine 12: 246-252.
26. Moss JW, Ramji DP (2016) Cytokines: roles in atherosclerosis disease progression and potential therapeutic targets. Future Med Chem 8: 1317-1330.
27. Ruscica M, Baragetti A, Catapano AL, Norata GD (2016) Translating the biology of adipokines in atherosclerosis and cardiovascular diseases: Gaps and open questions. Nutr Metab Cardiovasc Dis 88: 1054- 1057.
28. Buda AJ, Pinsky MR, Ingels NB Jr, Daughters GT, Stinson EB, et al. (1979) Effect of intrathoracic pressure on left ventricular performance. N Engl J Med 301: 453-459.
29. Romero-Corral A, Somers VK, Pellikka PA, Olson EJ, Bailey KR, et al. (2007) Decreased right and left ventricular myocardial performance in obstructive sleep apnea. Chest 132: 1863-1870.
30. Otto ME, Belohlavek M, Romero-Corral A, Gami AS, Gilman G, et al. (2007) Comparison of cardiac structural and functional changes in obese otherwise healthy adults with versus without obstructive sleep apnea. Am J Cardiol 99: 1298-1302.
31. Egan KJ, Knutson KL, Pereira AC, von Schantz M (2016) The role of race and ethnicity in sleep, circadian rhythms and cardiovascular health. Sleep Med Rev S1087-S1792.
32. Marin JM, Carrizo SJ, Vicente E, Agusti AG (2005) Long-term cardiovascular outcomes in men with obstructive sleep apnoea-

hypopnoea with or without treatment with continuous positive airway pressure: an obser- vational study. Lancet 365:1046-1053.

33. Turmel J, Series F, Boulet LP, Poirier P, Tardif JC, et al. (2009) Relationship between atherosclerosis and the sleep apnea syndrome: an intravascular ultrasound study. Int J Cardiol 132: 203-209.
34. Kuniyoshi FH, Garcia-Touchard A, Gami AS, Romero-Corral A, van der Walt C, et al. (2008) Day-night variation of acute myocardial infarction in obstructive sleep apnea. J Am Coll Cardiol 52: 343-346.
35. Doherty LS, Kiely JL, Swan V, McNicholas WT (2005) Long-term effects of nasal continuous positive airway pressure therapy on cardiovascular outcomes in sleep apnea syndrome. Chest 127: 2076-2084.
36. Bassetti CL, Milanova M, Gugger M (2006) Sleep-disordered breathing and acute ischemic stroke: diagnosis, risk factors, treatment, evolution, and long-term clinical outcome. Stroke 37: 967-972.
37. Valham F, Mooe T, Rabben T, Stenlund H, Wiklund U, et al. (2008) Increased risk of stroke in patients with coronary artery disease and sleep apnea: a 10-year follow-up. Circulation 118: 955-960.
38. Redline S, Yenokyan G, Gottlieb DJ, Shahar E, O'Connor GT, et al. (2010) Obstruc- tive sleep apnea-hypopnea and incident stroke: the Sleep Heart Health Study. Am J Respir Crit Care Med 182: 269-277.
39. Qureshi WT, bin Nasir U, Alqalyoobi, S, O'Neal WT, Mawri S, et al. (2015) Meta-Analysis of Continuous Positive Airway Pressure as a Therapy of Atrial Fibrillation in Obstructive Sleep Apnea. Am J Cardiol 116: e1767-e1773.
40. Peppard PE, Young T, Palta M, Skatrud J (2000) Prospective study of the association between sleep-disordered breathing and hypertension. N Engl J Med 342: 1378-1384.
41. Nieto FJ, Young TB, Lind BK, Shahar E, Samet JM, et al. (2000) Association of sleep-disordered breathing, sleep apnea, and hy- pertension in a large community-based study. Sleep Heart Health Study. Jama 283: 1829-1836.
42. Goncalves SC, Martinez D, Gus M, de Abreu-Silva EO, Bertoluci C, et al. (2007) Obstructive sleep apnea and resistant hypertension: a case-control study. Chest 132: 1858-1862.
43. Logan AG, Tkacova R, Perlikowski SM, Leung RS, Tisler A, et al. (2003) Refractory hypertension and sleep apnoea: effect of CPAP on blood pressure and barore ex. Eur Respir J 21: 241-247.
44. Oldenburg O, Lamp B, Faber L, Teschler H, Horstkotte D, et al. (2007) Sleep-disordered breathing in patients with symptomatic heart failure: a contemporary study of prevalence in and characteristics of 700 patients. Eur J Heart Fail 9: 251-257.
45. Parati G, Lombardi C, Castagna F, Mattaliano P, Filardi P, et al. (2016) Heart failure and sleep disorders. Nature Reviews Cardiology 13:389-403.
46. Stanchina ML, Ellison K, Malhotra A, Anderson M, Kirk M, et al. (2007) The impact of cardiac resynchronization therapy on obstructive sleep apnea in heart failure patients: a pilot study. Chest 132: 433-439.
47. Linz D, Linz B, Hohl M, Bohm M (2016) Atrial arrhythmogenesis in obstructive sleep apnea: Therapeutic implications. Sleep Medicine Reviews 87: e94
48. Kaneko Y, Floras JS, Usui K, Plante J, Tkacova R, et al. (2003) Cardiovascular effects of continuous positive airway pressure in patients with heart failure and obstructive sleep apnea. N Engl J Med 348: 1233-1241.
49. Linz D, Ukena C, Mahfoud F, Neuberger HR, Bohm M (2014) Atrialautonomic innervation: a target for interventional antiarrhythmic therapy? J Am Coll Cardiol 63: e24.
50. Ng CY, Liu T, Shehata M, Stevens S, Chugh SS, et al. (2011) Meta-analysis of obstructive sleep apnea as predictor of atrial fibrillation recurrence after catheter ablation. Am J Cardiol 108: 47-51.
51. Naruse Y, Tada H, Satoh M, Yanagihara M, Tsuneoka H, et al. (2013) Concomitant obstructive sleep apnea increases the recurrence of atrial fibrillation following radiofrequency catheter ablation of atrial fibrillation: clinical impact of continuous positive airway pressure therapy. Heart Rhythm 10: 331-337.
52. Yaggi H, Mohsenin V (2004) Obstructive sleep apnoea and stroke. Lancet Neurol 3: 333-342.
53. Minai OA, Ricaurte B, Kaw R, Mansour M, McCarthy K, et al. (2009) Frequency and impact of pulmonary hypertension in patients with obstructive sleep apnea syndrome. Am J Cardiol 104: 1300-1306.
54. Arias MA, Garcia-Rio F, Alonso-Fernandez A, Isabel Martínez, José Villamor (2006) Pulmonary hypertension in obstructive sleep apnoea: effects of continuous positive airway pressure: a randomized, controlled cross-over study. Eur Heart J 27: 1106-1113.
55. Sajkov D, Wang T, Saunders NA, Bune AJ, McEvoy RD (2002) Continuous positive airway pressure treatment improves pulmonary hemodynamics in patients with obstructive sleep apnea. Am J Respir Crit Care Med 2002; 165: 152-158.
56. McEnvoy RD, Antic NA, Heeley E, Luo Y, Luo Y, Ou Q, et al. (2016) CPAP for Prevention of Cardiovascular Events in Obstructive Sleep Apnea. N Engl J Med 375: 919-931.
57. Khayat R, Small R, Rathman L, Steven Krueger, Becky Gocke, et al. (2013) Sleep disordered breathing in heart failure: identifying and treating an important but often unrecognized comorbidity in heart failure patients. J Card Fail 19: 431-444.

Obstructive Sleep Apnea in Patients with Fibromyalgia: Report from a Fibromyalgia Clinic

Gail A Welsh[1], Mary O Whipple[1], Eric J Olson[2], Ann Vincent[1], Laura L Loehrer[1], Stephen S Cha[3] and Dietlind L Wahner-Roedler[1*]

[1]*Division of General Internal Medicine, Mayo Clinic, Rochester, Minnesota, USA*

[2]*Division of Pulmonary and Critical Care Medicine, Mayo Clinic, Rochester, Minnesota, USA*

[3]*Division Biomedical Statistics and Informatics, Mayo Clinic, Rochester, Minnesota, USA*

***Corresponding author:** Dietlind L Wahner-Roedler, Division of General Internal Medicine, Mayo Clinic, 200 First St SW, Rochester, MN 55905, USA
E-mail: wahnerroedler.dietlind@mayo.edu

Abstract

Objectives: Fatigue and unrefreshing sleep are symptoms of fibromyalgia and part of its diagnostic criteria. The literature is inconsistent regarding the prevalence of sleep disorders in fibromyalgia. The purpose of the study was to determine if obstructive sleep apnea (OSA) was more common in patients with fibromyalgia than in a general internal medicine clinic population.

Methods: The records of 500 patients seen in a fibromyalgia clinic who fulfilled diagnostic criteria for fibromyalgia were compared with 500 patients seen in a general internal medicine clinic who did not have the diagnosis of fibromyalgia. The presence of a diagnosis of OSA was abstracted from each record. Patients were matched for age, sex, and body mass index. Descriptive statistics were used to characterize the sample. Pearson χ^2 test and Fisher exact test were used for analysis.

Results: OSA was significantly more common in patients presenting to a fibromyalgia clinic compared with the patient population lacking the fibromyalgia diagnosis. This finding was independent of body mass index in overweight and moderately obese cohorts.

Conclusion: Patients with fibromyalgia should be screened for OSA because treatment of sleep disorders may help with symptoms of fatigue and unrefreshing sleep.

Keywords: Fibromyalgia patients; Sleep apnea; Sleep disturbances; Sleep problems

Abbreviations:

AHI: Apnea Hypopnea Index; BMI: Body Mass Index; BSQ: Berlin Sleep Questionnaire; CI: Confidence Interval; OSA: Obstructive Sleep Apnea; PSG: Polysomnography; REM: Rapid Eye Movement

Introduction

Obstructive sleep apnea (OSA) is the most common of all sleep-related breathing disorders. The estimated prevalence in North America is approximately 20% to 25% in males and 10% in females when OSA is defined as an apnea hypopnea index (AHI) greater than or equal to 5 events per hour, as determined by polysomnography (PSG) [1-3]. The strongest risk factor for OSA in both sexes is obesity, and prevalence of OSA increases with increasing body mass index (BMI) [3,4].

Sleep-related symptoms such as waking unrefreshed, fatigue, tiredness, and insomnia are common in patients with OSA; these are also common concerns for patients with fibromyalgia, a chronic condition characterized by widespread muscle pain and various symptoms such as cognitive difficulty, anxiety, and depression. Given the frequency with which sleep issues are reported, fatigue and waking tired or unrefreshed are included in the American College of Rheumatology diagnostic criteria for fibromyalgia [5]. PSG studies have been conducted in patients with fibromyalgia to delineate the physiologic basis of sleep-related symptoms, and distinctive patterns of alpha intrusion in non–rapid eye movement (REM) sleep have been described (phasic alpha, tonic alpha, and low alpha activity) [6-9].

The literature is inconsistent regarding the prevalence of sleep disorders in patients with fibromyalgia and the potential role of sleep disorders in fibromyalgia symptoms [7]. In a retrospective chart review of 23 women with fibromyalgia, Shah et al. [10] reported that a high percentage (83%) had an AHI greater than 15, indicating moderate sleep apnea. Their findings were also consistent with previous reports that suggested increased sleep latency and arousal index and reduced REM sleep in patients with fibromyalgia [11,12]. In another study of 28 women with fibromyalgia, 96% had sleep-disordered breathing [13]. The rates of sleep apnea reported in these studies, however, were significantly higher than that reported by Hamm et al. [14] who observed sleep apnea in 25% of patients with fibromyalgia, with 43% having alpha-delta intrusion. Similarly, Chen et al. [15] reported that 19% of females and 32% of males with fibromyalgia had documented sleep apnea. Although most published studies do not compare the prevalence of sleep apnea in patients with fibromyalgia vs individuals without chronic pain conditions, one controlled study showed no difference between patients and controls regarding the prevalence of sleep-disordered breathing [16]. However, patients with fibromyalgia did have greater sleep fragmentation than controls, which was consistent with the high rate of insomnia and unrefreshing sleep reported by patients with fibromyalgia [17].

Limited data describe the prevalence of fibromyalgia in patients with known sleep apnea. A study by Alvarez Lario et al. [18] reported no significant correlation between sleep apnea and the number of tender points in a sample of 30 patients with sleep apnea. In that study, only 1 patient had fibromyalgia. Another study reported that although OSA did not appear to be a significant problem in females with newly diagnosed fibromyalgia, fibromyalgia may be a marker of occult sleep apnea in males [19].

Research in animal models indicates that treatment of sleep disorders could have a positive impact on pain [20], and the same relationship potentially is present in patients with fibromyalgia. Strong evidence linking sleep apnea with fibromyalgia is lacking, but a case report describing a woman with a 10-year history of fibromyalgia suggests that treatment of sleep apnea could markedly reduce or eliminate symptoms of fibromyalgia for some patients [21].

The studies published to date have been conducted in relatively small groups of patients, and the reported associations between fibromyalgia and sleep apnea in men vs women differ substantially. Furthermore, although previous studies have confirmed the association between increased BMI and OSA, no reports describe a case-control study design in a large sample that allows evaluation of OSA prevalence in fibromyalgia, independent of BMI. The purpose of this study was to examine the frequency of OSA, the most common sleep-related breathing disorder, in patients presenting to a fibromyalgia clinic.

Methods

This study was approved by our institutional review board, and only patients who consented to use of their medical records for research were included in the study.

Setting

Patients included in this study were seen from December 2010 through October 2011 in the Fibromyalgia and Chronic Fatigue Clinic at a tertiary academic medical center in the United States.

Clinical design

We reviewed the charts of 500 consecutive patients who fulfilled the 2010 diagnostic criteria for fibromyalgia [5]. The following data were abstracted: age, sex, BMI, results of the Berlin Sleep Questionnaire (BSQ), results of an overnight oximetry test, results of a polysomnogram, and whether the patient had a previous or new diagnosis of OSA.

The BSQ was created during the 1996 Conference on Sleep in Primary Care held in Berlin, Germany, in which 120 US and German pulmonary and primary care physicians participated [22]. The questionnaire consists of 3 categories related to the risk of having OSA, including 1 introductory question and 4 follow-up questions concerning snoring, 3 questions addressing daytime sleepiness and 1 follow-up question about falling asleep while driving; and 1 question addressing the presence of hypertension. Patient BMI is also noted. Patients can be classified into high or low risk of OSA on the basis of their responses. Patients are considered high risk if 2 or more categories have positive scores (low risk is defined as only 1 or no categories with a positive score).

Overnight oximetry continuously records a patient's oxygen level with a pulse oximeter during sleep. An abnormal test is not diagnostic of OSA, but it can be useful to screen for patterns of desaturation and changes in heart rate suggestive of OSA and can prompt further diagnostic testing. All overnight oximetry tests in our study were reviewed by interpreters in the Pulmonary Function Lab at our institution and classified as normal or abnormal.

For PSG tests, OSA was defined as an AHI greater than 5 events per hour, with more than half of the disordered breathing events considered to be obstructive.

Controls

We used a random algorithm to select 1 matched control for each case from a pool of 21,944 outpatients seen in the general internal medicine division of our clinic during the same period; controls were matched by sex, age, and BMI. Charts of the controls were reviewed for a diagnosis of OSA. Patients with the diagnosis of fibromyalgia were excluded from the control pool.

Statistical Analysis

Descriptive statistics (mean, median, SD, and percent) were used to describe the sample. The Pearson χ^2 test and Fisher exact test were used for analysis and odds ratios and 95% confidence intervals (CI) were calculated for the overall sample and each BMI category.

Results

Of the 500 patients with fibromyalgia, 441 (88.2%) were women. Median age was 48 years (range, 18-82 years), and median BMI was 29.6 kg/m^2 (range, 15.6-64.3 kg/m^2). At presentation, 104 fibromyalgia patients (20.8%) had the diagnosis of OSA (Figure 1). Of the 396 remaining patients, 340 (85.9%) completed the BSQ and 191 (56.2%) had high risk of OSA; 146 (36.9%) underwent oximetry, and 63 (43.2%) had abnormal results. Forty-seven patients (11.9%) underwent PSG, and 32 (68.1%) received the diagnosis of OSA. Seventy-eight of 500 patients (15.6%) were advised to undergo PSG because of a high-risk BSQ score or an abnormal overnight oximetry test but were unable to stay for the evaluation.

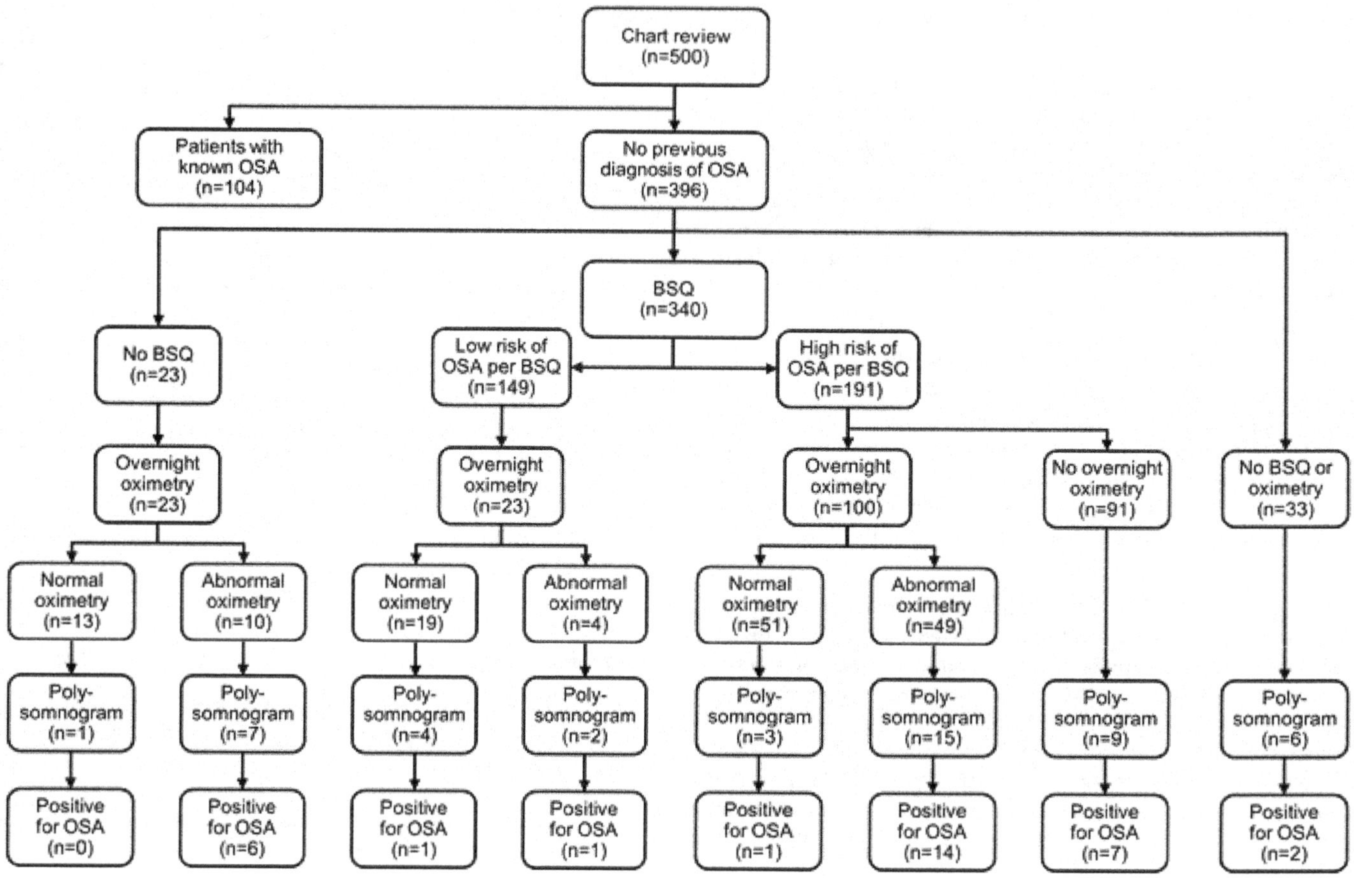

Figure 1: Summary of 500 Patients With Fibromyalgia Evaluated for OSA From December 2010 Through October 2011. BSQ indicates Berlin Sleep Questionnaire; OSA, obstructive sleep apnea.

The characteristics of the fibromyalgia and control cohorts (matched by sex, age, and BMI) are summarized in the Table 1. The Table further shows the percentage of OSA in the 2 groups, stratified by BMI category. In total, 104 (20.8%) in the fibromyalgia cohort had a previous diagnosis of OSA at initial presentation to fibromyalgia clinic, whereas 54 (10.8%) of the control group from the general internal medicine clinic had OSA, for an odds ratio of 2.17, 95% CI (1.52, 3.10). Among the 47 members of the fibromyalgia cohort who underwent PSG, 32 new cases were diagnosed. When including the 32 new cases of OSA in the fibromyalgia cohort, in total, 136 patients had a diagnosis of OSA, for a odds ratio of 3.09, 95% CI (2.19, 4.35). The higher rate of OSA in patients with fibromyalgia compared with controls was independent of increased BMI and this difference was statistically significant for two of the four BMI categories (25-29.9 kg/m^2 and 35.0 kg/m^2).

Variable	Controls (n=500)	Patients With Fibromyalgia (n=500)	Odds Ratio	95% CI		P Value[a]
				Lower Bound	Upper Bound	
Age, mean (SD), y	47.27 (12.97)	47.25 (12.98)				...
Female sex, No. (%)	441 (88)	441 (88)				...
BMI, mean (SD), kg/m^2	30.33 (8.35)	30.29 (7.71)				...

BMI categories, No. (%)						
<25.0 kg/m2	146 (29)	146 (29)				...
25.0-29.9 kg/m2	118 (24)	118 (24)				...
30.0-34.9 kg/m2	105 (21)	105 (21)				...
>35.0 kg/m2	131 (26)	131 (26)				...
OSA diagnosis, No. (%)	54 (11)	104 (21)	2.17	1.52	3.1	<0.001
BMI, <25.0 kg/m2	3 (2)	8 (5)	2.69	0.71	10.21	0.22
BMI, 25.0-29.9 kg/m2	5 (4)	17 (14)	3.48	1.28	9.52	0.012
BMI, 30.0-34.9 kg/m2	16 (15)	27 (26)	1.73	0.92	3.25	0.09
BMI, >35.0 kg/m2	30 (23)	52 (40)	1.82	1.14	2.9	0.005

Table 1: Characteristics of Fibromyalgia Cases and Controls and Prevalence of OSA (Stratified by BMI), [a]Controls were matched for age, sex, and BMI.

Discussion

Our study showed that the percentage of patients with OSA was significantly higher in patients presenting to a fibromyalgia clinic compared with a population of patients who did not have the diagnosis of fibromyalgia. Furthermore, additional cases of OSA were identified in a fibromyalgia population after screening with the BSQ and performing overnight oximetry studies.

This finding still holds true even when comparing cohorts matched by age, sex, and BMI. Medical conditions affecting prevalence of OSA, independent of BMI (or only weakly associated with BMI), include end-stage renal disease and postmenopausal status. The pathogenesis of OSA in patients with end-stage renal disease appears to be associated with factors such as pharyngeal narrowing associated with fluid overload [23]. Menopausal and postmenopausal women have an increased risk of OSA compared with premenopausal women, independent of age and BMI, with hormone replacement therapy appearing to reduce the risk [24,25]. We did not investigate the menopausal status or hormone replacement therapy use of any patients or controls enrolled in this study. However, because the 2 groups were matched for age and BMI, menopausal status and possible hormone replacement therapy use are unlikely causes of the observed differences in OSA.

Various substances and medications such as alcohol, benzodiazepines, and narcotics have been associated with OSA, and these factors may well exacerbate OSA in patients who are already at risk. Common medications used in patients with fibromyalgia that may affect sleep include anticonvulsants, psychostimulants, hypnotics, anti-parkinsonians, antidepressants, opiates, and anti-inflammatory agents [7]. We did not abstract patient medication usage, but we believe that the fibromyalgia patients were more likely to use medications such as opioids (which can potentially interfere with sleep) compared with the control group, thus contributing to the higher risk of OSA in the fibromyalgia cohort.

Some have evaluated the prevalence of sleep apnea in other rheumatologic conditions. Two abstracts described the risk of OSA in patients with rheumatoid arthritis. Holman et al. [26] reported a 45% prevalence of OSA in men with connective tissue diseases, including rheumatoid arthritis. The prevalence of OSA was high, regardless of BMI or the type of inflammatory disease. In a study from Japan, more than half of 96 patients with rheumatoid arthritis (mostly female) had OSA [27].

Strength of our study is the large number of patients in the fibromyalgia and control cohorts. In addition, the American College of Rheumatology's uniform diagnostic criteria for fibromyalgia was used to identify the fibromyalgia patients. We suspect that more patients in our fibromyalgia population had OSA than was recognized because 78 patients (15.6%) were noted to have high risk of OSA on the basis of their BSQ or an abnormal overnight oximetry but were unable to undergo further testing with PSG. A weakness of this study was that we did not review any PSG findings from the patients who had OSA diagnosed at another institution. Furthermore, we lacked follow-up on patients with fibromyalgia who were advised to have a local sleep study performed, based on our risk assessment. OSA very likely was underdiagnosed in the control population as well because the processes of evaluating OSA in the fibromyalgia clinic are different from those used in the general internal medicine practice. All patients presenting to our fibromyalgia clinic are screened with a BSQ unless they decline. If abnormal, overnight oximetry and/or PSG are pursued. General internal medicine clinic patients are not usually subjected to this level of rigorous screening. Also, clinicians are more likely to evaluate a female patient with fibromyalgia without a history of snoring for sleep apnea than a female patient without fibromyalgia, but with complaints of insomnia and fatigue.. Given that an additional 32 patients with fibromyalgia were diagnosed with OSA during their evaluation, our odds ratio of 2.17, 95% CI (1.52, 3.10) based on 104 patients with fibromyalgia and OSA at the time of their presentation to fibromyalgia clinic likely underestimates the true prevalence of OSA in fibromyalgia patients. Furthermore, because not all patients underwent PSG, we were unable to include odds ratios for upper airway resistance between the two cohorts. Future research with consistent screening in patients and controls would help clarify these issues.

Conclusion

Our results show a higher percentage of OSA in patients with fibromyalgia compared with general internal medicine patients. Clinicians who care for patients with fibromyalgia should be mindful of this association and consider appropriate screening and diagnostic studies if indicated.

References

1. Young T, Palta M, Dempsey J, Skatrud J, Weber S, et al. (1993) The occurrence of sleep-disordered breathing among middle-aged adults. N Engl J Med 328: 1230-1235.
2. Young T, Palta M, Dempsey J, Peppard PE, Nieto FJ, et al. (2009) Burden of sleep apnea: rationale, design, and major findings of the Wisconsin Sleep Cohort study. WMJ 108: 246-249.
3. Peppard PE, Young T, Barnet JH, Palta M, Hagen EW, et al. (2013) Increased prevalence of sleep-disordered breathing in adults. Am J Epidemiol 177: 1006-1014.
4. Young T, Skatrud J, Peppard PE (2004) Risk factors for obstructive sleep apnea in adults. JAMA 291: 2013-2016.
5. Wolfe F, Clauw DJ, Fitzcharles MA, Goldenberg DL, Katz RS, et al. (2010) The American College of Rheumatology preliminary diagnostic criteria for fibromyalgia and measurement of symptom severity. Arthritis Care Res (Hoboken) 62: 600-610.
6. Roizenblatt S, Moldofsky H, Benedito-Silva AA, Tufik S (2001) Alpha sleep characteristics in fibromyalgia. Arthritis Rheum 44: 222-230.
7. Roizenblatt S, Neto NS, Tufik S (2011) Sleep disorders and fibromyalgia. Curr Pain Headache Rep 15: 347-357.
8. Rizzi M, Sarzi-Puttini P, Atzeni F, Capsoni F, Andreoli A, et al. (2004) Cyclic alternating pattern: a new marker of sleep alteration in patients with fibromyalgia? J Rheumatol 31: 1193-1199.
9. Moldofsky H1 (2002) Management of sleep disorders in fibromyalgia. Rheum Dis Clin North Am 28: 353-365.
10. Shah MA, Feinberg S, Krishnan E (2006) Sleep-disordered breathing among women with fibromyalgia syndrome. J Clin Rheumatol 12: 277-281.
11. Horne JA, Shackell BS (1991) Alpha-like EEG activity in non-REM sleep and the fibromyalgia (fibrositis) syndrome. Electroencephalogr Clin Neurophysiol 79: 271-276.
12. Branco J, Atalaia A, Paiva T (1994) Sleep cycles and alpha-delta sleep in fibromyalgia syndrome. J Rheumatol 21: 1113-1117.
13. Gold AR, Dipalo F, Gold MS, Broderick J (2004) Inspiratory airflow dynamics during sleep in women with fibromyalgia. Sleep 27: 459-466.
14. Hamm C, Derman S, Russell IJ (1989) Sleep parameters in fibrositis/fibromyalgia syndrome. Arthritis Rheum 32:(Suppl): S70.
15. Chen LX, Baqir M, Schumacher HR (2004) Increased incidence of sleep apnea in fibromyalgia patients [abstract]. Arthritis Rheum 50: S494.
16. Jennum P, Drewes AM, Andreasen A, Nielsen KD (1993) Sleep and other symptoms in primary fibromyalgia and in healthy controls. J Rheumatol 20: 1756-1759.
17. Wolfe F, Ross K, Anderson J, Russell IJ, Hebert L (1995) The prevalence and characteristics of fibromyalgia in the general population. Arthritis Rheum 38: 19-28.
18. Alvarez Lario B, Teran J, Alonso JL, Alegre J, Arroyo I, et al. (1992) Lack of association between fibromyalgia and sleep apnoea syndrome. Ann Rheum Dis 51: 108-111.
19. May KP, West SG, Baker MR, Everett DW (1993) Sleep apnea in male patients with the fibromyalgia syndrome. Am J Med 94: 505-508.
20. Frange C, Hirotsu C, Hachul H, Araujo P, Tufik S, et al. (2014) Fibromyalgia and sleep in animal models: a current overview and future directions. Curr Pain Headache Rep 18: 434.
21. Sepici V, Tosun A, Köktürk O (2007) Obstructive sleep apnea syndrome as an uncommon cause of fibromyalgia: a case report. Rheumatol Int 28: 69-71.
22. Netzer NC, Stoohs RA, Netzer CM, Clark K, Strohl KP (1999) Using the Berlin Questionnaire to identify patients at risk for the sleep apnea syndrome. Ann Intern Med 131: 485-491.
23. Beecroft JM, Pierratos A, Hanly PJ (2009) Clinical presentation of obstructive sleep apnea in patients with end-stage renal disease. J Clin Sleep Med 5: 115-121.
24. Bixler EO, Vgontzas AN, Lin HM, Ten Have T, Rein J, et al. (2001) Prevalence of sleep-disordered breathing in women: effects of gender. Am J Respir Crit Care Med 163: 608-613.
25. Young T, Finn L, Austin D, Peterson A (2003) Menopausal status and sleep-disordered breathing in the Wisconsin Sleep Cohort Study. Am J Respir Crit Care Med 167: 1181-1185.
26. Holman AJ, DePaso WJ (2004) High prevalence of obstructive sleep apnea (OSA) in men with inflammatory arthritis [abstract]. Arthritis Rheum 50(9): A947.
27. Shimizu M, Tachibana N, Hagasaka Y, Goto M (2003) Obstructive sleep apnea in RA patients and effect of CPAP on RA activity. Arthritis Rheum 48 suppl: S114.

14

Parasomnia and Dissociative Disorders

Kader Semra Karataş[1]*, Mustafa Bilici[2] and Zerrin Pelin[3]

[1]*Department of Psychiatry Internal Medical Sciences, Rize Training and Research Hospital, Recep Tayyip Erdogan University, Rize, Turkey*
[2]*Psychology Department, Sabahattin Zaim University, Istanbul, Turkey*
[3]*Somnus Sleep Disorders Center, Neurology, Istanbul, Turkey*

Abstract

Objective: Parasomnias are Sleep Disorders characterized by abnormal behavioral and physiological events. Dissociative experiences that occur in dissociative Disorders can emerge at night and may be the cause of parasomnia. The aim of this study is to compare the Sleep characteristics of parasomnia patients with and without dissociative disorder in order to investigate whether dissociative experiences may continue while aSleep and to what extent they change parasomnia.

Method: Of patients who were evaluated after admission to the Center of Sleep Disorders (n: 2217) and polysomnography patients (n: 822), the study was conducted with 36 patients diagnosed with parasomnia according to the International Clasification of Sleep Disorder-2 diagnostic criteria. To patients diagnosed with parasomnia were evaluated with psychometric tests such as Dissociative Experiences Scale, Childhood Trauma Questionnaire, Pittsburg Sleep Quality Index, Iowa Sleep Experiences Survey, Hamilton Depression Rating Scale, Beck Depression Inventory, and Structured Clinical Interview for Dissociative Disorders. The patient group with parasomnia and dissociative disorder was called group I, and the patient group with parasomnia alone was called group II.

Results: Dissociative disorder was detected in 41.6% of patients with parasomnia. The difference in psychometric test scores between Group I and Group II was statistically significant. In polysomnographic examination, all subjects in Group I and Group II were superficial with Sleep delta wave.

Conclusion: Dissociative experiences and childhood trauma are more common in people with Parasomnia conditions. Patients with Parasomnia and Dissociative Disorder are more depressed, according to both the clinician's and their own views on the subject. Delta slow wave bursts are similar in both groups.

Keywords: Parasomnia; Dissociative Disorders; Depressive Disorders; Polysomnography; Childhood trauma

Abbreviations: PSG: Polysomnography, ST: Sleep Terror, SW: Sleepwalking, EEG: Electroencephalography, NREM: Non Rapid Eye Movement, CNS: Central Nervous System, SA: Sleep Activity, SL: Sleep Onset Latency, SP: Sleep Period, χ^2: Chi-Square Test, Z: Mann-Whitney U Test International Clasification of Sleep Disorder-2: ICSD-2, American Academy of Sleep Medicine: AASM, Motility: EMG Activity during Arousal Reaction, AHI + PLMI: Apnea Hypnoea Index + Periodic Leg Movement Index, NNW: Number of Nighttime Wakefulness, Min. O2: Minimum O2, SPT: Sleep Period Time, AI: Arousal Index, WASO: Wakeup After Sleep Onset, PWP: Peak Wave Period, SD: Standard Deviation

Introduction

Parasomnias are Sleep Disorders characterized by abnormal behavioral and physiological events that occur in various phases of Sleep. As a general rule, parasomnia can be seen upon any event that causes Sleep fragmentation, or in individuals with a predisposition to increased slow wave. Parasomnias are frequent in the general population, more than 30% of people have experienced at least one type of parasomnia during a period in their lives [1]. Although parasomnia is frequently seen during childhood, it subsides in the adulthood. Reduced N3 phase Sleep and Central Nervous System (CNS) maturation with age can be the reason behind the decreased parasomnia incidence in adulthood [1-3]. Although there are limited number of studies, parasomnia in the adulthood is mostly related to psychiatric diseases and medical conditions [2]. Studies on defining the correlation between psychiatric disorder and parasomnia in adulthood are insufficient. In most of the patients with parasomnia, bipolar Disorders, especially non-psychotic depressive disorder, and anxiety Disorders were reported [4]. Dissociative disorder is frequently observed alongside depressive Disorders [5]. In some individuals with dissociative amnesia, depressive symptoms can be seen together with self-harm, aggressive impulses, suicidal impulses and actions [6].

Reports on the fact that experiences grouped under the subject of post-traumatic arousal also continue during Sleep have brought a different perspective to the parasomnia studies. Reports on the facts that chronically recurring traumas since childhood are correlated with dissociative disorder [7] and people exposed to traumatic events are more dissociated than those who were not [8] have suggested that dissociative experiences of parasomnia patients that occur during daytime can also emerge at nighttime [9,10]. Heterogeneity in parasomnia etiology and the overlap between dissociative Disorders and parasomnias at the symptom level have caused the researchers to study the similarities between these diseases and whether or not there are separate diseases or different subtypes of the same disease. There are only a few studies on the correlation between parasomnia and dissociative Disorders.

***Corresponding author:** Kader Semra Karataş, Psychiatry Department, Rize Training and Research Hospital, Recep Tayyip Erdogan University, 53200, Rize, Turkey, E-mail: semra.karatas@erdogan.edu.tr

The goal of the study is to find the correlation between parasomnia and dissociative Disorder. Specific objectives include:

1) Determine whether stressor factors such as childhood traumas have an impact on parasomnia and if they manifest as behavioral symptoms in parasomnia,

2) Investigate the frequency of depressive mood in parasomnia and/or dissociative disorder patients,

3) If Sleep walking (SW) and Sleep teror (ST) are the answers to the thoughts in trauma-related deep wave Sleep, determine if parasomnia can be regarded as a variant of a dissociative process,

4) Identify if there is a correlation between overall Sleep quality, dissociative Disorders and parasomnia,

5) Study if parasomnia and dissociative disorder have common characteristics since similar arousal waves are observed in electroencephalography (EEG) of patients with parasomnia and patients who scored high in dissociative disorder.

Materials and Methods

Sample group

Target population of the study comprised patients admitted to Istanbul Erenköy Psychiatry and Research Hospital Center of Sleep Disorders between 11.10.2010-01.03.2012. Of patients admitted to the Center due to Sleep Disorders (n: 2217), patients with isolated symptoms such as respiratory problems in Sleep, hypersomnias, parasomnia, circadian rhythm Disorders, Sleep-related motility Disorders, teeth grinding, muscle cramps, were evaluated. Of admitted patients, those diagnosed with parasomnia based on International Clasification of Sleep Disorder-2 (ICSD-2) diagnostic criteria and who showed potentially aggressive behaviour towards the patients and others, those with severe social and familial problems, those who have Sleepiness and behavioural difficulties during the daytime, those suspected of having episodes or those whose Sleep Disorders cannot be properly diagnosed with the existing symptoms and meet the exclusion criteria (n: 822) were selected and polysomnographic examination was performed. Of the patients who underwent Polysomnography (n: 822), those diagnosed with Parasomnia (n: 36) based on clinical ICSD-2 diagnostic criteria and polysomnography examination were evaluated for whether or not they have dissociative disorder according to Structured Clinical Interview for Dissociative Disorders.

Exclusion criteria: Those younger than 18 years of age, having mental retardation, dementia, delirium and other amnestic disorder that can be detected through medical evaluation, with alcohol and drug addiction/abuse based on anamnesis, using psychotropic and mood stabilizer medication that affect the Sleep pattern, having bodily faults or growth retardation such that it affects polysomnography evaluation were not included in the study.

This study commenced upon obtaining permission from Istanbul Erenköy Psychiatriy and Research Hospital, Education Planning Committee (no: 33, 11.10.2010) in Turkey.

Data collection tool

A total of 36 patients who volunteered to participate in the study were informed about and included in the study. Informed consent forms were collected with signatures.

The patient group with parasomnia and dissociative disorder was called group I, and the patient group with parasomnia alone was called group II.

The clinician applied Structured Clinical Interview for Dissociative Disorders and Hamilton Depression Rating Scale to all patients. The scales Dissociative Experiences Scale, Iowa Sleep Experiences Survey, Pittsburg Sleep Quality Index, Childhood Trauma Questionnaire and Beck Depression Inventory were completed by all patients.

Structured Clinical Interview for Dissociative Disorders (SCID-D): SCID-D is a semistructured diagnostic interview for the assessment of dissociative Disorders according to the DSM-IV criteria. Instrument developed in 1984-1985 by an Associate Research Scientist in the Department of Psychiatry at Yale University. Marlein Steinberg recieved a grant that allowed for 3 years of testing. SCID-D has 8 sections of interview that psychiatric history, amnesia, depersonalization, derealization, identitiy confusion, identity alteration, associated features of identitiy confusion, follow-up on identitiy confusion and identitiy alteration. SCID-D is scored and interpretted in a concise and easy metod using a severity scale of the five dissociative symptoms. Interview begins with client's symptomatology, behaviours and intra-interviewing behaviours of dissociative Disorders. Interviewer transition is open – ended questions. The test uses a scale (1-4) to determine mild, moderate or severe symptomatology of each dissociative disorder symptoms. Each of the five symptoms has a severity scale of 4 and maximum score is 20. Validity is good to excellent in regard to the five dissociative symptoms and also dissociative Disorders. Test-retest reability indicates excellent reability with respect to the 5 Dissociative Disorders. The Turkish version of the scale has a reliability and validity and was studied by Sar et al. [11,12].

Dissociative Experiences Scale (DES)

DES was developed by Bernstein and Putnam in 1986. The overall DES score is obtained by adding up the 28 item scores and dividing by 28: this yields an overall score ranging from 0 to 100. It has been demonstrated that the scale differentiates patients with a chronic dissociative disorder and those with other psychiatric Disorders [13]. Patients who have DES avarage total score is 30 and up probably have dissociative Disorders in Turkish sample studies. The Turkish version of the scale was studied by Yargic and et al. has a reliability and validity [14]. The test-retest coefficient was calculated at close to 0.78 [13,14].

Hamilton Depression Rating Scale (HDRS)

The HDRS is a standard scale based on psychiatrists' assessments, and was developed in the late 1950s to measure depressive symptoms. The scale was initially designed to obtain a total score based on 17 of its 21 items. The 17 item version of the scale was modified by Max Hamilton. It has been used widely in research for initial and follow-up assessments of depressive symptoms. The scale was initially composed of open-ended questions directed to the patient by the evaluator. Afterward, the scale was modified to include standard questions for each item. Eight items are scored on a 5-point scale, ranging from 0=not present to 4=severe. Nine are scored from 0-2. Sum the scores from the first 17 items. 0-7=Normal 8-13=Mild Depression 14-18=Moderate Depression 19-22=Severe depression ≥ 23=Very Severe Depression. The Turkish version of the HDRS has sufficient internal consistency; split-half, test-retest, and inter-rater reliability; structural and similar scales validity; and was shown to be valid and reliable in the assessment of clinical depression. The test-retest coefficient was calculated at close to 0.85 [15].

Beck Depression Inventory (BDI)

Aeron T Beck originally developed BDI in 1961. In 1996 Beck developed a second version of the inventory. BDI has 21 items standard personality multible choise questionnaire test. BDI is a self reported analysis of depressive symptoms. It scored by summing the highest rating for each of the 21 item. Each item is then rated on a 4- point scale, ranging from 0 to 3, and the total score range from 0 to 63. The score ranging from 0 to 13 represent "minimal" depression; total score ranging from 14 to 19 represent "mild" depression while total scores from 20-28 are"moderate" and total scores from 29-63 are "severe". The Turkish version of the BDI has sufficient reliability and validity studied by Hisli [15,16].

Childhood Trauma Questionnaire (CTQ)-28

The CTQ-28 was developed as a screening tool for histories of abuse and neglect. The self-report includes a 28-item test that measures 5 types of maltreatment – emotional, physical, and sexual abuse, and emotional and physical neglect. Reliability for the CTQ is good with high internal consistency scores. Sexual Abuse, Emotional Neglect, Emotional Abuse, Physical Abuse have reported coefficients of 0.93-0.95, 0.88-0.92, 0.84-0.89, and 0.81-.086, respectively. Over a 3 ½ month period, the test-retest coefficient was calculated at close to 0.80. Factor analysis tests on the five-factor CTQ model showed structural invariance which demonstrate good validity. There cannot calculate cut off value about Turkish version. The Turkish researchers are evaluated CTQ-28 score as 5 points and up for sexual and physical abuse, 7 points and up for physical and emotioanl neglect according to their studies. The Turkish version of the CTQ is reliable and valid as its original form [17].

The Pittsburgh Sleep Quality Index (PSQI)

PSQI was developed by Dr. Daniel J. Buysse and coworkers at the University of Pittsburgh's Western Psychiatric Institute and Clinic in the late 1980s. The questionnaire has eighteen individual items which are used to generate seven composite scores. The results give numbers in seven categories: subjective Sleep quality, Sleep latency, Sleep duration, habitual Sleep efficiency, Sleep disturbances, use of Sleeping medication, and daytime dysfunction. Each component is scored between 0-3. Total score is between 0-21 that big values from 5 indicate poor Sleep quality, while small values from 5 indicate good Sleep quality. The Turkish version of PSQI was studied by Agargun and et al. in 1996 that has sufficient reliability and validity. The test-retest coefficient was calculated at close to 0.93[18].

Iowa Sleep Experiences Survey (ISES)

ISES was developed by Watson in 1999. In 2001 Watson described last formation of the survey. ISES determines various Sleep and dreamlike experiences frequency. ISES provides likert type measurement. Survey is diveded 2 section: General Sleep Experiences (GSE) and Lucid Dreaming (LD). The average of the points is obtained between all items. There is no validity or reliability in Turkish version. It is translated to Turkish. Total score of ISES is Cronbach alpha 0.87, 0.86 for GSE, and 0.83 for LR [19].

Polysomnography (PSG)

In polysomnographic examination, 6-channel EEG, 2 channel electrooculography, chin electromyography, oro-nasal air flow with nasal cannula, arterial oxygen saturation, respiratory effort with thoracoabdominal bands, and electrocardiography recordings were performed according to the international 10-20 mounting system of electrodes placed C4-A1, C3-O1-O2-A2, A1, A2, F4-A1, F3-A2. PSG were scored with RemLogic program. RemLogic is a full-feature software package that contains file management, collection and review services. Offers manual and automatic scoring opportunities. Scoring and reporting is done as specified by the American Academy of Sleep Medicine (AASM) rules. N7000 device used in multidirectional data collection is an extensive PSG amplificator with 32 channel application feature.

Analysis of polysomnographic recordings

The computer-aided evaluation of all parameters was checked manually (30 s epochs for Sleep staging). The following Sleep scoring data were included: Sleep period time (SPT), defined as time of Sleep onset to the end of Sleep, including all Sleep epochs and wakefulness after Sleep onset; wakefulness after Sleep onset (WASO), defined as time spent awake between the Sleep onset and the end of Sleep; total Sleep time (TST), defined as SPT minus WASO; number of nighttime wakefulness (NNW) was number of awakenings per hour SPT; Sleep latency defined as time between turning off the lights to the first epoch of any Sleep; Rapid Eye Movement (REM) latency, defined as time between Sleep onset to the first R EM epoch; minimum oxygen defined as minimum value of blood arterial oxygen saturation which measured by pulse oximeter; peak wave period (PWP) was, the duration of the dominant arousal wave at night. Arousal Index (AI) was calculated as number of nighttime arousals divided by TST. Sleep Efficiency (SE) was calculated as TST divided by SPT and TST divided by the time in bed. Apnea Hypopnea Index (AHI) defined as the number of apnea and hypopnea per hour in TST. Periodic Leg Movement Index (PLMI) was the ratio of number of movements that meet the criteria for periodic leg movement and the total Sleep period during which leg movements are recorded. Movement was EMG activity during arousal reaction. The percentage of TST in each Sleep stage (Non Rapid Eye Movement (NREM) 1-N1, NREM 2-N2, slow wave Sleep, including NREM 3).

Statistical Evaluation

In this study, statistical analysis was performed using SPSS 18.0 (Statistical Package for the Social Sciences). A p value < 0.05 was considered statistically significant. Since the group contained less than 30 members, non-parametric tests were used. Continuous variables were presented as mean and standard deviation, and categorical variables were presented as frequency and percentage. In the analysis, Mann Whitney U, Chi-square, Fisher exact Chi-square, Spearman correlation analysis of homogeneous of variance tests were used, and Levene test was used for the homogeneity of variance.

Results

86.7% of the patients in Group I were female and 13.3% were male and there was a statistical difference in the gender distribution between the two groups (χ^2:5.78, p: 0.01). 13.3% of the patients in Group I, 4.8% of the patients in Group II were divorced but no significant difference was observed between two groups (χ^2:1.37, p: 0.50). Education level was mostly high school and mean age distrubition and mean Body Mass Index is similiar in both groups (Table 1).

We determined of DES score was 42.65 ± 15.04 in a part of parasomnia patients (n=15). This was shown that these patients had probably dissociative Disorders also. According to SCID-D evaluation these patients diagnosed with dissociative disorder, dissociative amnesia was detected in 33.3%, dissociative fugue in 13.3%, and dissociative disorder that cannot be named otherwise in 53.4%. We found CTQ-28 score 11.14 ± 3.55 in Group I that indicated sexual or physical abuse and neglect too. We determined that Group I patients BDI score was 23.93 ± 6.2 (moderate depression), HDRS score was 16.26 ± 3.76

(moderate depression). Patients in Group I were depressed, according to both the clinician's and their own views on the subject. There were a statistically significant difference between the groups in terms of the total score of the clinical scales of DES, CTQ-28, BDI and HDRS scores (z: -5.06, p: 0.00, z: -2.78, p: 0.00; z: -3.49, p: 0.00, z: -4.03, p: 0.00) (Table 2).

Subjective Sleep quality, the primary component of PSQI, Sleep latency, the secondary component of PSQI, and Sleep Disorders, the fifth component of PSQI were statistically different in two groups (z: -2.19, p: 0.03, z: -3.26, p: 0.00, z: -2.95, p: 0.01).

ISES GSE subgroup scores were 3.59±1.29 and 2.45±0.89 and total scores were 5.55 ± 2.16 and 4.33 ± 1.77 for Group I and Group II and statistical difference was detected between the two groups (z:-2.60, r: 0) (Table 2).

PWP of arousals duration were 32.36 ± 19.89 second in Group I, 18.23 ± 18.95 second in Group II. NNW were 1.84 ± 0.91 per hour in Group I, 1.13 ± 1.02 per hour in Group II. Statistical difference in the duration of waves where the Sleep is superficial and NNW was detected between the two groups (z:-3.37, r: 0; z:-2.55, p: 0.01). N1 mean ratio was 5.30 ± 1.71% in Group I patients and 3.19 ± 1.78 in Group II patients. There were statistical difference between two groups (z:-3.10, p: 0.001). In all of the patients who had parasomnia, Sleep arousals were with delta waves. In group I, 12 patients (80%) and in group II, 13 patients

	Group I (n=15)		Group II (n =21)		χ^2	p
	n	%	n	%		
Gender						
Female	13	86.7	10	47.6	5.78	0.01
Male	2	13.3	11	52.4		
Marital status						
Single	3	20.0	7	33.3	1.37	0.5
Married	10	66.7	13	61.9		
Divorced	2	13.3	1	4.8		
Education level						
Illiterate	1	6.7	0	0.00	1.99	0.57
Primary education	2	13.3	2	9.5		
High school	6	40.0	9	42.9		
License school	6	40.0	10	47.6		
	Mean ± SD		**Mean ± SD**		z	
Age	34.73 ± 11.11		35.19 ± 11.17		-0. 145	0.89
Height	1.59 ± 0.07		1.68 ± 0.11		-2.142	0.03
Weight	62.60 ± 9.79		9.57 ± 11.86		-1.526	0.13
BMI	24.46 ± 3.74		24.38 ± 2.71		0.42	0.68

z: Mann-Whitney *U* Test, SD: Standard Deviation, χ^2: Chi-Square test

Table 1: Demographic Characteristics of the Groups and Their Comparison

Variables	Group I (n=15)	Group II (n = 21)	z	p
DES	42.65 ± 15.04	5.38 ± 4.20	-5.06	0
CTQ-28	11.14 ± 3.55	7.80 ± 2.21	-2.78	0
PSQI				
Subjective Sleep quality	2.06 ± 0.79	1.42 ± 0.74	-2.19	0.03
Sleep latency	1.80 ± 0.56	1.19 ± 0.40	-3.26	0
Sleep period	1.40 ± 1.18	1.04 ± 0.86	-0.81	0.42
Habitual Sleep efficiency	2.53 ± 0.99	2.42 ± 1.07	-0.29	0.77
Sleep disturbances	2.53 ± 0.51	2.00 ± 0.44	-2.95	0
Use of Sleeping medication	2.13 ± 1.30	1.42 ± 1.46	-1.55	0.12
Daytime dysfunction	2.20 ± 0.77	1.66 ± 0.85	-1.9	0.06
Total Points	14.66 ± 3.51	11.19 ± 3.21	-2.76	0
ISES				
GSE	3.59 ± 1.29	2.45 ± 0.89	-2.6	0.01
LR	1.96 ± 1.40	1.97 ± 1.16	-0,38	0.7
Total Points	5.55 ± 2.16	4.33 ± 1.77	-1.96	0.05
BDI	23.93 ± 6.25	11.57 ± 10.78	-3.49	0
HDRS	16.26 ± 3.76	7.57 ± 5.47	-4.03	0

z: Mann-Whitney U test, DES: Dissociative Experiences Scale, CTQ-28: Childhood Trauma Questionnaire-28, PSQI: Pittsburg Sleep Quality Index, ISES: Iowa Sleep Experiences Survey, GSE: General Sleep Experience, LR: Lucid Dreams, BDI: Beck Depression Inventory, HDRS: Hamilton Depression Rating Scale

Table 2: Identifier Properties of the Clinical Features of Group

Variables	Group I (n=15)	Group II (n = 21)	z	p
PWP	32.36 ± 19.89	18.23 ± 18.95	-3.37	0
Movement	1.00 ± 0.00	0.95 ± 0.21	-0.85	0.39
SL	10.77 ± 11.10	9.21 ± 10.21	-0.79	0.43
SPT	410.69 ± 15.74	422.22 ± 34.02	-0.85	0.39
TST	371.94±37.11	383.65±46.81	-1.11	0.27
WASO	38.12 ± 38.32	38.25±36.99	-0.02	0.98
NNW	1.84±0.91	1.13 ± 1.02	-2.55	0.01
Min O2	91.93 ± 2.84	89.34 ± 8.32	-0.87	0.38
	Mean ± SD	**Mean ± SD**	**z**	**p**
N1	5.30 ± 1.71	3.19±1.78	-3.1	0
N2	62.45 ± 6.25	59.99 ± 13.39	-0.13	0.89
N3	24.06±6.55	30.63 ± 21.65	-0.67	0.5
REM	8.06 ± 6.25	7.89 ± 7.75	-0.27	0.78
SE	88.24 ± 8.41	89.07 ± 9.54	-0.45	0.65
Arousals	23.26 ± 26.55	60.33 ± 93.47	-0.9	0.37
AI	3.84 ± 4.23	11.04 ± 16.34	-0.75	0.45
AHI+PLMI	8.03 ± 14.62	4.08 ± 4.81	0.35	0.65
	n=15 %	**n=21%**	χ^2	**p**
Alpha wave	12 80	1361.9	0.29	0.29
Delta wave	15 100	21100		

z: Mann-Whitney U Test, χ^2: Chi-square test, SD: Standard Deviation, PWP: Peak Wave Period, Movement: EMG activity during Arousal reaction, SL: Sleep Latency, SPT: Sleep Period Time, TST: Total Sleep Time, WASO: wakeup after Sleep onset, NNW: Number of Nighttime Wakefulness, Min. O2: Minimum O2, SE: Sleep Efficiency, AI: Arousal Index, AHI + PLMI: Apnea Hypnoea Index+ Periodic Leg Movement Index

Table 3: Comparison of Sleep Parameters of the Groups.

(61.9%) Sleep arousals had also with alpha wave in addition to delta wave. There was no statistical difference between these ratios (Table 3).

Discussion

This study aimed at discribing correlation between parasomnia and dissociative disorder. We found NREM parasomnia and dissociative disorder more commen in females. Schenck et al. showed that dissociative disorder and NREM parasomnia occur more frequently in women, and men who have SW and ST [20]. The other research was emphasized that Sleep-related dissociative Disorders are more frequently observed in females [1]. It stated that dissociative Disorders are mostly observed in women in the other study [21]. In our study there were no association among age distrubition, marital status, education level and BMI. It was reported that there is not sufficient information on demographic data such as gender and weight in parasomnia [22]. Higher ratio of females in Group I suggested that dissociative Disorders are frequently observed in females. Further studies is necessaray make clear among sociodemografic datas, parasomnia and dissociative Disorders.

We determined a part of the patients of parasomnia had dissociative Disorders too and called Group I. Patients who diagnosed with dissociative disorder was detected dissociative amnesia in 33.3%, dissociative fugue in 13.3%, and dissociative disorder that cannot be named otherwise in 53.4%. In our study in Group I had also sexual or physical abuse and neglect.

The correlation among dissociation, childhood neglect and abuse were shown in both prospective and retrospective studies [23-25]. Personality dissociation that develops to protect oneself from intense anxiety in the face of danger or intense stress can manifest itself in the form of dissociative amnesia, dissociative fugue, depersonalization, SW and ST [26]. Some authors report that Sleep-related aggressive behavior can be correlated with dissociative identity disorder in particular, dissociative fugue or dissociative disorder that cannot be named otherwise [8,20]. It is emphasized that the dissociative experiences during the daytime for those exposed to traumatic events can also occur at night and can be a cause of parasomnia [9,27]. It is known that undesired repressed traumatic experience re-emerges in deep wave phase [28]. If SW and ST are the answers to the thoughts in trauma-related deep wave Sleep, parasomnia can be accepted as the variant of a dissociative process and can be hypothesized that it disrupts Sleep by forming an arousal situation. In our study, significant high scores in Group I DES and CTQ-28 can be correlated with dissociation, childhood traumas and recurring traumas and Sleep-related experiences.

We found patients in Group I were depressed, according to both the clinician's and their own views on the subject in our study. It reported that depressive and dissociative Disorders are frequently observed together [5]. In some patients with dissociative amnesia, depression symptoms can accompany [6]. It was reported that in some patients with major depressive disorder that may be associated with Sleep disorder, EEG may have alpha intrusions in delta wave Sleep, and especially this finding can be seen in treatment-resistant major depressive disorder [29]. Whether the presence of an alpha delta wave pattern with a wake-up reaction in PSG evaluations in patients with depressive disorder, or the ability of patients with alpha delta patterns to develop a depressive disorder in PSG studies is debatable. Pelin et al. reported a case of dissociative disorder and parasomnia in a patient with psychometric examination and depressive disorder [30]. These findings suggest that depressive symptomatology may be more frequent in patients with parasomnias and dissociative Disorders than patients with parasomnia alone.

Zadra et al. were reported that NREM parasomnia episodes can be alpha, theta and delta wave or a combination of them without full awakening [31]. It was emphasized that, in PSG examination, hypersynchronous delta wave activity is seen at the beginning of NREM parasomnia episode [32], and that spectral wave power and slow delta waves were seen before the beginning of parasomnia episodes [8]. In our study, Group I had Sleep quality failure, delayed Sleep latency and Sleep Disorders, with subjective evalution of Sleep. And also polysomnographic evaluation of Sleep pattern showed us NNW and N1 phase percentage extent, presence of delta slow wave activity at the beginning of NREM parasomnia episodes, support NREM parasomnia. Moreover, additional alpha wave activity in 80% of the patients in Group I and 61.9% of Group II support NREM parasomnia nature. The presence of a certain hierarchy of arousals suggests that the first developing autonomic/subcortical activation is cortical and often motor activation may be a consequence of the arousal order. Parrino et al. based on AASM definition, emphasized that other than the arousal reaction in the Sleep, K-complex and delta bursts can be seen and these can arise due to autonomical functions. Besides the Sleep-like features of the delta burst and K-complex, their effect on cerebral activation is attracting interest [33]. Although slow EEG components such as delta wave bursts and K-complex, and traditional arousals such as fast rhythms are different in EEG, they may participate in the complex of cerebral activation. The fact that arousal reactions of all patients took place in slow wave component support that these waves may have affect the cerebral activation. Studying traumatic experiences that can cause dissociative disorder under the subject of increased arousal [9,10] supports the fact that these experiences continue during the Sleep [9]. A more meaningful superficial Sleep transition in Group I patients with dissociative Disorders may be due to the fact that traumatic experiences hold an important place in their etiology. As long as Sleep-related dissociative disorder diagnosis is not made, it can be considered that arousal parasomnias such as SW and ST originate from the dissociative Disorders and is a protector dissociative mechanisms. SW and ST can develop due to reduced cortical inhibition during Sleep. In our study, the number of the night arousal, arousal wave duration, and elevation in N1 phase percentage suggest that parasomnia and dissociative disorder together contribute to arousal reactions.

The limitations of our study are as follows:

1) Studies that will be conducted in a wider group of patients will provide results that will yield more reliable results.

2) The fact that we cannot perform PSG two nights in a row is another limitation of our study.

References

1. Thorpy MJ, Plazzi G (2010) The parasomnias and other Sleep related movement Disorders (1st edn.). Cambridge University Pres, NY, USA.
2. Guilleminault C, Kirisoglu C, Bao G, Arias V, Chan A, Li K (2005) Adult chronic Sleepwalking and its treatment based on polysomnography. Brain 128: 1062-1069.
3. Matwiyoff G, Lee-Chiong T (2010) Parasomnias: an overview. Indian J Med Res 131: 333-337.
4. Abad VC, Guilleminault C (2006) Sleep and psychiatry. Dialogues Clin Neurosci 7: 291-303.
5. Agargun MY, Kara H, Ozer OA, Selvi Y, Kıran U, Kıran S (2003b) Nightmares

and dissociative experiences: the key role of childhood traumatic events. Psychiatry Clin Neurosci 57: 139-145.

6. Kritchevsky M, Chang J, Squire LR (2004) Functional amnesia: clinical description and neuropsychological profile of 10 cases. Learning and Memory 11: 213-226.
7. Lowenstein RJ, Putnam FW (2007) Dissociative Disorder. Kaplan MD, Sadock BJ (eds.). Comprehensive textbook of psychiatry, 8 edtn, Solar Printing House, Ankara.
8. Foote B, Smolin Y, Kaplan M, Legatt ME, Lipschitz D (2006) Prevalence of dissociative Disorders in psychiatric outpatients. Am J Psychiatry 163: 623-629.
9. Agargun MY, Kara H, Ozer OA, Selvi Y, Kıran U, Ozer B (2003a) Clinical importance of nightmare disorder in patients with dissociative Disorders. Psychiatry Clin Neurosci 57: 575-579.
10. Aydın H (2009) 7. Psychiatric Disorders and Sleep ınternational biological psychiatry congress, Edirne, Turkey.
11. Steinberg M (1994) Structured clinical ınterview for dsm-ıv dissociative Disorders (SCID-D), Revised. Washington, DC, American Psychiatric Press.
12. Sar V, Tutkun H, Yargıc LI (1996) DSM-IV Structured opinion score for dissociative Disorders (scıd-d) english version. Clinical psychotherapy unit, Istanbul type faculty of psychiatry.
13. Carlson EB. Putnam FW. Ross CA (1993) Validity of the dissociative experiences scale in screening for multiple personality disorder: a multicenter study. Am J Psychiatry 150: 1030-1036.
14. Yargıc LI, Tutkun H, Sar V (1995) The reliability and validity of the Turkish version of the dissociative experiences Scale. Dissociation 8: 10-13.
15. Akdemir A, Turkcapar MH, Orsel SD, Demirergi N, Dag I, Ozbay ME (2001) Reliability and validity of the Turkish version of the hamilton depression rating scale. compr psychiatry 42: 161-165.
16. Kilinc S, Torun F (2011) Depression rating scales used in clinical practice in Turkey. Dirim Type Newspaper 86: 39-47.
17. Sar V, Ozturk E, Ikikardes E (2012) Validity and reliability of the Turkish version of childhood trauma questionnaire. Turkiye klinikleri J Med Sci 32: 1054-1063.
18. Aydemir O, Koroglu E (2007) Clinical factors used in psychiatry. 3 edtn, Hekimler yayin birligi, Ankara.
19. Kucukgoncu S, Aktar E, Erginbas E, Bestepe EE, Calikusu C, Algin F, Erkoc S(2010) Relationship between dissociative experiences, abnormal Sleep experiences, and Sleep quality in undergraduate students. Dusunen Adam 23: 77-84.
20. Schenck CH, Milner DM, Hurwitz TD, Bundlie SR, Mahowald MW (1989) Dissociative Disorders presenting as somnambulism: polysomnographic, video and clinical documentation (8 cases). Dissociation 4: 194-204.
21. Sar V, Akyuz G, Kundakci T, Kiziltan E, Dogan O (2004) Childhood trauma, dissociation, and psychiatric comorbidity in patients with conversion disorder. Am J Psychiatry 161: 2271-2276.
22. Aslan S, Yetkin S, Albayrak FS, Gulcat Z, Maral I, Aycan S, Sutcigil L, Özgen F, Aydin H (2005) Symptoms of hipersomnia are widespread in an urban area of Ankara. Klinik Psikiyatri 8: 172-179.
23. Lewis DO, Yeager CA, Swica Y, Pincus JH, Lewis M (1997) Objective documentation of child abuse and dissociation in 12 murderers with dissociative identity disorder. Am J Psychiatry.154: 1703-1710.
24. Isaaca M, Chand PK (2006) Dissociative Disorders and conversion Disorders: to define boundaries. Current Opinion in Psychiatry 19: 61-66.
25. Sar V (2011) Epidemiology of dissociative Disorders: An overview. Epidemiology research international 10: 1-8.
26. Nijenhuis ER, Van der Hart O (2011) Dissociation in trauma: a new definition and comparison with previous formulations. J trauma dissociation 12: 416-445.
27. Tuncel D, Orhan FO (2009) Parasomniler: tani, siniflama, klinik özellikleri. Current Approaches in Psychiatry 1:280-296.
28. Sar V (2006) The scope of dissociative Disorders: an international perspective. Psychiatr Clin N Am 29: 227-244.
29. Jaimchariyatam N, Rodriguez CL, Budur K (2011) Prevalence and correlates of alpha-delta Sleep in major depressive Disorders. Innov Clin Neurosci 8: 35-49.
30. Pelin Z, Karatas S, Kesebir S (2012) Jactatio corporis nocturna and dissociative disorder: a case report. Turkish J Psyc 23 :141-144.
31. Zadra A, Pilon M, Joncas S, Rompré S, Montplaisir J (2004) Analysis of postarousal EEG activity during somnambulistic episodes. J Sleep Res.13: 279-284.
32. Jaar O, Pilon M, Carrier J, Montplaisir J, Zadra A (2010) Analysis of slow-wave activity and slowwave oscillations prior to somnambulism. Sleep 33: 1511-1516.
33. Parrino L, Smerieri A, Rossi M, Terzano MG (2001) Relationship of slow and rapid EEG components of CAP to ASDA arousals in normal Sleep. Sleep 24: 881-885.

Reduced Apnea-Hypopnea Index in Patients with Severe Sleep Apnea Syndrome as Determined by Cervical Collar and Mandibular Advancement Device Combination Therapy

Florim Delijaj[1*], **Gustaf Levin**[2], **Eva Lindberg**[3] **and Eugen Wang**[4]

[1]*Department of Public Health and Caring Sciences (IFV), Uppsala Centre for Clinical Research Sormland (CKFD), Eskilstuna and Department of Primary Care, Tunafors Family Center, Sormland County Council, Sweden*

[2]*Department of Surgery, ENT Clinic in Eskilstuna, Sormland County Council, Sweden*

[3]*Department of Medical Sciences, Respiratory, Allergy and Sleep Research, Uppsala University, Sweden*

[4]*Department of Surgery Sciences, Uppsala University and Center for Clinical Research, Sormland, Uppsala University, Eskilstuna, Sweden*

[*]**Corresponding author:** Delijaj F, Department of Public Health and Caring Sciences (IFV), Uppsala Centre for Clinical Research Sormland (CKFD), Eskilstuna and Department of Primary Care, Tunafors Family Center, Sörmland County Council, Sweden, E-mail: Florim.Delijaj@dll.se

Abstract

Study Objectives: In patients with severe obstructive sleep apnea syndrome (OSAS), continuous positive airway pressure (CPAP) is first-line therapy. Compliance to CPAP is sometimes a problem, and mandibular advancement device (MAD) is then an alternative. However, this alternative is often not effective. It was hypothesized that patients suffering from OSAS would have a freer airway, resulting in a decreased apnea-hypopnea index (AHI), through use of a cervical collar (CC) to extend the neck. To study the effect of this new therapy, a randomized crossover study was conducted to compare MAD monotherapy with CC/MAD combination therapy.

Methods: Eight patients with severe OSAS (AHI>30) who had ceased to use CPAP were enrolled in the randomized crossover study. Four patients started with MAD and four with CC/MAD for one week followed by a wash-out period and then cross-over. Polygraphic sleep recordings were performed at baseline and after each therapy.

Results: The baseline AHI was 51.5 ± 22.5. AHI was reduced to 30.4 ± 23.2 through MAD monotherapy, and to 14.9 ± 10.2 through CC/MAD combination therapy. The effect of the combination therapy was statistically significantly ($p=0.018$) better than that of the monotherapy. Four patients were achieved an AHI<10/h through use of the combination therapy.

Concusions: The study showed a significant reduction in AHI scores in patients with severe OSAS through use of the CC/MAD combination therapy as compared to the MAD monotherapy. This first report indicates a new possibility for treating severe OSAS in non-compliant CPAP users.

Keywords: Cervical collar; CC/MAD combination therapy; Non-compliant CPAP users; Obstructive sleep apnea

Abbreviations AHI: Apnea-Hypopnea Index; CC: Cervical Collar; CPAP: Continuous Positive Airway Pressure; CMSC: Cervico Mandibular Support Collar; MAD: Mandibular Advancement Device; ODI: Oxygen Desaturation Index; OSAS: Obstructive Sleep Apnea Syndrome; ΔAHI: The difference in AHI

Introduction

Obstructive sleep apnea syndrome (OSAS) is a common disease in the adult population [1]. OSAS is also associated with increased risk for occupational and road accidents as a result of fatigue and daytime sleepiness [2,3]. Furthermore, patients with untreated moderate and severe OSAS run an increased risk of cardiovascular morbidity [4-6]. CPAP is the most effective treatment for patients with severe OSAS; however, 29%-83% of patients use CPAP for less than 4 hours a night due to the practical difficulties of using the CPAP device [7]. Wolkove et al. found significant problems with CPAP compliance in long-term treatment. Among 80 patients who participated in their study, 15% had abandoned CPAP after 10 months, and 31% never commenced therapy after the initial diagnosis [8]. Oral therapy such as use of a mandibular advancement device (MAD) has been shown to be an effective treatment for mild to moderate OSAS [9-11]. The main function of MAD is to protrude the mandible forward, causing the airway to remain open during sleep [9]. MAD therapy is also an alternative when patients reject CPAP or when CPAP is not tolerated for various reasons [12]; however, the effect is less powerful than that achieved with CPAP [13].

There are different causes of OSAS, and being overweight and sleeping in the supine position play significant roles. Obese patients show an increase in pharyngeal tissue, which constitutes an anatomical basis for respiratory obstruction during sleep [14]. The supine sleeping position generates mandibular retraction and tongue collapse, which have the same result [15]. Skinner et al. [16] compared the effectiveness of a cervicomandibular support collar (CMSC) with standard CPAP. The CMSC's function was to prevent downward displacement of the mandible as well as to maintain the head in slight extension during sleep. Their study could not demonstrate that the CMSC used as a single therapy was an effective treatment [16].

Finding a treatment to prevent collapse of the airway during sleep is an interest resulting from knowledge of conditions in the upper respiratory airway that is associated with OSAS. An important aspect is that extending the neck and pulling out the mandible reduce mechanical barriers in the upper airways. Our hypothesis was that patients suffering from severe OSAS would have a freer airway through use of a cervical collar (CC) to extend the neck. The knowledge that the function of MAD is to protrude the mandible forward, causing the airway to remain open during sleep, has led to the hypothesis that CC and MAD would have a synergistic effect. To study this effect with the CC, a pilot randomized crossover study was conducted to compare MAD monotherapy with CC/MAD combination therapy in patients with severe OSAS.

Materials and Methods

Ethics statement

This study was approved by the Stockholm Ethics Committee (2012/1084-31/4). The patients agreed to participate and gave their written informed consent. The patients received detailed information and were instructed to discontinue the treatment in the event of discomfort or other complications. They were informed they could cease participation whenever they wished.

Patients

Eight patients with severe OSAS were included in the study. They had all been prescribed CPAP therapy at the ENT clinic at the County Central Hospital (Malarsjukhuset) in Eskilstuna, Sweden but had ceased CPAP-treatment due to intolerance. The inclusion criteria were: severe OSAS (AHI>30/h), BMI less than 35, non-pregnant, and no medical history of whiplash, rheumatic disease, or osteoporosis. Patients with fibromyalgia, psychiatric and neurological disorders, and with alcohol and drug abuse problems as well as patients being treated with different kinds of sedative were also excluded. To identify the study population, a total of 166 patients who had failed follow-up during the last two years were contacted by telephone. Of these 166 patients, 131 still used their CPAP, 8 patients could not be reached, and 27 patients had ceased CPAP treatment due to discomfort (e.g., dry mouth or nose, runny nose, headache). Of these 27 patients, 16 agreed to be included in the study, and 12 (10 men and 2 women) met the inclusion criteria. Four patients dropped out at the onset of the study. Eight patients completed the study; all of them were men aged 56.1 ± 10.2 (mean ± SD).

Study design

Patients underwent a physical examination that included measurements of blood pressure, cardiac, nose-throat and thyroid status prior to the study. They were recorded using polygraphy to obtain baseline values for sleep-disordered breathing and to ensure that they still had an AHI of >30/h. Patients were then randomized into two groups: starting with MAD monotherapy or with combination CC/MAD therapy. Patients had to choose between two envelopes containing letter A or B. The devices (MAD or CC/MAD) were used for a period of one week until the patients felt comfortable with the treatment. Then each patient underwent full-night polygraphy. Patients could choose any sleep position they wished. After sleep registration, the patients slept without any treatment for at least one week (washout period). Then a crossover to the other treatment condition was made.

Mandibular advancement device (MAD)

Each patient received a MAD from a dental specialist at Malarsjukhuset in Eskilstuna. The MAD was individually adapted according to construction bites. The device was adjusted after a 1-month habituation period in patients with side effects.

Cervical collar (CC)

In our study, a neck collar (Vista CC) that already existed on the market was used, Figure 1. It is intended for indications of various diseases such as traumatic cervical injury, cervical disc herniation and other neck problems. The main reason we chose the Vista CC was its design, which allows adjustment of the elevation level to achieve sufficient effect, i.e., extending the neck. The CC has six height settings to choose from, and adjustment between them is easy. All patients were instructed to select the highest level for the CC during polygraphy.

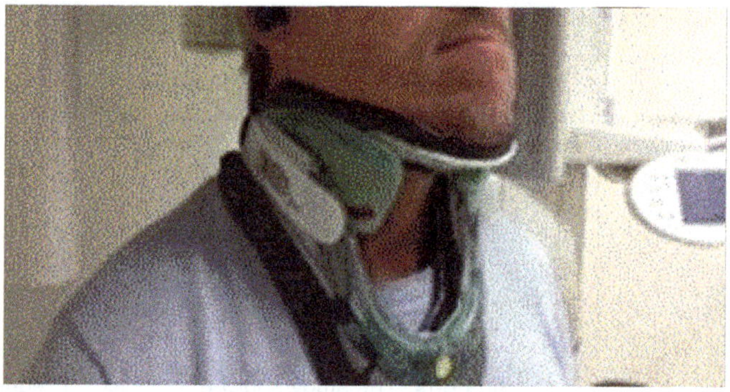

Figure 1: The neck collar (Vista CC) used in the study. CC were adjusted in the highest elevations level in combination with MAD, holding the mandible in a forward position. Anterolateral view.

Polygraphy

Polygraphy was performed in patients' homes with Embletta PDS recorder equipment (Medcare, Reykjavik, Iceland). RemLogic 3.2 analysis software (Embla Systems LLC, Thornston, CO) was used. All sleep recordings were evaluated and scored manually by the same experienced sleep technician. The patients filled in standardized questionnaires about sleep time (time of sleep onset and awakenings) and sleep quality. Sleep time was defined when the recording showed a continuous curve of smooth breathing in combination with non-body-movements or the presence of apnea/hypopnea. Apneas, hypopneas and desaturations were scored according to the criteria of the American Academy of Sleep Medicine [17]. Obstructive apnea was defined as a decrease in respiratory airflow of more than 90% for more than 10 seconds with preserved respiratory movement in the thoracic or abdominal wall. Hypopnea was defined as a reduction in nasal pressure signal of 50% or more from baseline for >10 sec in combination with an oxygen desaturation (OD) of >3% (4B Rule). OD was defined as a reduction in saturation of at least 3% from baseline.

AHI was defined as the total sum of apneas and hypopneas divided by registration/sleep time.

Analysis

Differences in baseline measurements between treatment groups were analyzed using t-tests. In the primary analysis, paired t-tests were used to test mean differences between MAD monotherapy and CC/MA combination therapy. To test for violation of the normal distribution assumption we used the Shapiro-Wilks test, with a p-value of 0.08 (MAD) and 0.10 (CC/MAD) respectively, indicating they both follow a normal distribution.

However, considering the small sample the Wilcoxon signed rank test was also used to test the difference between treatment periods. As is common, we set the significance level (α) generally at 0.05. That together with the small sample size (n=8), causes the power of the test to be fairly low.

The power of the t- test and the Wilcoxon signed rank test of no difference in AHI between MAD and MAD/CC was 0.23 and 0.20 respectively. The existence of a carryover effect was examined by conducting a t-test on the difference between treatment groups using measures from both treatment periods.

Results

Four patients started with MAD (Group A), and four started with CC/MAD (Group B). The characteristics of both groups were comparable. The demographic data are shown in Table 1. The mean of baseline AHI for both groups was more than 51; for four patients among them, AHI ranged from 57-96.

Variables	Group		p-value
	A	B	
Age	55.5 ± 2.9 (54-60)	56.7 ± 19.8 (38-72)	0.88
BMI	28.7± 3.7 (26.8-34.3)	28.8 ± 3.2 (24.4-32.1)	0.97
AHI	45.3 ± 16.4 (30.8-57.4)	57.5 ± 28.5 (36.1-96.7)	0.49
Data are presented as mean ± SD (range)			

Table 1: Demographic data and baseline values for AHI from the two randomized.

All eight patients completed both treatments. No severe adverse event was reported during the study. The outcome data for each patient are shown in Table 2.

Patient No	Random Type	Baseline	MAD	CC/MAD	
		AHI	AHI	AHI	ΔAHI
1	A	30.8	21.3	12.3	-9.0 (-18.5)
2	B	96.7	45.8	27.4	-18.4 (-69.3)
3	B	36 .1	7.7	8.2	0.5 (-27.9)
4	A	31.6	9.7	5.9	-3.8 (-25.7)
5	A	57.4	61.6	29.7	-31.9 (-27.7)
6	B	61.2	63.7	22.6	-41.1 (-38.6)
7	B	36.3	10.8	4.6	- 6.2 (-31.7)
8	A	61.6	22.8	8.1	-14.7 (-53.5)
Mean ± SD		51.5 ± 22.5	30.4 ± 23.2	14.9 ± 10.1	-15.5 ± 36.1 (-36.5 ± 79.8)
A= MAD monotherapy, B= CC/MAD combination therapy					

Table 2: AHI scores for each patient.

There was a clear reduction in mean AHI with CC/MAD combination therapy compared to MAD monotherapy (-15.5 ± 36.0) (p=0.018) and compared to baseline (-36.5 ± 79.8) (Figure 2). In two patients, AHI decreased to < 10/h with MAD monotherapy, and four patients achieved an AHI<10/h with the CC/MAD combination.

One patient's AHI was somewhat higher with CC/MAD than with MAD, but both values were <10/h. The greatest reduction in AHI (-69.3 index points) was shown in a patient with baseline AHI 96.7.

In case of violation of the normality assumption the t-test was complemented with the Wilcoxon signed ranks test for the difference in AHI between MAD and CC/MAD, which resulted in a p-value of 0.016.

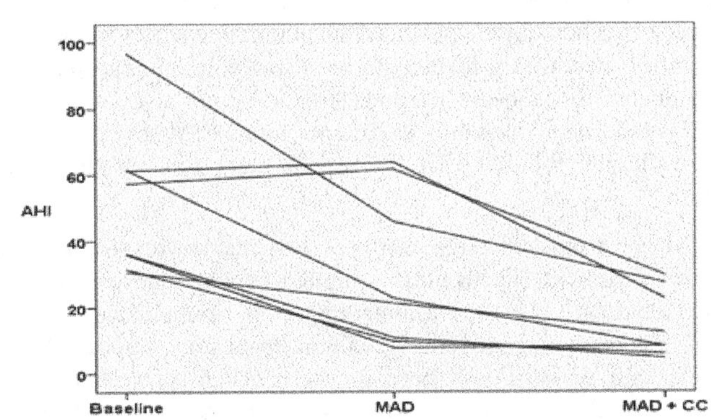

Figure 2: AHI score at baseline and after treatment with MAD and with MAD in combination with CC.

The baseline oxygen desaturation index (ODI) was 50.3. Table 3 shows that the mean ODI decreased significantly from 31.2 with MAD to 16.5 with CC/MAD (p=0.027).

The reduction patterns for ODI and AHI show approximately the same numerical trend. There was a clear reduction in AHI in both the supine and non-supine positions. Baseline AHI in the non-supine position was 34.4.

Supine sleep time was longer with CC/MAD compared to MAD and baseline (p=0.005). BMI did not change significantly between recordings. Average oxygen saturation showed small improvements with CC/MAD (p=0.957).

Polygraphy data	Baseline	MAD	CC/MAD	p-Value
Apnea + Hypopnea/h (AHI)	51.5 ± 22.5 (30.8-96.7)	30.4 ± 23.2 (7.7-63.7)	14.9 ± 10.1 (4.6-29.7)	0.018
Body mass index	28.5 ± 3.2 (24.4-34.3)	29.2 ± 4.8 (24.4-35.9)	29.3 ± 3.4 (25.0-35.9)	0.391
Oxygen Desaturation Index (ODI)	50.3 ± 22.6 (29.4-98.3)	31.2 ± 21.6 (9.7-57.6)	16.5 ± 12.9 (4.9-41.3)	0.027
Average Oxygen Saturation	89.6 ± 3.6 (82.6-94.7)	90.3 ± 2.5 (85.9-94.6)	90.8± 2.5 (87.8-94.9)	0.957
Total sleep time (min)	377 ± 38.5 (313-422)	427 ± 67.7 (332-504)	349 ± 43.8 (282-422)	0.006
Supine sleep time (%)	69.6 ± 35.8 (7.2-100)	62.8 ± 33.3 (14.7-94.5)	71.8 ± 28.9 (32.8-100)	0.005
AHI supine position	59.3 ± 18.3 (32.1-91.9)	46.6 ± 29.4 (7.5-82.9)	18.2 ± 11.2 (5.6-36.9)	0.009
AHI non-supine position	34.4 ± 36.0 (0.0 -102)	20.3 ± 18.8 (6.6-61.8)	2.9 ± 2.0 (0-5.5)	0.04
Data are presented as mean ± SD (range), n=8, age: mean 56.1 ± 10.1 (38-72). p-Value were analyzed using t-tests. (Wilcoxon signed ranks test for the difference in AHI between MAD and CC/MAD resulted in a p-value of 0.016).				

Table 3: The relevant values for recorded polygraphic data.

Discussion

The present study showed a significant reduction in AHI scores in adults with severe OSAS using CC/MAD combination therapy compared to using MAD monotherapy.

The difference was even greater compared to baseline AHI and ODI. Four patients were achieved an AHI<10/h using CC/MAD combination therapy. All patients were achieved an AHI<5/h when they sleep in a non-supine position in combination with CC/MAD. To confirm this hypothesis, further studies using polysomnography must be conducted to delineate sleep stages. Our study also showed that AHI was reduced significantly in patients with CC/MAD combination therapy, despite the fact that they spent more time in the supine position.

CPAP is the most effective treatment for patients with severe OSAS; however, treatment effectiveness is limited by compliance with long-term treatment [7,8,18]. Maintaining this compliance requires intensive education, motivational enhancement and support [19,20]. Patients with severe OSAS need to use CPAP to prevent the risks associated with the disease. MAD is an alternative to CPAP but unfortunately does not have the same effect in patients with severe OSAS [13]. MAD has the best effect in patients with mild to moderate OSAS [9-11]. Pharyngeal surgery is another option for treatment; however, long-term studies have shown suboptimal results. The surgery is also associated with some risk of side effects [21,22]. There is therefore a need for alternative forms of treatment for patients with severe OSAS who cannot use CPAP.

As far as we know, our study is the first to investigate the effect of neck extension in combination with MAD. We found that the treatment was effective in reducing AHI and ODI in patients with severe OSAS. The strength of this study includes its randomized crossover design, which offers more data than a study performed with a limited number of patients. However, there are a number of limitations to this pilot study that should be considered. Most importantly, all recordings were performed with polygraphy, and sleeping time could therefore only be estimated by the manual evaluation of sleep by sleep technicians and standardized questionnaires. In addition, hypopneas were defined according to the AASM scoring rules 2007 that have later been updated. However, identical scoring rules were used before and after each treatment period. CC/MAD may cause discomfort, which could reduce sleep time and thus the AHI. However, the AHI for polygraphy in this study was based on recording times obtained while patients slept. Another limitation of the study is the small number patients, although we did perform extensive data analysis for each patient. Given that the present investigation is based on eight patients, it should be considered a pilot study. A larger, randomized, and placebo-controlled multicenter study is therefore warranted. Gender is also an issue, as the present study included only male participants. This is related to the way we identified our patients. There were no women who met our inclusion criteria.

Our results showed a significant reduction in AHI scores in adults with severe OSAS after using CC/MAD combination therapy for one week. To confirm the patients' compliance with long-term treatment using this concept, follow-ups will be carried out. The Vista CC was not made specifically for treating patients with OSAS, and construction could therefore be optimized.

Skinner et al. [16] compared the effectiveness of a cervicomandibular support collar (CMSC) with standard CPAP. Their study did not demonstrate that CMSC was an effective treatment. We believe that the Vista collar that was used in the present study provides higher elevation of the head than the CMSC does, thus enabling freer airways. Another possibility is that a cervical collar is only effective in the combination with MAD.

We have not found any similar previous studies, though many have tested different positioning methods. Head extension using a CC provides more space in the upper airway. The MAD moves the mandible forward, and the CC provides an additional effect by closing the mouth and thus increasing the degree of protrusion. This increases the airway space between the tongue and the posterior pharyngeal wall.

In conclusion, the present randomized crossover pilot study showed a significant reduction in AHI in patients with severe OSAS through the use of CC/MAD combination therapy as compared to MAD monotherapy. Although the study has several limitations, this first promising report may lead to new therapy using a CC for this group of patients-patients with severe OSAS who are difficult to treat owing to non-compliance with CPAP therapy. Further studies are needed to confirm the benefits of this new CC/MAD combination therapy and also CC treatment as monotherapy for OSAS cases of varying severity.

Conflict of Interest

The authors declare no financial support or other benefit that could be interpreted as a conflict of interest.

Acknowledgments

This study was supported by the Research and Development Center, Sormland County Council, Sweden. We are thankful to Fredrik Granstrom for his contribution to the statistical analysis and to Ronnie Jonsson for his work as sleep technician at the Department of Clinical Physiology MSE, including his scoring of the sleep recordings.

References

1. Peppard PE, Young T, Barnet JH, Palta M, Hagen EW, et al. (2013) Increased prevalence of sleep-disordered breathing in adults. Am J Epidemiol 177: 1006-1014.
2. Lindberg E, Carter N, Gislason T, Janson C (2001) Role of snoring and daytime sleepiness in occupational accidents. Am J Respir Crit Care Med 164: 2031-2035.
3. Horstmann S, Hess CW, Bassetti C, Gugger M, Mathis J (2000) Sleepiness-related accidents in sleep apnea patients. Sleep 23: 383-389.
4. Peker Y, Hedner J, Norum J, Kraiczi H, Carlson J (2002) Increased incidence of cardiovascular disease in middle-aged men with obstructive sleep apnea: a 7-year follow-up. Am J Respir Crit Care Med 166: 159-165.
5. Yaggi HK, Concato J, Kernan WN, Lichtman JH, Brass LM, et al. (2005) Obstructive sleep apnea as a risk factor for stroke and death. N Engl J Med 353: 2034-2041.
6. Wang X, Ouyang Y, Wang Z, Zhao G, Liu L, et al. (2013) Obstructive sleep apnea and risk of cardiovascular disease and all-cause mortality: a meta-analysis of prospective cohort studies. Int J Cardiol 169: 207-214.
7. Richard W, Venker J, den Herder C, Kox D, van den Berg B, et al. (2007) Acceptance and long-term compliance of nCPAP in obstructive sleep apnea. Eur Arch Otorhinolaryngol 264: 1081-1086.
8. Wolkove N, Baltzan M, Kamel H, Dabrusin R, Palayew M (2008) Long-term compliance with continuous positive airway pressure in patients with obstructive sleep apnea. Can Respir J 15: 365-369.
9. Doff MHJ, Hoekema A, Wijkstra PJ, van der Hoeven JH, Huddleston Slater JJR, et al. (2013) Oral appliance versus continuous positive airway pressure in obstructive sleep apnea syndrome: a 2-year follow-up. Sleep 36:1289-1296.
10. Rose EC, Barthlen GM, Staats R, Jonas IE (2002) Therapeutic efficacy of an oral appliance in the treatment of obstructive sleep apnea: a 2-year follow-up. Am J Orthod Dentofacial Orthop 121: 273-279.
11. Marklund M, Sahlin C, Stenlund H, Persson M, Franklin KA (2001) Mandibular advancement device in patients with obstructive sleep apnea : long-term effects on apnea and sleep. Chest 120: 162-169.
12. Lavigne GJ, Goulet JP, Zuconni M, Morrison F, Lobbezoo F (1999) Sleep disorders and the dental patient: an overview. Oral Surg Oral Med Oral Pathol Oral Radiol Endod 88: 257-272.
13. Okuno K, Sato K, Arisaka T, Hosohama K, Gotoh M, et al. (2014) The effect of oral appliances that advanced the mandible forward and limited mouth opening in patients with obstructive sleep apnea: a systematic review and meta-analysis of randomised controlled trials. J Oral Rehabil 41: 542-554.
14. Schwab RJ, Kim C, Bagchi S, Keenan BT, Comyn FL, et al. (2015) Understanding the anatomic basis for obstructive sleep apnea syndrome in adolescents. Am J Respir Crit Care Med 191: 1295-1309.
15. Farronato G, Storti E, Cuzzocrea ML, Lucchese A, Cossellu G, et al. (2013) Three-dimensional changes of the upper airway in patients with obstructive sleep apnea syndrome after a non-adjustable oral appliance treatment. Minerva Stomatol 62: 107-116.
16. Skinner MA, Kingshott RN, Jones DR, Taylor DR (2004) Lack of efficacy for a cervicomandibular support collar in the management of obstructive sleep apnea. Chest 125: 118-126.
17. Iber C, Ancoli-Israel S, Chesson A, Quan S (2007) The AASM manual for the scoring of sleep and associated events: rules, terminology and technical specifications.
18. McArdle N, Devereux G, Heidarnejad H, Engleman HM, Mackay TW, et al. (1999) Long-term use of CPAP therapy for sleep apnea/hypopnea syndrome. Am J Respir Crit Care Med 159: 1108-1114.
19. Bahammam AS, Alassiri SS, Al-Adab AH, Alsadhan IM, Altheyab AM, et al. (2015) Long-term compliance with continuous positive airway pressure in Saudi patients with obstructive sleep apnea. A prospective cohort study. Saudi Med J 36: 911-919.
20. Lai AYK, Fong DYT, Lam JCM, Weaver TE, Ip MSM (2014) The efficacy of a brief motivational enhancement education program on CPAP adherence in OSA: a randomized controlled trial. Chest 146: 600-610.
21. Hultcrantz E, Johansson K, Bengtson H (1999) The effect of uvulopalatopharyngoplasty without tonsillectomy using local anaesthesia: a prospective long-term follow-up. J Laryngol Otol 113: 542-547.
22. Esclamado RM, Glenn MG, McCulloch TM, Cummings CW (1989) Perioperative complications and risk factors in the surgical treatment of obstructive sleep apnea syndrome. The Laryngoscope 99: 1125-1129.

Revision of Estimation Method for an Established Morphometric Model for Prediction of Obstructive Sleep Apnea

Oommen Nainan[1]*, Jayan B[2], Chopra SS[3] and Mukherjee M[4]

[1]Graded Specialist-Orthodontics & Dentofacial Orthopedics, Naval Institute of Dental Sciences, India
[2]Department of Dental Surgery, Armed Forces Medical College, India
[3]Classified Specialist-Orthodontics & Dentofacial Orthopedics, Corps Dental Unit, India
[4]Classified Specialist-Periodontology, Military Dental centre, India

Abstract

Background: The morphometric model (MM) provides a rapid, accurate and reproducible method for predicting whether patients in an ambulatory setting are at risk for obstructive sleep apnea (OSA).

Introduction: The aim of this study was to estimate mean MM scores in a mixed Indian population and to test a revision of the method for making intraoral measurements.

Methods: A total of 60 subjects were included in the study and were divided into two groups of 30 subjects each; Group 1: Patient group; Group 2: Control group. A comparative cross-sectional study design was employed and MM value as suggested by Kushida was estimated by applying their clinical rule. The measurements in our study were made on study models to ensure precise and accurate measurement of these anatomic distances, thus ensuring a greater accuracy for the morphometric model.

Results: The comparison of morphometric model values between OSA and non OSA groups showed an extremely statistically significant difference. The average predictive morphometric model value for OSA in this sample of Indian patients is only slightly lesser than that observed by Kushida

Conclusions: The results of this study could facilitate the early recognition of OSA and support the available diagnostic setup. This revised methodology may be used to widen the reach of the morphometric model from the sleep physician's clinic to the Dental operatory.

Keywords: Obstructive sleep apnea; Morphometric model; Polysomnography; Predictors; Clinical rule

Introduction

Obstructive sleep apnea (OSA) is characterized by repetitive obstruction of the upper airway during sleep, resulting in oxygen desaturation and sleep fragmentation. Even though OSA is fairly common, it often remains undiagnosed in primary care practice. While overnight polysomnography (PSG) is considered the 'gold standard' for the diagnosis of OSA, the need for accurate, quantitative diagnostic criteria is further compounded by the significant cost incurred with routine PSG. However, the lack of a simple, non-invasive, repeatable method has been an obstacle for the early recognition of OSA patients. The limited number of sleep laboratories available restricts the proper identification of OSA and may lead to underestimation of the magnitude of the problem and under-treatment, with undesirable public and personal health consequences.

Common symptoms of the condition have limited predictive value in identifying patients with OSA [1]. The morphometric model is a useful screening test to investigate the possibility of OSA in patients during initial office visits. The most commonly used predictive model is the morphometric model given of the Stanford Sleep Disorders Clinic and Research Centre, California (hereafter referred to as the Stanford Morphometric Model-SMM), which provides a rapid, accurate and reproducible method for predicting whether patients in an ambulatory setting are at risk for OSA [2]. This clinical morphometric model combines measurements of the oral cavity with body mass index and neck circumference and was tested on Caucasian patients, where it was found that patients with values equal to or more than 70, typically had OSA. There is no data available on the applicability of the predictive model to Indian subjects.

The key step in the management of OSA is to firmly establish the diagnosis. The Dental Practitioner in general and the Orthodontist in particular, now has an ever increasing role in the recognition of a patient who may be at risk for a sleep disorder. We carried out a pilot study with the aim of estimating mean SMM scores in a mixed Indian population. The method used in the original study by Kushida for intra-oral measurements, was found to be subjective and difficult to standardize for a group. A revision of the method for making intraoral measurements was also tested with an objective to provide increased usefulness to clinicians tackling this significant disorder, in many countries. The results of this study could facilitate the early recognition of OSA and support the available diagnostic setup. Based on the intra oral findings, orthodontists may request a polysomnographic evaluation when OSA is suspected and the final diagnosis of sleep disorder, its severity and the evaluation of comorbidities are made by a physician according to polysomnographic findings.

***Corresponding author:** Oommen Nainan, Graded Specialist-Orthodontics & Dentofacial Orthopedics, Naval Institute Of Dental Sciences, INHS Asvini Campus, Colaba, Mumbai 400005, Maharashtra, India;
E-mail: droommennainan@yahoo.in

Material and Methods

This multi-disciplinary study was undertaken at the Division of Orthodontics and Dentofacial Orthopedics, Armed Forces Medical College, Pune, India. The research protocols were reviewed and approved by the Institutional Ethical Committee of the hospital. Informed consent under witness was obtained from each participant at enrollment after each subject was explained the nature and purpose of the study. To detect a clinically significant difference with 80% power, α=0.05 and a ratio between two groups of 1:1, 60 adult Indians aged 18 years and above were recruited for this study [3]. A comparative cross-sectional study design was employed. The total of 60 subjects included in the study was divided into two groups of 30 subjects each; Group 1: Patient (test) group; Group 2: Control group.

The patient sample (test group) consisted of 30 randomly selected PSG diagnosed OSA patients referred by the Department of Respiratory Medicine, Military Hospital, Cardio-Thoracic Centre, Pune, India, for the analysis of craniofacial morphology. PSG performed was level I, using a 16-channel polygraph (Sleep Scan Analysis VISION, Bio-logic Systems Corp, USA). For the purpose of this study, only one variable- the number of apneas and hypopneas was utilized. There was no prior knowledge of the patient to be seen and there was no regular pattern of days to examine the patients. For the test group, the patients who satisfied the following criterion were included in the study: age - 18 years and above; polysomnographic evidence of OSA (defined as an apnea/hypopnea index (AHI) of $\geq$ 5/hour of sleep) and the presence of at least ten teeth in each arch. AHIs were calculated using using the "recommended" (AHI_{Rec}) AASM hypopnea scoring criteria. Apnoea was defined as cessation of airflow for atleast 10 seconds with oxygen desaturation of more than 3%. Hypopnoea was defined as a reduction of 30% or greater in airflow from baseline for more than 10 seconds with associated drop in oxygen saturation of 4% or more and arousal as per the recommendations of American Academy of Sleep Medicine Task Force, 2001.

The control group consisted of 30 randomly selected adults attending the dental outpatient department, with an Angle's Class I molar relation and no history of sleep obstructed breathing. The control group was matched with the patient sample to the best extent possible for age, gender, height and weight. For the control group, the subjects who satisfied the following criterion were included in the study: age - 18 years and above; subjects with Angle's Class I occlusion, Epworth Sleepiness Scale (ESS) score <9 (to exclude daytime sleepiness); no reported snoring by family members and the presence of at least ten teeth in each arch. Snoring frequency, snoring intensity and ESS was used as a questionnaire for selection of subjects in the control group.

The exclusion criteria for both groups were: edentulous subjects; subjects with hypothyroidism; subjects with history of orthodontic treatment; subjects with history of reconstructive/orthognathic surgery; subjects with craniofacial deformity, such as cleft lip and / or palate; subjects with history of pharyngeal surgery and subjects with patient-specific disorders (such as neuromuscular disorders).

Each of the groups consisted of 19 men and 11 women. Data collection was divided into three sections as follows:

a. Medical and sleep history including an ESS.

b. Clinical examination with anthropomorphic recordings of the subject's height, weight and neck circumference. Neck circumference (NC) in centimetres, was measured with a tape measure, at the level of the cricothyroid cartilage in upright awake subjects. For each subject, obesity was expressed as body mass index (BMI) [4].

c. Study model analysis: Measurements were taken from the maxillary and mandibular study models using a pair of digital callipers (Workzone, Global tronics GmbH & Co, Germany), with a resolution of 0.01 mm.

Upper and lower dental arch study models were obtained with alginate dental impression material and dental stone. The following measurements were recorded on the study models [2,5]. All the measurements were carried out by the principal investigator.

1. Maxillary intermolar width [Mx]: Distance between the mesiobuccal cusp tips of the crowns of the maxillary right and left permanent first molars (Figure 1).
2. Mandibular intermolar width I [Mn]: Distance between the mesiobuccal cusp tips of the crowns of the mandibular right and left permanent first molars (Figure 2).
3. Overjet [OJ]: Horizontal overlap of the crowns of the maxillary and mandibular central incisors, in millimetres.
4. Palatal height [P]: To standardize measurement of palatal depth/ height, models were trimmed until the distal contact point of the upper first molars showed up on the edge. Distance from the mid-deepest part of the palate to the line connecting the left and right distolingual cusp tips of the upper first molars was taken as palatal depth (Figure 3).

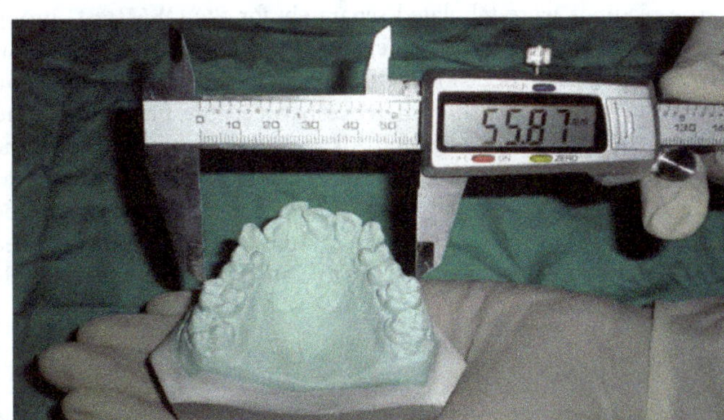

Figure 1: Measurement of maxillary intermolar width on study model.

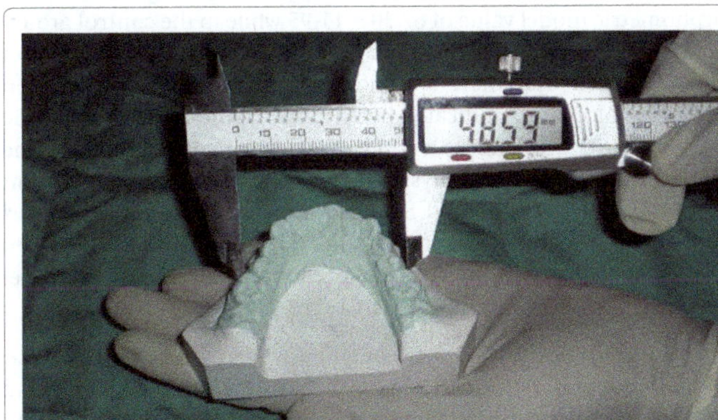

Figure 2: Measurement on mandibular intermolar width on study model.

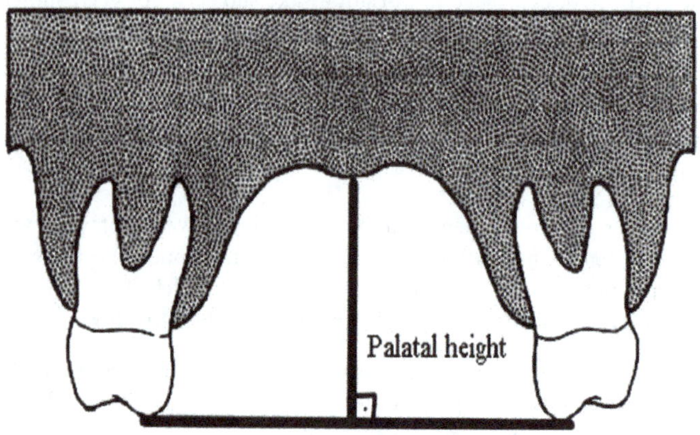

Figure 3: Measurement of palatal height/depth.

SMM score was calculated by applying the clinical rule as follows:

P+ (Mx-Mn) + 3 x OJ + 3 x (BMI – 25,0) x (NC / BMI)

where P=palatal height in millimeters, NC=neck circumference in centimetres, measured at the level of cricothyroid membrane, Mx=distance between the mesial surfaces of the crowns of the maxillary molars in millimetres, MN=distance between the mesial surfaces of the crowns of the mandibular molars in millimeters, OJ=overjet, horizontal overlap of the crowns of the maxillary and mandibular central incisors in millimeters, BMI=body mass index (kg/m^2).

Data compilation and statistical analysis

The readings were tabulated separately for the OSA (test) group and control group. The measurement of 20 randomly selected casts was repeated on separate occasions with a 2-week interval, for evaluation of intra-operator error. The difference between the first and second measurements was not significant. All measurements obtained in the study were expressed as mean ± standard deviation (SD). The data was analysed using MATLAB version 1.0 and Excel 2007. To determine the correlation between OSA severity as indicated by apnea/hypopnea index [AHI] and Stanford morphometric model, linear and multiple regression models were applied.

Results

Stanford morphometric model values were calculated for all the subjects. The comparison of morphometric model values between OSA and non OSA groups showed an extremely statistically significant difference (P<0.0001) with the OSA group having an average morphometric model value of 67.30 ± 11.95 while in the control group, it was 55.43 ± 7.80, as shown in Table 1. The results of the regression analysis showed that there was no significant correlation between the severity of OSA as indicated by AHI and Stanford morphometric model value in this sample of Indian OSA patients (Table 1). The results of the regression analysis indicate that there is no significant correlation between AHI and Stanford morphometric model in this sample of Indian OSA patients. The line diagram for the distribution of patient's AHI versus the calculated Stanford morphometric model value is depicted graphically in Chart 1.

The average age was 53.6 ± 9.42 years. While the two groups had no significant difference in terms of height, the OSA patients were found to be significantly heavier than control subjects with a resulting statistically significant increase in BMI (P<0.05), as shown in Table 2. The patients in the test group also had a statistically significant increase in neck circumference (P<0.05), when compared to the controls. The neck circumference in the test group ranged from 34 to 45 cms with an average of 41.11 ± 2.05 cms for men and 37.55 ± 3.53 cms for women. Table 2 presents the mean of general physical examination measurements of the two groups. All patients in the test group had varying degree of OSA, as confirmed by overnight polysomnography and symptoms of snoring and excessive daytime sleepiness. OSA severity was defined by the AHI. The AHI ranged from 5.6 per hour to 86.4 per hour with an average of 42.04 ± 26.14 events per hour. In the test group, the ESS recorded a statistically significant increase (P<0.05) and ranged from 9 to 20 with an average of 13 ± 2.85 events per hour.

The comparison of mean intraoral values between OSA and controls is summarised in Table 3. Overjet was found to be larger in the controls when compared with the OSA sample, but analyses failed to detect

S No	Parameter	Patients with OSA (Test Group) (n=30)	Patients without OSA (Control Group) (n=30)	P value (<0.05)
1	Age,yrs	53.6 ± 9.42	53.6 ± 9.422	—
2	ESS score	13 (± 2.85)	3.26 (± 0.94)	<0.0001*
3	Weight,kg	80.10 (± 12.5)	67.13 (± 6.78)	<0.0001*
4	Height,mtrs	1.64 (± 0.01)	1.64 (± 0.09)	1
5	Body Mass Index, kg/m2	29.47 (± 4.57)	24.84 (± 1.87)	<0.0001*
6	Neck Circumference, cm	39.80 (± 3.16)	36.10 (± 2.59)	<0.0001*
7	Maxillary intermolar distance, mm	53.05 (± 3.57)	51.58 (± 3.26)	<0.01*
8	Mandibular intermolar distance, mm	46.51 (± 3.93)	44.48 (± 2.87)	0.208
9	Palatal Height, mm	24.1 (± 1.74)	20.75 (± 2.01)	<0.05*
10	Overjet,mm	1.97 (± 1.92)	2.80 (± 1.76)	0.086
11	AHI, events/hr	42.04 (± 26.14)		
12	Morphometric Model Value	67.30 (± 11.95)	55.43 (± 7.80)	<0.0001*
13	Corelation between AHI & SMM			0.209

Table 1: Comparison of Study Group Characteristics & Correlation Between Smm Values & Ahi.

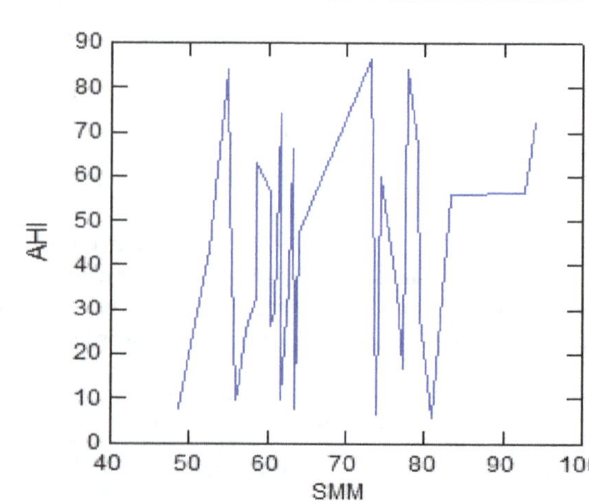

Chart 1: Line Diagram For The Distribution of Patient's Ahi Versus Calculated Stanford Morphometric Model Values.

S no	Parameter	Test Group (n=30)		Control Group (n=30)		df (n-1)	P value (<0.05)
		Mean	SD	Mean	SD		
1	Ht in mtrs	1.64	0.01	1.642	0.09	29	1
2	Wt in kgs	80.1	12.5	67.13	6.78	29	<0.0001*
3	BMI(kg/m^2)	29.47	4.57	24.84	1.87	29	<0.0001*
4	NC in cms	39.8	3.16	36.1	2.59	29	<0.0001*
5	ESS	13	2.85	3.26	0.94	29	<0.0001*
6	AHI	42.04	26.14			29	

Ht - height; Wt - weight; BMI - body mass index; NC - neck circumference; ESS - Epworth sleepiness scale; AHI - apnoea hypopnoea index.
*P ≤ 0.05 = statistically significant.

Table 2: Comparison of Mean of General Physical Characteristics between Test and Control Groups.

S no	Parameter	Test Group (n=30)		Control Group (n=30)		df (n-1)	Regression coefficient	P value (<0.05)	R value (<0.01)
		MEAN	SD	MEAN	SD				
	Column 1	Column 2	Column 3	Column 4	Column 5	Column 6	Column 7	Column 8	Column 9
1	Mx	53.05	3.57	51.58	3.26	29	0.061	<0.05*	<0.01**
2	Mn	46.51	3.93	44.48	2.87	29	-1.875	0.208	≥ 0.01
3	OJ	1.97	1.92	2.8	1.76	29	0.06	0.086	≥ 0.01
4	P	24.1	1.74	20.75	2.01	29	0.043	<0.05*	<0.01**

Mx - maxillary intermolar width; Mn - mandibular intermolar width; OJ - overjet;
P - depth of palate;
*P ≤ 0.05 = statistically significant.
**R < 0.01 = statistically significant.

Table 3: Comparison of Mean of Intraoral Measurements between Test and Control Groups.

statistically significant differences (P>0.05). Statistically significant differences were found between the groups for the measurements of palatal height/ depth (P<0.05).

Discussion

Different clinical prediction rules have been described in the literature. Scientists have used various factors to predict a person's risk of having OSA, based on their demographics, symptoms and body-mass index. Using these factors, scientists have been able to correctly identify 76% to 96% of patients who have OSA and 13% to 54% of patients who do not have OSA [6]. A comprehensive comparative effectiveness review carried out by the U.S. Department of Health and Human Services has concluded that of the available models, the morphometric model by Kushida gave near perfect discrimination between OSA and non-OSA subjects [7].

Sleep problems are common among primary care patients. A study conducted in an Indian population estimated the prevalence of sleep-disordered breathing (SDB) among middle-aged urban Indian men to be at 19.5% and that of obstructive sleep apnea-hypopnea syndrome (SDB with excessive daytime sleepiness), to be 7.5% [8]. Many studies have been done assessing craniofacial characteristics in OSA patients using cephalometrics, computed tomography, magnetic resonance imaging and acoustic reflection. Although there is controversy in the results, craniofacial alterations most closely related to the occurrence and severity of OSA are: retroposition of the maxilla, shortening of the mandibular body, inferiorly displaced hyoid bone, retrognatism, dental occlusion class II and narrow, arched hard palate [9,10].

No data are available on the applicability of the predictive SMM in patients with OSA from the Indian subcontinent and a Medline search confirms that this is the first study evaluating the correlation between SMM values and the severity of OSA, from this country. There has been only one previous Indian study in which a diagnostic model was derived and validated for the prediction of OSA in subjects presenting with non-sleep-related complaints [11]. The results of our study indicate that the relatively easier morphometric measurements afforded by the SMM enable faster screening for OSA in a primary health care setting. Other studies worldwide have also validated the applicability of SMM in identifying OSA in clinical practice, with the separation value between subjects with or without OSA being 70 [12,13].

An important aspect in medical research is to understand and improve existing measurement frameworks and methodology. In the original study, measurements were made in the mouth. The measurements in our study were made on study models to ensure precise and accurate measurement of these anatomic distances, thus ensuring a greater accuracy for the morphometric model. Plaster study models were used for the intraoral measurements in this study, since they are a standard component of orthodontic records and they are fundamental to diagnosis and treatment planning, case presentations, evaluation of treatment progress and results, besides record keeping [14]. The dental arch dimensions were measured on study models made of dental stone, by means of digital vernier callipers. Compared to dividers, studies have shown that by using sliding manual/digital vernier callipers, accurate measurements could be made from the study models in all three dimensions [15]. Although some new methods like geometric morphometrics provide excellent possibilities for morphological analysis, distance measurements on dental casts were calculated because most dental practitioners are familiar with the method used in this study.

On comparing the SMM values in this pilot study, we have been able to demonstrate statistically significant differences between the two groups. The comparison of morphometric model values between OSA and non-OSA groups showed a highly statistically significant difference, with the OSA group having an average SMM value of 67.30 while in the control group, it was 55.43. The average morphometric model value in this sample of Indian OSA patients is only slightly lesser than that observed by Kushida who found that patients with values equal to or more than 70, typically had OSA [2]. The fact that the populations under study in our group and in the study by Kushida, belong to different origins (Indian and North-Americans) and that there was no standardization to account for ethnicity may explain the differences between both studies.

The method used by Kushida and in subsequent studies for measurement of palatal depth was found to be subjective and difficult to standardize for a large group. The palatal height as suggested in the study by Kushida was measured with the tongue in a relaxed position and the maxillary and mandibular incisor tips subtending an angle of 20 degrees from the mandibular condyle. A new method for measurement of palatal depth was resorted to, because it is difficult to measure palatal depth with 20 degrees mouth opening and from the dome of the tongue in all cases. In order to standardize the measurement of palatal depth in this study, the study models were trimmed until the distal contact point of the upper first molars showed up on the edge. Distance from the mid-deepest part of the palate to the line connecting the left and right distolingual cusp tips of the upper first molars was taken as palatal depth. In the present study, statistically significant differences were found between the two groups for the measurements of palatal height/depth ($P<0.05$) with the mean palatal depth in patients being greater than the mean palatal depth of the controls.

The minimum age of the subjects in this study was chosen on the basis of previous studies which have reported that molar and canine arch widths do not change after 13 years of age in females and 16 years of age in males [16]. Therefore, it was assumed that the arch widths of the subjects studied were fully developed. The strength of the present study is the inclusion of a relatively large group of Indian patients with OSA, who underwent a limited hospital-based sleep study, matched with control subjects for age and gender. This study highlights the importance of matching subjects for age to prevent any age-related morphological changes from confounding the results.

Study Limitations

This is a cross-sectional study based on enrolment of patients attending one hospital clinic. As expected, the patients in this study only represent at best the patients attending this clinic. Further research is necessary to generalise the results to the general population and other ethnicities. Another limitation of this study was that PSG was not carried out for the controls, due to ethical considerations and the prohibitive expense of the procedure. This is usually the case with studies incorporating normal controls who do not exhibit any symptoms of OSA.

Conclusion

1. The SMM proposed by Kushida is applicable to this selected sample in clinical practice.
2. The average predictive morphometric model value for OSA in this sample of Indian patients is slightly lesser than that observed by Kushida.
3. The revised approach for making intraoral measurements was tested and validated in this case study, performed in a real and mature measurement framework.

Our immediate objectives were to better formalize the use of the morphometric model by restructuring existing measurement frameworks and to augment the existing approach. This revised methodology may be used to widen the reach of the morphometric model from the sleep physician's clinic to the dental operatory.

References

1. Hoffstein V, Szalai JP (1993) Predictive value of clinical features in diagnosing obstructive sleep apnoea. Sleep 16: 118-122.
2. Kushida CA, Efron B, Guilleminault C (1997) A predictive morphometric model for the obstructive sleep apnoea syndrome. Ann Intern Med 127: 581-587.
3. Dupont WD, Plummer WD (1997) PS power and sample size program available for free on the internet. Controlled Clin Trials 18: 274
4. Revicki DA, Israel RG (1986) Relationship between body mass indices and measures of body adiposity. Am J Public Health 176: 992-994.
5. Sayin MO, Turkkahraman H (2004) Comparison of dental arch and alveolar widths of patients with Class II division 1 malocclusion and subjects with Class I ideal occlusion. Angle Orthod 74: 356-360.
6. Lee RW, Chan AS, Grunstein RR, Cistulli PA (2009) Craniofacial phenotyping in obstructive sleep apne--a novel quantitative photographic approach. Sleep 32: 37-45.
7. Ethan M Balk, Denish Moorthy, Ndidiamaka Obadan (2011) Diagnosis and treatment of obstructive sleep apnea in adults. Agency for Healthcare Research and Quality.
8. Udwadia ZF, Doshi AV, Lonkar SG, Singh CI (2004) Prevalence of sleep-disordered breathing and sleep apnea in middle-aged urban Indian men. Am J Respir Crit Care Med 169: 168-173.
9. Lowe AA, Santamaria JD, Fleetham JA, Price C (1986) Facial morphology and obstructive sleep apnea. Am J Orthod Dentofac Orthop 90: 484-491.
10. Jayan B, Prasad BNBM, Kotwal A, Kharbanda OP, Chowdhury SKR, et al. (2007) The role of cephalometric analysis in obese and non obese urban Indian adults with obstructive sleep apnea syndrome: A Pilot Study. Indian J Sleep Med 2: 59-63.
11. Sharma SK, Malik V, Vasudev C, Banga A, Mohan A, et al. (2006) Prediction of obstructive sleep apnea in patients presenting to a tertiary care center. Sleep Breath 10: 147-154.
12. Soares MC, de Azeredo Bittencourt LR, Zonato AL, Gregorio LC (2006) Application of the Kushida morphometric model in patients with sleep-disordered breathing. Bras J Otorrinolaringol 72: 541-548.
13. Jung DG, Cho HY, Grunstein RR, Yee B (2004) Predictive value of Kushida Index and acoustic pharyngometry for the evaluation of upper airway in subjects with or without obstructive sleep apnea. J Korean Med Sci 19: 662-667.
14. Santoro M, Galkin S, Teredesai M, Nicolay OF, Cangialosi TJ (2003) Comparison of measurements made on digital and plaster models. Am J Orthod Dento facial Orthop 124: 101-115.
15. Singh SP, Goyal A (2006) Mesiodistal crown dimensions of the permanent dentition in North Indian children. J Indian Soc Pedod Prev Dent 24: 192-196.
16. Knott VB (1972) Longitudinal study of dental arch widths at four stages of dentition. Angle Orthod 42: 387-394.

Self-Management Techniques for Excessive Daytime Sleepiness Used by Participants in a Narcolepsy Advocacy Group

Lois E Krahn[1*] **and Eve R Rogers**[2]

[1]*Sleep Medicine, Mayo Clinic Arizona, Phoenix, Arizona, USA*

[2]*Sleep Medicine, Columbus, Ohio, USA*

***Corresponding author:** Lois E Krahn, Sleep Medicine, Mayo Clinic Arizona, Phoenix AZ, United States, E-mail: Krahn.Lois@Mayo.edu

Abstract

Study objectives: Excessive daytime sleepiness (EDS) interferes with functioning and causes distress for narcoleptic patients. Self-management techniques are believed to an important part of a comprehensive treatment plan for patients with narcolepsy. Relatively little is known about how behavioral tactics are perceived and which techniques are used more often. This study examined behavioral techniques used for EDS in a non-clinical sample.

Methods: A survey developed by the authors listing 16 different possible behavioral tactics plus write in options was distributed at a national Narcolepsy Network conference.

Results: Data were analyzed for 44 respondents who self-identified as having narcolepsy. Walking around a room was the most commonly used tactic identified by 73% of respondents. Napping ranked second, with scheduled and unplanned naps endorsed to the same degree. Talking, fidgeting and eating tied for third most cited. On a visual analog scale 0-10 with 10 high, the absolute effectiveness of behavioral techniques were rated as 7.2 and effectiveness relative to optimized prescription medication was lower at 5.3. Only 66% of respondents recalled ever having been counseled by a health care provider to try self-management techniques.

Conclusions: Walking around and naps were identified as the most used self-management options. Respondents viewed behavioral techniques to have moderate value. Relatively few participants recalled being encouraged by health care providers to supplement prescription approaches with self-management strategies. Healthcare providers need more familiarity with behavioral techniques for managing excessive daytime sleepiness so they can counsel patients to explore these interventions.

Keywords: Narcolepsy; Sleepiness; Hypersomnolence; Behavioral techniques

Introduction

Self-management techniques, increasingly an area of focus within health care, have not been examined closely for patients with excessive daytime sleepiness (EDS). EDS is an omnipresent symptom of narcolepsy that can limit functioning and cause distress. Especially prior to the diagnosis of a specific sleep disorder, sleepy persons experiment with behavioral tactics to cope symptoms. After diagnosis many persons employ self-management techniques to augment other therapies in the context of a multimodal treatment plan.

Relatively little information is available regarding how patients view self-management techniques for managing excessive daytime sleepiness. After interviewing 20 patients Rogers listed behavioral approaches that patients utilized to cope with EDS and cataplexy [1]. Her 1984 paper does not report which tactics are more commonly utilized. Garma and Marchand in 1994 studied patients with narcolepsy who returned for follow-up after deciding to discontinue stimulant medications. This study found that, because they preferred to rely on napping, 6 of these 13 patients stopped medications [2]. In their 2007 review of behavioral techniques of narcolepsy Broughton and Murray commented that patients sought to avoid hypnogenic situations, specifically sedentary behaviors, boredom, overly warm situations and slow rhythmic stimulation. Consciously increasing stimulation was described as "very effective" with examples of patients preferring to stand rather than sit, move about as much as possible, increase background noise, seek a cooler environment, and go outside to a more stimulating environment [3]. Several trials have produced data that scheduled naps are efficacious in reducing EDS [4,5]. Little is known about how persons with EDS attributed to narcolepsy rank specific tactics relative to one another or compared with medications.

This study was designed to solicit data regarding the participants' perception of behavioral techniques. A non-clinical population was targeted to reach people who use self-management techniques in addition to or potentially in place of medical interventions. Questions were designed to investigate the frequency that an individual used various techniques and a global assessment of the usefulness of behavioral interventions in the management of EDS associated with narcolepsy.

Methods

This study was approved by the Institutional Review Board of the Mayo Clinic. The authors developed a survey titled "The effectiveness of self-management strategies used to manage excessive daytime sleepiness associated with narcolepsy". Respondents were presented with a list of 16 self-management techniques used for EDS. The 16 tactics were selected based on information gathered from patients with narcolepsy in the course of clinical practice as well as the published reports by Rogers, Garam and Broughton [1-3]. In addition the survey included multiple spaces for the respondents to write in additional behavioral tools and comments. Three additional questions utilizing a visual analogue scale (VAS) addressed the global value of behavioral techniques and whether health providers had discussed the potential role of non-pharmacologic tactics. The survey was distributed in a hard copy format at the annual meeting of the Narcolepsy Network, a national patient advocacy organization formed in 1984. Self-reported demographic and clinical data included demographics and basic disease characteristics. Participants who self-identified as having narcolepsy were asked to provide their age at the onset of symptoms, age of diagnosis and whether they had cataplexy. Respondents indicated their implied consent to participate by returning a completed form. Data was analyzed looking at the frequency each tactic was endorsed for self-management of EDS.

Results

The study group consisted of 44 respondents who self-identified as having narcolepsy. The respondents were 66% female, with an average age of 45 (range 19-89). The mean age of onset of narcoleptic symptoms was 17 years (range 7-60) and mean age of diagnosis age 32 years (range 17-65). Twenty-nine (66%) participants had narcolepsy associated with cataplexy. There was no statistically significant difference between respondents with and without cataplexy in the survey results. A response rate to the survey cannot be calculated since the number of attendees diagnosed with narcolepsy is not tracked. Narcolepsy Network conferences draw persons with narcolepsy as well as family members, friends and healthcare professionals.

	Rank Order	Frequency	Percentage Endorsed (%)
Walking around	1	33	75
Naps, scheduled	2	31	70
Naps, unscheduled	2	31	70
Talking to Someone	3	28	64
Fidgeting	3	28	64
Eating	3	28	64
Exercise (working out)	4	27	61
Listening to upbeat music	4	25	57
Drinking a cold beverage (not caffeine or alcohol)	5	23	52
Caffeinated beverage	6	20	46
Blast of cold air	7	18	41
Hot bath/shower	8	16	36
Smoking tobacco	8	5	11
Caffeine pills	9	3	7

Table 1: Behavioral techniques most often used for ED.

All respondents identified multiple techniques with a mean of 7 different tactics per respondent (range 3-13). Table 1 displays the survey data concerning preferred behavioral techniques.

The most highly endorsed tactic was physical exertion in the form of simply walking around. The second most frequently noted was napping. Respondents endorsed relying on planned naps as often as unscheduled naps. Several respondents wrote in comments that their work or school schedule prevented them from napping as much as they would like.

Working out and listening to upbeat music, tactics that represent increased stimulation, all fell in the mid-range. Caffeinated beverages were ranked considerably higher than caffeine in a pill or other formulation. No respondent endorsed nicotine in either a smokeless or other formulation i.e. transdermal nicotine. Using stimulating substances like tobacco and caffeine pills were least used of inventory of tactics. Several respondents commented that the resulting heightened alertness was too transient to be of benefit.

Overall no differences were observed based on age or gender, although there was a trend that younger patients utilized music (possibly with a convenient device like a MP3 player) more than older ones. No respondent identified simply a single technique; all endorsed a variety of tactics. Respondents wrote in a variety of additional techniques as listed in Table 2.

Keeping a regular sleep schedule
Pinching
Utilizing self-hypnosis
Massaging
Tickling
Utilizing biofeedback
Avoiding anti-inflammatory foods
Knitting
Listening to books on tape while driving
Yelling at self
Splashing water on face

Table 2: Other tactics written in by respondents.

Only 29 (66%) respondents could recall ever discussing behavioral techniques with a health provider. The VAS (0 never, 10 frequently) measuring how often health care providers had encouraged use of self-management techniques generated a mean of 3.8. Participants also provided a global impression of the effectiveness of behavioral techniques yielding a mean score of 7.2 on the VAS.

Details were not collected concerning current or past prescription medications used by the respondents. The complexity of multiple possible medications, varying doses, polypharmacy and long duration of therapy meant that collecting this information and correlating it with the behavioral techniques was deemed impractical. Nearly all respondents were currently using prescription medications for their narcoleptic symptoms and they were asked to compare their experience of the effectiveness of medications with behavioral tactics in general using the VAS. The mean VAS score was 5.3 when asked to compare a global impression of behavioral tactics relative to optimized prescription medications. Several participants commented that behavioral techniques were previously of greater importance prior to starting sodium oxybate.

Discussion

A wide variety of behavioral tactics were endorsed as useful for the management of EDS in this population. Physical activity in the form of walking around was the most cited tactic. This finding supports Broughton and Murray's observations that narcoleptic patients rely on physical stimulation to manage symptoms. These data indicate that persons with narcolepsy dealing with EDS use physical activity to address EDS with napping as a second choice. Standing up and walking around in a work or school environment may be more socially acceptable and convenient than taking a nap. Several factors including employment or school schedule likely dictate how often a person can manage EDS with napping. One respondent commented that once retired he could at last take scheduled naps making this self-management tactic more feasible. Conceivably patients select a specific behavioral technique based on their circumstances. Which raises a key question - can time be taken for a planned nap? These data suggest that the respondents' circumstances more often were conducive to walking around.

Respondents commented that they valued behavioral techniques as a means to augment prescription medication. The degree to which self-management tactics could allow for reductions in medication dose or extend the dosing intervals is not known. Having confidence in a variety of coping strategies may enhance a patient's sense of control over EDS and increase self-esteem. Accordingly patients should be encouraged to try behavioral tactics as part of a comprehensive treatment [6]. However, in order to counsel patients adequately, health care providers must have familiarity with self-management techniques [3].

This study had several shortcomings. The diagnosis of narcolepsy was based on patient self-report. In the interest of keeping the survey brief, specific data about the prescription agents, doses, and duration of prescription medication use was not collected. Comparing various medications, combinations of agents, doses and dosing intervals was impractical. Data are not available to compare the efficacy of specific behavioral techniques to specific prescription medications. Numerous patients volunteered that self-management techniques had relatively more value before they were started on medications, specifically sodium oxybate. The survey did not seek to assess if particular techniques were favored in any particular setting or time of day.

The study design solicited input concerning behavioral techniques for EDS with the assumption that subjects had already awakened for the day and were struggling to optimize alertness. The questions did not seek to address the scenario where a patient is regaining alertness after the primary nocturnal sleep episode or a nap. Different tools, such as alarm clocks and vibrating devices, may be used in this setting. Hot showers and baths were included in this survey although when endorsed by respondents it was unclear if these were utilized to prevent drowsiness or regain alertness.

Conclusions

This project sought to solicit the perception of persons who identify as having narcolepsy regarding self-management techniques for EDS. Walking around and naps were identified as the most commonly used self-management options. Relatively few patients recalled being encouraged by health care providers to supplement prescription approaches with self-management strategies. Subsequent investigations should be undertaken to generate more data about the relative efficacy, timing and application so that these techniques can be optimized for persons with narcolepsy.

Acknowledgement

The authors wish to thank the leaders and members of the Narcolepsy Network for their interest and invaluable assistance with this study.

References

1. Rogers AE (1984) Problems and coping strategies identified by narcoleptic patients. J Neurosurg Nurs 16: 326-334.
2. Garma L, Marchand F (1994) Non-pharmacological approaches to the treatment of narcolepsy. Sleep 17: S97-102.
3. Broughton RJ, Murray BJ (2006) The Behavioral Management of Narcolepsy. In: Bassetti C, Billiard M, Mignot E (eds.) Narcolepsy and Hypersomnia. New York: Informa Healthcare.
4. Guilleminault C, Stoohs R, Clerk A (1993) Daytime somnolence: therapeutic approaches. Neurophysiol Clin 23: 23-33.
5. Mullington J, Broughton R (1993) Scheduled naps in the management of daytime sleepiness in narcolepsy-cataplexy. Sleep 16: 444-456.
6. Krahn LE, Hershner S, Loeding LD, Maski KP, Rifkin DI, et al. (2015) Quality measures for the care of patients with narcolepsy. J Clin Sleep Med 11: 335.

18

Short Blue Light Pulses (30 Min.) in the Morning are Able to Phase Advance the Rhythm of Melatonin in a Home Setting

Geerdink M[1*], Beersma DGM[1], Hommes V[2] and Gordijn MCM[1,3]

[1]*Department of Chronobiology, GeLifes, University of Groningen, The Netherlands*

[2]*Philips Consumer Lifestyle, Drachten, The Netherlands*

[3]*Chrono@Work B.V., Groningen, The Netherlands*

[*]**Corresponding author:** Geerdink M, Department of Chronobiology, GeLifes, University of Groningen, The Netherlands, E-mail: m.geerdink@rug.nl

Abstract

It is known that light in the morning is able to induce phase advances of the endogenous clock, however most studies have tested the phase advances in highly controlled laboratory conditions. At home the environmental lighting is more variable. In theory, a high intensity short morning-light pulse in the short-wavelengths-range (blue light) should be capable of inducing phase advances. If this is also true in a home setting, this could be a firm basis supporting light treatment in late chronotypes who suffer from a late sleep phase. In a study carried out in summer, 11 normal to relatively late (habitual midsleep 4:15-6:09 hours) chronotypes (age range 23-27 years, 4f/7m) participated in two conditions: (1) 1 baseline day followed by 3 consecutive days of 30 min. blue morning-light pulses, (2) 1 baseline day followed by 3 consecutive days of 60 min. blue light pulses. Blue light was applied by use of the Philips GoLite BLU (HF3320, blue leds, intensity at the cornea 2306 melanopic-lux, 300 lux, 3.65 W/m^2). During all four evenings, subjects were asked to protect themselves from light exposure (<10 lux). The response of the melatonin rhythm, calculated as a shift in dim light melatonin onset (DLMO), to a single 30 min. light pulse varied between subjects and resulted in a non-significant phase advance of 15 (±48) min. (t10 = 1.04; P = 0.33), and a significant advance of 30 (±41) min. to a single 60 min. light pulse. (t10 = 2.40; P < 0.05). After 3 days of light exposure both in the 30- and in the 60 min. light pulses condition significant phase advances of DLMO were observed; 49 (±58) min. (t10 = 2.80; P < 0.05) and 59 (±29) min. (t10 = 6.9; P < 0.001) respectively. No significant differences were found in the DLMO shifts between conditions. In addition there was a trend for a lower sleepiness score directly after waking up after using light for 3 days in both conditions (t10 = 3.38; P = 0.096, 60 min. and (t10 = 4.10; P = 0.070, 30 min.). A prelimin.ary analysis of actimetry data indicated some support for an effect on sleep timin.g. The data support the conclusion that light pulses of 30 min. in the morning on three consecutive days, in a home setting, in combination with dim light during the evenings, can be part of an efficient phase advancing chronotherapy protocol.

Keywords: Blue light; Home-setting; Melatonin; Phase advance; Light therapy; Late chronotypes; Sleep

Introduction

In humans, the endogenous clock, located in the Suprachiasmatic Nuclei (SCN) in the hypothalamus, is responsible for generating oscillations with a period of approximately 24 hours in physiological, behavioural and psychological variables. In order to keep these circadian rhythms entrained to the natural alternation of light and darkness, this clock needs to be synchronized daily.

Light is the main synchronizer, also called 'Zeitgeber', for entrainment of our clock; the exposure of light induces phase shifts of our clock resulting in either a delaying (biological rhythms shift to a later clock time with light exposure in the evening) or advancing (biological rhythms shift to an earlier clock time with light exposure in the morning) direction [1,2]. Since light is a potent Zeitgeber, the use of light therapy to treat circadian rhythm sleep disorders is a potentially effective treatment [3-5]. However, most studies have tested the phase shifting effects of light in highly controlled laboratory conditions. At home, the situation is completely different.

Subjects are exposed to a highly variable environment with large fluctuations in daytime light exposure, natural light exposure in the sleeping room etc. The current study was set up to test whether short pulses of light in the morning, in such a highly varying environment, are able to induce significant phase advancing shifts of circadian rhythms within 1-3 days to make it useful to treat late timing of biological clocks and sleep phases.

The sleep-wake cycle in humans is one of the rhythms that show a clear 24h pattern; the generation of this 24-rhythm is partly under control of the biological clock [6-8]. If exposed to a regular light-dark cycle, the sleep-wake cycle will be entrained; in other words, sleep would occur at the same phase of the light-dark cycle each day.

In reality, sleeping out of phase with the external light-dark cycle, especially sleeping late, is very common in our civilized society and is related to health problems [9-12]. A large number of people may therefore benefit from a correction of their clock and sleep timing. Because light is so effective in phase shifting the clock, it is often proposed as the most effective method to advance a late sleep phase [3-5]. However there is no general accepted protocol for the optimization of light therapy.

There are several factors that are important in optimizing light therapy. One is, like the correct timing of light. Phase response curves (PRC's) have been measured to quantify the induced phase shift of the biological clock as a function of the time at which the subject is exposed to light. The most complete phase response curve (PRC) in humans has been published by Khalsa and colleagues [13]. The authors found the maximum phase advance when applying the center of a long 6.7-hour light pulse 9 hours after the start of the rise of melatonin, also known as the 'dim light melatonin onset' (DLMO). In a laboratory study of St. Hilaire and coworkers [14] a PRC with a hour white light pulse was tested. The results revealed that also for pulses of 1 hour the largest phase advances are found when timing the center of the light pulse around 9 hours after DLMO.

The intensity and duration of light exposure are other important factors in optimizing light therapy; both these factors contribute in a non-linear, dose dependent manner to the magnitude of a phase shift [15]. Constructed a dose response curve for light intensity with long (5 hours) light pulses. They found that high intensity full spectrum white light doses (9500 lux) generated the largest phase shifts.

Under these conditions, saturation of the logistic regression curve occurred already at one tenth (1000 lux) of the intensity of a maximum dose. This dose still generated a phase shift of 90% of the maximum. Under natural circumstances people are not dark adapted and they may need higher light intensities to show similar phase shifts.

The dose response curve for the duration of a light pulse is also not linear. The 1h light pulses in the study of St. Hilaire et al. [16] in humans elicited a maximal phase advance of 1.2h, which is 44% of the response of 2.7h generated by the 6.7h light exposure in the study of Khalsa et al. [13]. Such dimin.ishing responses to extended stimulation are considered the result of adaptation processes; therefore the beginning of a light pulse is most important for the phase shifting effects [17].

In addition to timing, intensity and duration, a fourth important factor that can be used to optimize light therapy are the spectral characteristics of the light source. There is accumulating evidence that both light-induced phase shifts-as well as the suppression of melatonin-are most sensitive to light with short wavelengths: 440-490 nm, or blue light [18-23]. This sensitivity to blue light is due to the protein melanopsin, located in the "intrinsically photosensitive retinal ganglion cells" (ipRGC's) [24,25]. This photopigment is most reactive to ~480 nm light [25-27].

In a recent study, a comparison was made between the PRC obtained by Khalsa and colleagues [13] to 6.7h full spectrum white light with the PRC to blue light pulses (monochromatic 480 nm light) of similar duration (6.5) [28]. Although the blue light pulse contained only 0.4% of the energy of the full spectrum white light pulse, no significant differences could be found in the magnitude of the phase shifts.

Since blue light is very effective in shifting our circadian system, it may potentially decrease the intensity and duration of light therapy needed for an optimal effect and therefore improve therapy compliance, and final treatment success.

Therefore the hypothesis of this study is, whether optimally timed, short light pulses of 30 min. per day with a high blue photon density, applied by the subjects themselves at home, are able to shift the circadian rhythm of melatonin. If so, it can be an effective tool in the treatment of a delayed biological clock and sleep phase.

Material and Methods

Subjects

Subjects were recruited from the student population of the University of Groningen, the Netherlands, via newspaper- and internet advertisements. Thirteen healthy subjects (seven men and six women, mean age (±SD) 23.9 ± 1.9 years) were selected and completed the protocol. During the analysis, two subjects were excluded due to non-compliance and possible improper timing of the light pulses as a consequence; analysis is performed on 11 subjects (4f/7m, mean age (±SD) 24.1y ± 1.6y, range age 23-27y).

Selection of subjects was based on the following criteria: Subjects had to be healthy without suffering from depressed mood (Beck Depression Inventory-II, Dutch version, (BDI-II_NL) < 8; [29,30], did not report sleep disturbances, were non-smokers, did not consume too many drinks with caffeine (no more than 8 units per day) or alcohol (no more than 10 units per week), did not work in night shifts, did not cross more than two time zones in the preceding three months and were not colour blind (tested with an Ishihara colour blindness test). Female subjects were only included if they were using hormonal contraceptives. Chronotype was determined using the habitual mean midsleep (hMS, this is the clock time at the midpoint between sleep onset and sleep end), based on 7 days of data weighted for day of the week (Munich Chronotype Questionnaire (MCTQ)) [31].

Subjects were selected if their habitual midsleep was between 4:15 and 6:09 hours, indicating normal to moderately late chronotype for the age category of 20-30 years (based on the MCTQ 2008 NL database, Gordijn et al. unpublished) [17]. This selection was on the premise that inducing possible phase advances of endogenous rhythms and sleep would be more advantageous for relatively late people. The average hMS in the selected subjects in this study was (±SD) 5:00 ±35 min. All subjects were Dutch citizens from birth and fluent in Dutch. All subjects gave written informed consent and were compensated for their participation. The experimental protocol was approved by the Medical Ethics Committee of the University Medical Center Groningen.

Melatonin profiling day

In order to estimate the optimal timing of the blue light pulses, the experiment started with a 'melatonin profiling day' in our human time isolation facility centre, Groningen (NL). Subjects arrived 10 hours before their habitual midsleep and left 5 hours after their habitual midsleep (used as an individual reference time). They collected a total number of twelve saliva samples in dim light (<10 lux) during the evening or in darkness during short moments of awakening in the night and early morning. Saliva was collected by chewing on a cotton swab (Salivette®, Sarstedt BV, Etten-Leur, NL).

At least 1 ml. of saliva per sample was collected every hour during the time subjects were awake and every two hours during scheduled sleep time. The saliva samples were centrifuged and frozen at -80°C for further analysis. Melatonin concentration was assessed by radioimmunoassay (RK-DSM; Bühlmann Laboratories, Alere Health, Tilburg, The Netherlands). The inter assay variance was 11.3% for the low concentrations and 12.2% for the high concentrations. The intra assay variance was 10.7% for the low concentrations and 10.0% for the high concentrations.

A bimodal skewed baseline cosine function was fitted through the individual data points [32]. The maximum value of the fitted curve of each individual was set at 100% and used to normalize each curve. Dim Light Melatonin Onset (DLMO) was calculated as the moment at which the melatonin rhythm crosses the 25% value of this fitted maximum by linearly interpolating the raw values preceding and following the 25% value. The average DLMO time on the melatonin profiling day was 22:20 (±0:15 SEM).

Experimental design

Subjects participated in two experimental conditions in a random order: a 30 min.ute and a 60 min.ute blue light pulse condition. The first experimental condition started at least one and not more than 2 weeks after the 'melatonin profiling day'. This allowed for full recovery from the sleep interruptions during that day. Each condition consisted of 4 consecutive days, starting with 1 baseline evening/night followed by 3 mornings with light pulses (Figure 1).

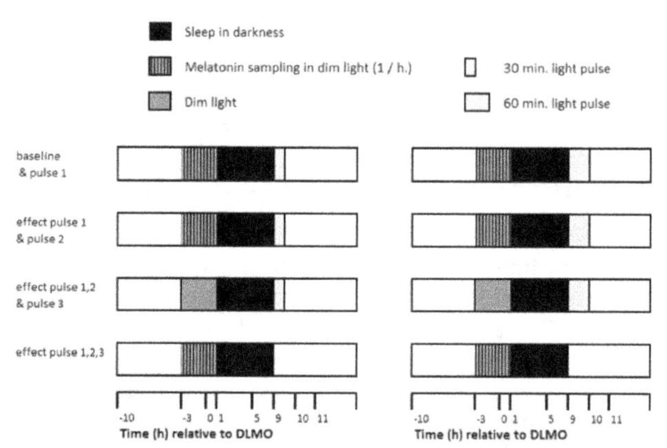

Figure 1: Schedule of the experimental design (melatonin profile day is not shown). The 2 experimental weeks are shown by the columns. Experimental days of an experimental week are indicated by bars. An experimental week consisted of 1 baseline day and 3 test days with 3 light pulses.

There was at least 1 week and not more than 2 weeks of no interventions in between conditions. All light pulses and measurements were conducted at home. During the week prior to each condition, subjects were asked to schedule their sleep according to their habitual sleep timin.g. This was checked with actigraphy and data from 8 subjects was available. During the week before starting the experiment hMS was on average (±SD) 2 min. (±13) earlier than the hMS calculated from the MCTQ questionnaire.

From these data it seems fair to conclude that the participants had consistent sleep habits prior to the start of the experiment. During each experimental condition, subjects received instructions when to go to sleep, when to stay in dim light and how and when they had to expose themselves to the blue light pulses. Sleep timing during the experimental weeks was adjusted to the timing of the light pulses in order to allow for 8 hours of sleep (Figure 1). Effect of the light pulses on the melatonin rhythm was measured by analyzing saliva samples collected after 1 pulse i.e., on the 2nd evening and after 3 pulses i.e., on the 4th evening and compared to melatonin pattern at the baseline evening i.e., 1st evening. During these evenings, subjects were required to collect the saliva samples themselves (Figure 1, starting at -3 and ending +1 hours relative to DLMO calculated from the melatonin profiling day) in dim light (<10 lux).

This resulted in 5 samples per evening. Subjects were asked to write down the exact timing of each saliva sample collection; no single timing point deviated more than 5 min. from the time point in the instructions. Subjects already knew how to collect saliva, because they had prior experience during the melatonin profiling day in the lab. At home, they were instructed to stay in dim light starting one hour prior to the first sample, and not change posture 5 min. prior to and during collection of the sample. They were not allowed to drink anything else than water, nor to eat during the sampling period, starting one hour prior to the first sample. They were instructed to rinse their mouth 15 min. prior to each sample.

Light exposure

Subjects were asked to expose themselves to either the 30 min. or 60 min. high intensity blue light pulses by sitting in front of the GoLite Blu lamp with an angle of 45° (Philips GoLite BLU HF3330, peak transmission at 470 nm, intensity at the cornea 2306 (m (elanopic)-lux (See Lucas et al. [33] for an explanation of the unit 'm-lux'), 300 lux, 3.65 W/m^2)) during 3 consecutive mornings. Light exposure was scheduled 9h after DLMO (Figure 1), as determin.ed from the melatonin profiling day. Because the average DLMO time on the melatonin profiling day was 22:20 (±0:15 SEM), light exposure started at 07:20 (±0:15 SEM) on average.

During all four evenings of each condition, including the one evening without saliva collection, subjects were asked to stay in dim light (<10 lux).

Rest-activity and light measurements

In order to quantify the timing and quality of the 24 hours profile of rest and activity, subjects wore an activity monitor, called Actiwatch® (AW2, Philips/Respironics, Fypro, Geffen, NL), on the non-domin.ant wrist during the experimental weeks. The AW2 is an activity-recording device that measures wrist movements to quantify the rest-activity cycle and it records environmental light exposure. The device has the appearance and the weight of a watch (without a clock). Subjects were asked to wear the AW2 all day and night.

While analyzing the data of all 13 subjects, we carefully inspected the sleep offset times of the AW2 data. We excluded 2 individuals who did not wake up within one hour of the instructed wake-up time. We concluded that these subjects did not comply with the instructions, and could not have had their light exposure at the proper time.

In addition, to measure properly light exposure and to be able to check for compliance of the light treatment the subjects wore either a Lightwatcher (Object Tracker, Vienna, Austria) or a Daysimeter (Lumen Tech Innovations, New York, USA). Unfortunately, because of failure of devices, the differences between devices and the way of wearing the devices, a complete data analysis of environmental light exposure in a quantitative way was not succesful.

In those cases where we could analyze whether subjects received a light pulse at the proper time, compliance was 100% in the 60-min. light pulse condition (10 subjects) and on average 87% in the 30-min. light pulse condition (1 pulse could not be recognized in 4 out of 7 subjects). Since this was a within study and compliance in the observed data was 100% in the 60-min. condition, it was concluded that the missing pulses in the 30 min. condition were most likely due to not wearing the device in the proper direction, more than that subjects did not obey the rules.

Questionnaires

Each morning of the experimental days, subjects were asked to complete a sleep diary. The diary consisted of a list of questions about sleep timin.g, sleepiness and sleep quality. Subjects rated their sleep quality with marks (from 0 = Very bad to 10 = Excellent). Subjective ratings of sleepiness were scored with the Karolinska sleepiness scale (KSS) (Akerstedt and Gillberg, 1990). Ratings on the KSS range from 1 to 9, with 1 meaning very alert and 9 meaning very sleepy. Subjects had to rate their sleepiness immediately after waking up and after the experimental light exposure.

Statistical analysis

For the differences in timing of DLMO, sleep onset, sleep offset, sleepiness and sleep quality between conditions, a repeated-measures ANOVA was used with one factor for condition (2 levels; 30 min. and 60 min.) and one factor for the number of pulses (4 levels; 0-3). If the factor 'condition' or the interaction of 'condition *pulses' was significant, a 'simple contrasts' test (equal to a paired sample T-test) was included to the ANOVA to see how many pulses were needed to see significant differences between conditions.

The conditions were also tested separately for the effects of the number of pulses. This was done with a repeated-measures ANOVA with one factor for the number of pulses and 'simple contrast tests' were used to compare the number of pulses to zero pulses (baseline day). The significance level was defined as p = 0.05. All parameters were tested two-tailed.

Results

DLMO shifts

The salivary melatonin level rose in the evenings of all three nights in the two conditions (Figure 2). The 25% level of the maximum fitted value (definition of DLMO, see methods) is indicated by the black horizontal lines. The median DLMO times in the condition with 30 min. light pulses were 23:02h (baseline day i.e., 0 pulses), 22:47h (2nd day i.e., after 1 light pulse) and 22:24h (4th day i.e., after 3 light pulses). The median DLMO times in the condition with the 60 min. light pulses were 23:23h (0 pulses), 22:50h (after 1 light pulse) and 22:08h (after 3 light pulses). See also Figures 2A and 2B.

Exposure to one 30 min. light pulse, actually timed 8.4 (SD 1.2) hours after baseline DLMO the night before, did result in a non-significant phase advance of the melatonin rhythm of 15 (±15 min. SEM) (t10 = 1.04; P =0.33). Exposure to one 60 min. light pulse, timed 8.2 (SD 0.8) hours after baseline DLMO the night before, resulted in a significant phase advance of 30 (±12 min. SEM) (t10 = 2.40; P < 0.05).

The actual timing of the first light pulses in the 30 min. blue light pulse condition and the 60 min. blue light pulse condition, although both a bit earlier than the scheduled 9h after DLMO, did not significantly differ from each other (t = 0.90; df = 10; P = 0.39). After 3 days of light exposure both 60- and 30 min. light pulses were able to elicit significant phase advances of the melatonin rhythm; a phase advance of 49 (±17 min. SEM) (t10 = 2.80; P < 0.05) resulted from exposure to three 30 min.

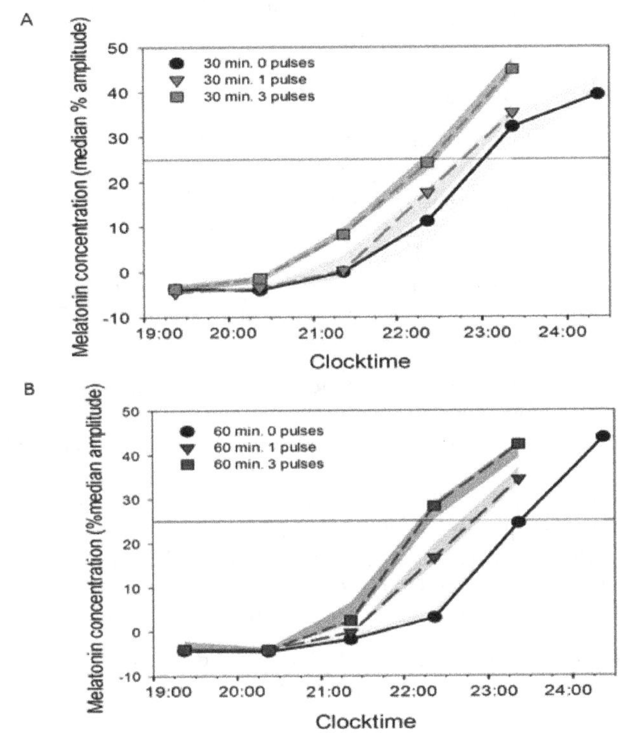

Figure 2: The ascending part of the melatonin curve during three different nights. The 25% of the amplitude is indicated by the horizontal black lines. A: 30-min. light pulse condition. B: 60 min. light pulse condition. Symbols represent the median values within the groups. Shaded areas represent the 45-55% percentile intervals.

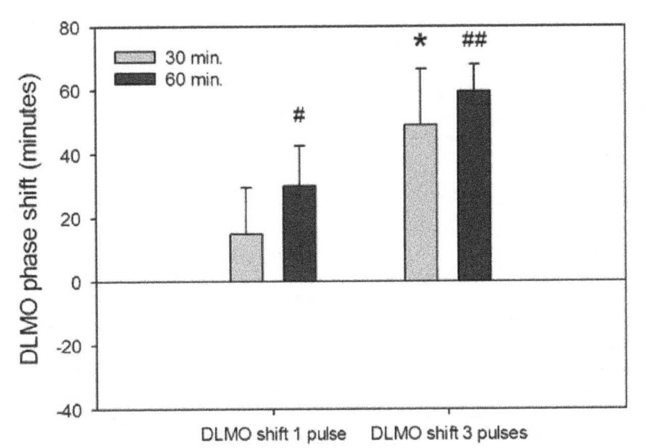

Figure 3: The shift in DLMO in min. on day 2, i.e., after one light pulse and on day 4, i.e., after three light pulses compared to baseline. Positive values mean phase advances, negative delays. Significant shifts are indicated by $^{*\#}$P < 0.05; $^{\#\#}$P < 0.001.

light pulses and a phase advance of 59 (±8.7 min. SEM) (t10 = 6.9; P < 0.001) from exposure to three 60 min. light pulses (Figure 3). Interestingly, no significant differences were found between the DLMO shifts after 30 min. light pulses and 60 min. light pulses: neither the shifts after one pulse ($F_{1,10}$ = 0.96; P = 0.35) nor after three consecutive days with light pulses ($F_{1,10}$ = 0.291; P = 0.65) were found to be significantly different from each other (Figure 3).

Sleepiness patterns over the week

In order to see possible differences in the decline in sleep inertia, participants were asked to provide their sleepiness scores with the Karolinska Sleepiness Scale (KSS score) 5 min. after waking up, as well as 30 min. after waking up or after using the GoliteBLU lamp for 30 or 60 min. The decline in sleep inertia was found to be significant on all days, however no differences in sleep inertia decline were found for the interaction of the number of pulses and conditions (Pulses X Condition $F_{3,8}$ = 0.81; P = N.S).

There were small trends for different KSS scores immediately after waking up after 2 and 3 pulses. In the 60 min. condition there was a trend for a lower KSS score immediately after waking up after 3 pulses 5.9 (±0.5 SEM) (t_{10} = 3.38; P = 0.096) compared to baseline KSS score 6.4 (±0.5 SEM). A similar trend for a decline in sleepiness immediately after waking up was observed in the 30 min. light condition; after 2 pulses the KSS score was on average 6.6 (±0.5 SEM) (t_{10} = 4.23; P = 0.067) and after 3 pulses 6.1 (0.6 SEM) (t_{10} = 4.10; P = 0.070), compared to the average baseline KSS score 7.6 (0.5 SEM).

The sleepiness scores in the 30 min. and 60 min. light pulse conditions were not significantly different from each other, not immediately after waking up ($F_{1,10}$ = 2.89; P = 0.12), nor after using the GoliteBLUE lamp ($F_{1,10}$ = 0.98; P = 0.35).

Sleep timing

To optimize the timing of the light pulses and to allow for 8 hours of sleep per night, subjects received individual instructions when to go to bed and when to wake up. Therefore, sleep timing was influenced by scheduled sleep and wakeup times. However, subjects were allowed to sleep and wake up earlier (not later) if they wanted.

After the experiment, the actual sleep timing was determined from data from the Actiwatch (AW2) that subjects wore on all experimental days, or from the sleep diary, if data from the AW2 was not available, which was the case for 4 out of 11 subjects. Sleep timing data, i.e., average (±SE) sleep onset and sleep offset times for the baseline night and for the nights after one, two or three light pulses are shown in Table 1.

Sleep times in the 30 min. and 60 min. light conditions were not significantly different from each other, not for sleep onset ($F_{1,10}$ = 0.17; P = 0.69), nor for sleep offset ($F_{1,10}$ = 1.90; P = 0.20). Both experimental conditions resulted in a significantly earlier sleep onset compared to baseline (Table 1), though this was obtained later i.e., after 3 pulses in the 30 min. light pulse condition and already after 1 pulse in the 60 min. condition.

Sleep parameter	Condition	N	Baseline	1 light pulse	2 light pulses	3 light pulses
Sleep onset (h:min.)	60 min.*	11	0:42 (0:16)	0:00 (0:19)*	0:12 (0:18)*	0:00 (0:13)*
Sleep offset (h:min.)	60 min.	11	7:24 (0:15)	7:24 (0:16)	7:24 (0:16)	7:24 (0:15)
SOL (min.)	60 min.	7	4.3 (2.6)	4.3 (2.4)	8.7 (3.2)	17.3 (5.4)
Duration (h.)	60 min.*	7	5.8 (0.2)	6.5 (0.1)*	6.3 (0.2)	6.2 (0.2)
Awakenings/h.	60 min.	7	4.3 (0.4)	4.2 (0.4)	4.5 (0.4)	3.8 (0.4)
WASO (min.)	60 min.	7	44.4 (4.3)	50.1 (2.6)	55.0 (5.4)	41.3 (7.7)
SQR (Dutch marks)	60 min.	11	6.4 (0.3)	6.4 (0.5)	6.5 (0.3)	6.4 (0.4)
Sleep onset (h:min.)	30 min.*	11	0:36 (0:14)	0:24 (0:23)	0:06 (0:22)	0:00 (0:12)*
Sleep offset (h:min.)	30 min.	11	7:36 (0:19)	7:30 (0:17)	7:30 (0:15)	7:30 (0:16)
SOL (min.)	30 min.*	7	20.6 (3.5)	6.7 (3.0)*	9.1 (3.2)	10.7 (3.3)
Duration (h.)	30 min.*	7	5.9 (0.2)	6.2 (0.2)	6.1 (0.3)	6.4 (0.1)*
Awakenings/h.	30 min.	7	4.6 (0.4)	4.3 (0.4)	4.2 (0.4)	4.3 (0.5)
WASO (min.)	30 min.	7	50.0 (3.7)	48.9 (3.9)	55.3 (9.3)	53.7 (7.9)
SQR (Dutch marks)	30 min.	11	5.8 (0.5)	6.3 (0.3)	6.4 (0.5)	6.3 (0.3)
Italic parameters = Conditions are significantly different P < 0.05				Italic numbers = Significantly different from baseline P < 0.05		
WASO = min. awake after sleep onset			SOL = Sleep onset latency		SQR = Sleep quality rating	

Table 1: Sleep parameters with either 30 or 60 min. light pulses.

Sleep quality

Objective sleep quality was analysed from the data of the AW2's (Table 1). Due to failures of the AW2's in data collection, data on sleep quality of only 7 subjects (2f/5m) could be analysed. Objective sleep quality measures were sleep onset latency (SOL), sleep duration (Duration), the number of awakenings per hour (Awakenings/h) and min. awake after sleep onset (WASO). The subjective sleep quality rating (SQR) was asked for in the sleep diary on experimental days (Table 1).

The 30 min. and 60 min. conditions were only found to be significantly different for sleep onset latency (SOL) ($F_{1,6}$ = 10.9; $P < 0.05$). This difference may have been caused by the longer sleep onset latency on the baseline day in the 30 min. condition. For the other sleep quality parameters there were no significant differences between conditions: sleep duration ($F_{1,6}$ = 0.50; P = 0.51), number of awakenings/h ($F_{1,6}$ = 0.29; P = 0.61), WASO ($F_{1,6}$ = 1.15; P = 0.33), SQR ($F_{1,10}$ = 0.45; P = 0.52).

Compared to baseline, sleep duration was longer for the 60- and 30 min. conditions on the 2nd and 4th day respectively. Sleep onset latency was shorter on the second day (after one light pulse) in the 30 min. condition compared to the baseline day. Again, this may have been caused by the longer sleep onset latency of the baseline day in the 30 min. condition.

Discussion

This study demonstrates that three optimally timed, high blue light intensity, short pulses (30 min.), applied in a home situation, accompanied by dim light prior to sleep, are able to significantly phase advance the melatonin rhythm. The phase shifting effects of these three short blue light pulses are not significantly different from the effects of the positive control condition with three longer (60 min.) blue light pulses. The effects on the sleep-wake rhythm and morning sleepiness were also not significantly different between the 30-min. and the 60-min. blue light pulse conditions.

The idea that short light pulses are able to influence the circadian system is not new. However, up till now the positive findings were based on the effects of short light pulses mostly in highly controlled lab conditions. A dose response study of light pulse duration by Chang and colleagues (2012) revealed that the melatonin rhythm can be phase-delayed by a single light pulse in the evening of only 12 min. A more recent study of Gabel and colleagues (2013) showed that the melatonin rhythm can also be phase-advanced by a single blue light pulse in the morning of only 20 min.

Both these studies were carried out with subjects living in a controlled situation with a dimly lit environment outside the light exposure period. In a recent other home setting study [34] the effects of 30-45 min. of bright white light were tested in 10 subjects suffering from Delayed Sleep Phase Disorder. In that study, light was administered in one out of four different conditions, including a control condition, at waking up in a protocol wherein subjects received instructions to wake up one hour earlier each day until the preferred rising time was reached during a 2-week period. Unfortunately possible effects of the treatment on DLMO could be assessed in only 4 subjects and no statistical effect of light was observed in this small group. Analysis of actigraphy data on sleep parameters during the second week of treatment did not show a significant difference between the four conditions.

In our study we asked the subjects to stay in dim light during the evenings, both to be able to accurately estimate the onset of melatonin, and to prevent a possible counteracting effect of evening light exposure on the phase shifting effect of the morning light pulse. It is possible that protection to evening light by itself has played a role in the observed phase advance, but this has not been tested. Nevertheless, it seems unlikely that an almost one hour phase advance is the result of four consecutive dim light evenings alone.

The current study confirms the results of the controlled lab studies [16,35] and supports the conclusion that a combination of short light pulses of 30 min. in the morning and dim light in the evening is also capable of advancing the melatonin rhythm when applied in a home situation with no real control over environmental light. This is the situation in which light treatment for circadian rhythm sleep/wake disorders predominantly will take place.

The main focus of the present study was to test the effects of short blue light pulses on the melatonin rhythm. Therefore the setup of the study was not meant to test the effects on sleep, and actimetry data could be obtained in only 7 out of 11 subjects. For this reason, the results on the effects of the experimental conditions on sleep should be interpreted with caution.

Nevertheless, in addition to the shift in the melatonin rhythm there was also a small, but significant shift (30-40 min.) in sleep onset time. This shift was not significantly different for the 30- and 60 min. light pulse conditions. The shift in sleep onset time might reflect a shift in the circadian pacemaker, or be the effect of the shift of the melatonin rhythm, or the fact that the participants were instructed to wake up earlier than that they normally did (higher sleep pressure in the evening), or a combination.

Another finding was a trend for a reduction of sleepiness in the morning. Not only after light exposure, but even directly at waking up, probably resulting from a shift of the circadian pacemaker influencing sleep propensity and daytime alertness [8].

In contrast to the previous lab study of Gabel et al. [35], who showed a significant phase advance after 120-min. light pulse, the current home study shows more individual variation in phase advances in response to shorter light pulses, resulting in a non-significant phase advance after 130-min. light pulse? The larger variation may result from the different environmental circumstances, as the lighting conditions are variable at home while more constant in the lab.

In addition, due to less controlled conditions, both in light exposure and in accurate timing of saliva collection, the estimation of DLMO may be more variable by itself, resulting in the non-significant shift after one day with a 30-min. light pulse in this study.

Indeed, light in the morning is not the only factor responsible for the phase-advancing effects of light. The studies of Hébert et al., Chang et al. and Giménez et al. [36-38] revealed that the 'light history' is also important for the responsiveness to light. Participants in lab conditions with dim light environments are more dark adapted and are therefore more sensitive to light (Hebert et al., Chang et al.) [37].

Even in a real-life setting, but with a reduction in blue light exposure through blue reducing contact lenses, it is possible to influence the non-image forming responses to light (Giménez et al.) [38].

Another important factor for an optimal substantial phase advance is the complete pattern of light-dark exposure during the rest of the day (Appleman et al., Burgess et al.) [39,40]. Especially low light levels in the evening are essential for an optimal phase advance. It is even possible to phase advance the melatonin rhythm without extra light in the morning.

When subjects are forced to sleep 2-3 hours earlier than they normally do, in other words, if they do not receive light in the evening their melatonin rhythm can also be phase advanced (Gordijn et al., Sharkey et al.) [41,42].

Although the subjects were told to dim their lights during the experimental evenings of the current study, there may have been variation in these evening light settings. Besides, there were no light restrictions during the remaining part of the day, and this study was carried out in summer.

Therefore, the light exposure patterns between individuals and between days must have been very different and these differences in prior light history may have influenced the phase shifts.

It is against this background of varying daytime and evening time light exposure that we still found significant phase advances with three days of only 30 min. extra blue light exposure in the morning. This emphasizes the conclusion that blue light therapy in the morning is potentially highly effective as a treatment for circadian rhythm sleep disorders with a late sleep phase.

A limitation of this home study is the lack of objective compliance data for all subjects both to the light therapy/dark instructions and to the strict timing of the collection of saliva for melatonin analysis. The data that were obtained supported the fact that subjects indeed followed instructions to a large extent, but a 100% certainty is not possible.

For a follow-up study, it is interesting to specifically monitor the extra light that is received during the light therapy session in relation to environmental light conditions over the whole day, to investigate whether this indeed plays a role in the efficacy of morning light treatment. The attempt to do this in the current study failed due to technical problems. Also the lack of a control condition without experimental light exposure is a limitation of the study.

Expectations of subjects have been demonstrated to influence light treatment effects in depression studies (Putilov & Danilenko, Flory et al., Knapen et al.) [43-45] and it is possible that the instructions of sleep scheduling or being admitted to the study protocol by itself influenced the observed effects.

Although an optimal 'placebo light' condition to control for expectations and for the effects of the experimental conditions is not possible in studies on the effects of light therapy, including a control condition with a 'placebo lamp' with the same visual brightness in a next study is definitely needed.

From the current study it is clear that optimally timed, short duration, high intensity blue light pulses of 30 min. have high potential to be effective when used in a light therapy design for phase advancing the circadian system. This includes both a proper instruction of when and how long to use the light, as well as when to protect from light, e.g. in the evening. A light therapy protocol for clinicians would benefit from a more easy instruction for the timing of light than in the current study where timing of light was relative to DLMO.

Since the phase angle of DLMO and sleep seems to be highly variable, especially in late chronotypes, this issue should be solved in additional experiments. Also to be able to generalize the effects of these short blue light pulses to the population, larger groups- and more variation within participants is needed.

Finally, to be clinically relevant, it still needs to be demonstrated whether also the sleep-wake rhythm and sleep architecture will improve in response to blue light therapy and if morning sleepiness at waking up can indeed be reduced with a longer treatment protocol.

References

1. Daan S, Pittendrigh CS (1976) A Functional analysis of circadian pacemakers in nocturnal rodents II. The Variability of Phase Response Curves. J comp Physiol 106: 253-266.
2. Beersma DGM, Daan S (1993) Strong or weak resetting by light-pulses in humans. J Biol Rhythms 8: 340-347.
3. Barion A, Zee PC (2007) A clinical approach to circadian rhythm sleep disorders. Sleep Med 8: 566-577.
4. Morgenthaler TI, Lee-Chiong T, Alessi C, Friedman L, Aurora RN, et al. (2007) Practice parameters for the clinical evaluation and treatment of circadian rhythm sleep disorders. Sleep 30: 1445-1459.
5. Bjorvatn B, Pallesen S (2009) A practical approach to circadian rhythm sleep disorders. Sleep Med Rev 13: 47-60.
6. Borbély AA (1982) A two-process model of sleep regulation I. Physiological basis and outline. Human Neurobiol 1: 195-204.
7. Daan S, Beersma DGM, Borbély AA (1984) Timing of human sleep-Recovery process gated by a circadian pacemaker. Am J Physiol 2: R161-R178.
8. Dijk D, Czeisler CA (1994) Paradoxical timing of the circadian rhythm of sleep propensity serves to consolidate sleep and wakefulness in humans. Neurosci Lett 166: 63-68.
9. Roenneberg T, Kuehnle T, Juda M, Kantermann T, Allebrandt K, et al. (2007) Epidemiology of the human circadian clock. Sleep Med Rev 11: 429-438.
10. Roenneberg T, Allebrandt KV, Merrow M, Vetter C (2012) Social Jetlag and Obesity. Curr Biol 22: 939-943.
11. Wittman M, Dinich J, Merrow M, Roenneberg T (2006) Social jetlag: Misaligments of biological and social time. Chronobiol Int 23: 497-509.
12. Touitou Y (2013) Adolescent sleep misalignment: a chronic jetlag and a matter off public health. J Physiology Paris 107: 323-326.
13. Khalsa SBS, Jewett ME, Cajochen C, Czeisler CA (2003) A phase response curve to single bright light pulses in human subjects. J Physiol London 549: 945-952.
14. St Hilaire MA, Gooley JJ, Khalsa SBS, Kronauer RE, Czeisler CA, et al. (2012) Human phase response curve to a 1h pulse of bright white light. J Physiol 13: 3035-3045.
15. Zeitzer JM, Khalsa SBS, Boivin DB, Duffy JF, Shanahan TL, et al. (2005) Temporal dynamics of late-night photic stimulation of the human circadian timing system. Am J Physiol Reg I 289: R839-R844.
16. Chang AM, Santhi N, St Hilaire M, Gronfier C, Bradstreet DS, et al. (2012) Human responses to bright light of different durations. J Physiol 590: 3103-3112.
17. Beersma DGM, Comas M, Hut RA, Gordijn MCM, Rueger M, et al. (2009) The progression of circadian phase during light exposure in animals and humans. J Biol Rhythms 24: 153-160.
18. Thapan K, Arendt J, Skene DJ (2001) An action spectrum for melatonin suppression: evidence for a novel non-rod, non-cone photoreceptor system in humans. J Physiol 535: 261-267.
19. Lockley SW, Brainard GC, Czeisler CA (2003) High sensitivity of the human circadian melatonin rhythm to resetting by short wavelength light. J Clin Endocr Metab 88: 4502-4505.
20. Warman VL, Dijk DJ, Warman GR, Arendt J, Skene DJ (2003) Phase advancing human circadian rhythms with short wavelength light. Neurosc Lett 342: 37-40.
21. Wright HR, Lack LC, Kennaway DJ (2004) Differential effects of light wavelength in phase advancing the melatonin rhythm. J Pineal Res 36: 140-144.
22. Brainard GC, Sliney D, Hanifin JP, Glickman G, Byrne B, et al. (2008) Sensitivity of the human circadian system to short-wavelength (420-nm) light. J Biol Rhythms 23: 379-386.
23. Brainard GC, Hanifin JP, Warfield B, Stone MK, James ME, et al. (2015) Short-wavelength enrichment of polychromatic light enhances human melatonin suppression potency. J Pineal Res 58: 352-361.

24. Berson DM, Dunn FA, Takao M (2002) Phototransduction by retinal ganglion cells that set the circadian clock. Science 295: 1070-1073.

25. Hattar S, Liao HW, Takao M, Berson DM, Yau KW (2002) Melanopsin-containing retinal ganglion cells: Architecture, projections and intrinsic photosensitivity. Science 295: 1065-1070.

26. Enezi J, Revell V, Brown T, Wynne J, Schlangen L, et al. (2011) A "Melanopic" spectral efficiency function predicts the sensitivity of melanopsin photoreceptors to polychromatic lights. J Biol Rhythms 26: 314-323.

27. Bailes HJ, Lucas RJ (2013) Human melanopsin forms a pigment maximally sensitive to blue light (lambda(max) approximate to 479 nm) supporting an activation of G(q/11) and G(i/o) signaling cascades. P Roy Soc B-Biol Sci 280: 1759.

28. Rüger M, St Hilaire MA, Brainard GC, Khalsa SS, Kronauer RE, et al. (2013) Human phase response curve to a single 6.5h. pulse of short-wavelength light. J Physiol 591: 353-363.

29. Beck AT, Steer RA, Ball R (1996) Comparison of Beck Depression Inventories-IA and –II In psychiatric outpatients. J Pers Asses 67: 588-597.

30. Beck AT, Steer RA, Brown GK (2002) Beck Depression Inventory-II. Dutch version. Swets Test Publishers, Lisse.

31. Roenneberg T, Wirz-Justice A, Merrow M (2003) Life between clocks: Daily temporal patterns of human chronotypes. J Biol Rhythms 18: 80-90.

32. Van Someren EJW, Nagtegaal E (2007) Improving melatonin phase estimates. Sleep Med 8: 590-601.

33. Lucas RJ, Peirson SN, Berson DM, Brown TM, Cooper HM, et al. (2014) Measuring and using light in the melanopsin age. Trends Neurosc 37: 1-9.

34. Saxvig IW, Wilhelmsen-Langeland A, Pallesen S, Vedaa Ø, Nordhus IH, et al. (2014) A randomized controlled trial with bright light and melatonin for delayed sleep phase disorder: Effects on subjective and objective sleep. Chronobiol Int 31: 72-86.

35. Gabel V, Maire M, Reichert CF, Chellappa SL, Schmidt C, et al. (2013) Effects of artificial dawn and morning blue light on daytime cognitive performance, well-being, cortisol and melatonin levels. Chronobiol Int 30: 988-997.

36. Hébert M, Martin SK, Lee C, Eastman CI (2002) The effects of prior light history on the suppression of melatonin by light in humans. J Pineal Res 33: 198-203.

37. Chang AM, Scheer FAJL, Czeisler CA (2011) The human circadian system adapts to prior light history. J Physiol 589: 1095-1102.

38. Giménez MC, Beersma DGM, Bollen P, Linden ML, Gordijn MCM (2014) Effects of a chronic reduction of short-wavelength light input on melatonin and sleep patterns in humans: Evidence for adaptation. Chronobiol Int 31: 690-697.

39. Appleman K, Figueiro MG, Rea MS (2013) Controlling light-dark exposure patterns rather than sleep schedules determines circadian phase. Sleep Med 5: 456-461.

40. Burgess HJ (2013) Evening ambient light exposure can reduce circadian phase advances to morning light independent of sleep deprivation. J Sleep Res 22: 83-88.

41. Gordijn MCM, Beersma DGM, Korte HJ, Van den Hoofdakker RH (1999) Effects of light exposure and sleep displacement on Dim Light Melatonin Onset. J Sleep Res 8: 163-174.

42. Sharkey KM, Carskadon MA, Figueiro MG, Zhu Y, Rea MS (2011) Effects of an advanced sleep schedule and morning short wavelength light exposure on circadian phase in young adults with late sleep schedules. Sleep Med 12: 685-692.

43. Putilov AA, Danilenko KV (2005) Antidepressant effects of light therapy and "natural" treatments for winter depression. Biol Rhythm Res 36: 423-437.

44. Flory R, Ametepe J, Bowers B (2010) A randomized, placebo-controlled trial of bright light and high-density negative air ions for treatment of Seasonal Affective Disorder. Psychiat Res 177: 101-108.

45. Knapen SE, van der Werken M, Gordijn MCM, Meesters Y (2014) The duration of light treatment and therapy outcome in seasonal affective disorder. J Affect Disorders 166: 343-346.

19

Sleep Apnea-hypopnea Syndrome Associated with Rett Syndrome: Respiratory pattern in the Awake State and Nocturnal Polysomnographic Study

Eusebi Chiner *, **Jose N Sancho-Chust, Esther Pastor, Pedro Landete, Cristina Senent and Patricia Pérez-Ferrer**

Pneumology Section, Hospital Universitario San Juan de Alicante, Alicante, Cta Alicante-Valencias/n. 03550, Sant Joan d'Alacant, Spain

***Corresponding author:** Dr. Eusebi Chiner Vives, Sección de Neumología, Hospital Universitari de Sant Joan d'Alacant, Cta Alicante-Valencia s/n 03550 Sant Joan d'Alacant, Spain, E-mail: chiner_eus@gva.es

Abstract

A 14-year old girl with Rett syndrome was studied. The patient had roncopathy, sleepiness, decreased activity and performance, corrected kyphoscoliosis, obesity, retrognathia, ojival palate and dental malocclusion. Nocturnal polysomnography (PSG) showed a moderate obstructive and apparently central sleep apnea-hypopnea syndrome (SAHS) with associated hypoventilation, corrected by continuous positive airway pressure of 11 cm H_2O. Respiratory monitoring in the awake state showed a characteristic pattern of episodes of hyperventilation with hypocapnia followed by central apnea and accompanying desaturations. We conclude that patients with Rett syndrome should be studied using PSG in order to rule out SAHS since multiple predisposing factors are often also present.

Keywords: Rett syndrome; Nocturnal respiratory pattern; Awakening respiratory pattern; Sleep apnea-hypopnea syndrome; Cardiorespiratory function; CPAP; Treatment

Introduction

Rett syndrome (RTT) is a severe, progressive neurodevelopmental disorder that appears in early childhood and affects females almost exclusively. It is characterized by progressive cerebral atrophy, autism, manual stereotypes, dementia, acquired microcephaly, apraxia of gait and a tendency to suffer epileptic crises [1]. It has occasionally been described in association with sleep apnoea-hypopnoea syndrome (SAHS). We report the case of a 14-year old patient with RTT, studied from the respiratory point of view in the awake state and when sleeping using polysomnography (PSG), who was treated with continuous positive airway pressure (CPAP).

Case Report

A 14-year old girl diagnosed at the age of 33 months as having RTT was seen in the Pneumology Outpatients' Clinic due to suspicion of SAHS. Her parents reported snoring with pauses of apnoea during the night for several years which had become worse in the last 1-2 years.

At the same time the patient exhibited excessive sleepiness during the day, a decrease in her normal activity and attention at school together with an increase in weight. On physical examination, dental malocclusion and malposition, Mallampati IV, retrognathia and ojival palate were found.

Conventional diagnostic PSG was done during the first night followed by monitoring when the patient was awake the following morning. During sleep, there was an efficiency of 71.4%, 13.2 arousals/hour and destructuration of the sleep architecture, with a decrease in the percentage of deep sleep and REM stage (REM: 6%, stage 1: 17%, stage 2: 32%, stage 3-4: 45%), together with multiple central and obstructive respiratory events (predominantly hypopnoeas) which determined an apnoea-hypopnoea index (AHI) of 18.6 events/hour together with an oxyhemoglobin (SpO_2) desaturation index of 26/hour,

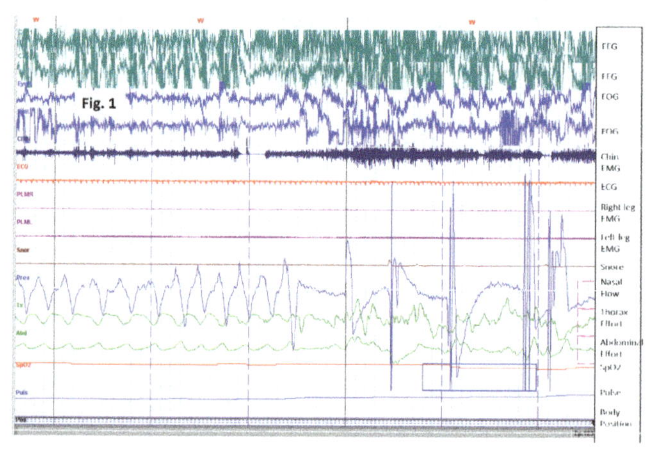

Figure 1: Characteristic respiratory pattern recording in the awake state. Hypopnoeas and central apnoeas; Irregular respiration, alternating periods of hyperventilation and central apnoea. Abbreviations: EEG: Electroencefalogram. EOG: Electrooculogram. EMG: electromyogram. SpO_2: oxygen saturation measured by pulse oxymetry

minimum SaO_2 of 82% and T90 (percentage of sleep time with oxygen saturation below 90% (T90) defined as the ratio between time in minutes with saturation values under 90% divided by the total sleep time of 100 minutes) of 22% associated to hypoventilation component. When the patient was awake, the ventilatory pattern was monitored for one hour, together with the analysis of end tidal expired CO_2 ($EtCO_2$, Nellcor™ N-85 Portable Pulse Oximetry Monitor with Microstream®). An irregular ventilatory pattern was seen with sudden changes in tidal volume and episodes of hyperventilation with hypocapnia reaching a mean $EtCO_2$ of 20, followed by central apnoeas and SaO_2 desaturations (Figure 1).

During the first half of the second night, adjustment was made with non-invasive ventilation using BIPAP® with values of IPAP of 12 cm H_2O and EPAP of 3 cm H_2O. Both central and obstructive respiratory events were seen to persist as well as pathological desaturations (Figure 2A). During the second half of the night, a recording was made of the CPAP levels which eventually reached 11 cm H_2O and the respiratory events practically ceased, with the sleep pattern returning to normal together with the number of arousals and the SaO_2 levels remained above 90% (Figure 2A and B). Nocturnal CPAP was maintained at 11 cm H_2O using a nasal mask. At subsequent check-ups, good tolerance and adaptation were found, together with an improvement in the patient's sleepiness during the day, degree of physical activity and performance at school.

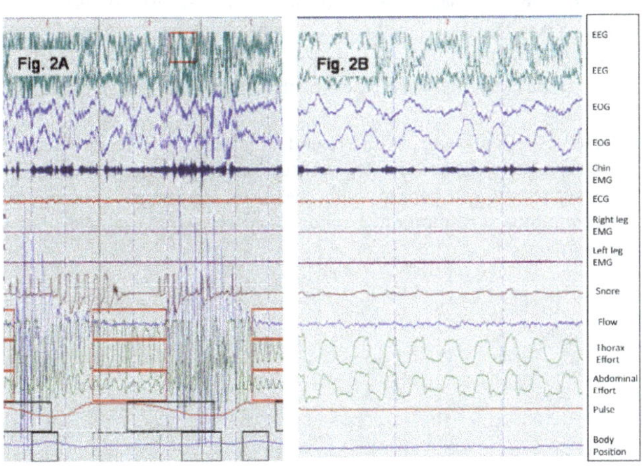

Figure 2: Nocturnal polysomnographic recordings: (2A) recording during sleep showing episodes of obstructive apnea accompanied by desaturation of hemoglobin and arousals; (2B) normalization of respiratory events during sleep by treatment with CPAP. Abbreviations: EEG: Electroencefalogram. EOG: Electrooculogram. EMG: electromyogram. SpO_2: oxygen saturation measured by pulse oxymetry

Discussion

The genetic basis of RTT consists of mutations or deletions of methyl-CpG-binding protein 2 (MeCP2) whose gene is located in the long arm of chromosome X (Xq28), which are described in 90% of the cases [1]. This protein acts in particular in the hypocampus, cortex and cerebelum, and plays an important part in modulating the activity of genes and neurons involved in social interactions. The phenotype spectrum of its mutation includes mental retardation, epilepsy, Angelman-like phenotype syndrome and autism.

RTT implies an alteration of the interactions between the autonomic, peripheral and central nervous systems, and hypofunction of neurotransmitters (glutamate, gamma-aminobutyric acid (GABA), serotonine or noradrenaline) has been postulated [2]. It has been suggested that altered expression of neuropeptide antagonists, such as substance P and methionine-encephalin, is the cause of the respiratory manifestations in this disease [2].

Patients show an immature sleep pattern with no reduction in the total sleep time and daytime sleep seen in normal children [3]. Periodic respiratory dysfunction, electroencephalographic (EEG) alterations, spasticity, eating disorders, retarded growth, cardiac disautonomy, constipation, dystonia and scoliosis are quite common. The degree of kyphoscoliosis tends to increase with growth, and at an age of around 16-20 years 43% of patients exhibit a severe degree or have already been operated on.

The respiratory pattern is characteristic, as it was in our patient. After a period of normal respiration with no hypoxemia, there is a period of hyperventilation with hypocapnia and prolonged periods of central apnea of up to 19 seconds accompanied by Valsalva manoeuvres and hypoxemia, with SaO2 desaturations of up to 50% [4]. Respiratory alkalosis and hypoxemia reported as a result of hypoventilation may contribute to brain damage [5]. Furthermore, hyperventilation is accompanied by an increase in blood pressure with an increase in vagal tone and decrease in heart rate. EEG shows theta 3-5Hz waves throughout the cerebral cortex [6]. Other respiratory patterns have also been described such as those of Biot or Cheyne-Stokes, being more severe the younger the child [7]. These events do not occur during sleep, when the respiration is regular during both NREM and REM sleep; the efficiency and architecture of sleep are maintained, with only lower values of SaO2 in the REM stage described, but these are within the normal range [8]. Therefore, patients with RTT do not have alterations in the system controlling ventilation and the alterations described when the patient is awake are due to an abnormality in the cortical influence of ventilation and alterations in the autonomic control of respiration. It has also been suggested that there is an autonomic alteration, due to longer QT intervals and a decrease in heart rate variability, with a greater incidence of sudden death [9].

Few studies have been done on respiratory disorders during sleep. Rohdin et al. [10] monitored 12 RTT girls in their home showing apnoea, hypoventilation or shallow breathing in wakefulness, but the authors did not specified the type of respiratory alteration during sleep. Weese-Mayer et al. [11] studied 47 girls with RTT and determined that, although the breathing and heart rate appeared more regular during the night, some irregularities could appear at home. Recently d'Orsy et al. [12] studied a 3-year-old girl showing central apnoeas not only during awake, but also during sleep. Some authors hypothesize that breathing dysregulation in RTT results from disturbances in mechanisms that modulate the respiratory rhythm, acting either alone or in combination with more subtle disturbances in rhythm and pattern generation [13].

Our patient could have had nocturnal hypoventilation due to her kyphoscoliosis despite the fact that it had been corrected, but what was most striking were the clinical symptoms suggesting SAHS and the predisposing factors. Normalization of the ventilatory pattern by means of CPAP and not BIPAP® supports the fact that the hypoventilation component was due to the severity of the obstruction of the upper airway, which was the main cause of SAHS and the apparently central apnoeas were obstructive in origin, normalizing the nocturnal respiratory pattern with CPAP. In these cases only the response to CPAP distinguishes the true central apneas from obstructive apneas. In our case, it is possible that the espiratory airway pressure (EPAP) applied during the titration was insufficient to overcome the obstructive apneas and had gotten a good response to the BIPAP increasing the EPAP. If respiratory events had persisted, switching to adaptive servo ventilation could be the best treatment option [14]. Given that SAHS in the child population may present neuropsychiatric alterations such as hyperactivity, attention deficit, etc., these may cause the neurological symptoms of the disease to worsen even more, as occurred in our patient.

We conclude that to perform a nocturnal polygraphic recording with monitorization of respiratory variables in patients with RTT may be essential for diagnosis and treatment of SAHS, which may be associated with RTT since there are many potential predisposing factors. Daytime monitorization of the ventilation pattern may reveal characteristic alterations that appear when the patient is awake.

References

1. Weaving L, Ellaway CJ, Gécz J, Christodoulou J (2005) Rett syndrome: clinical review and genetic update. J Med Genet 42: 1-7.
2. Glaze DG (2005) Neurophysiology of Rett syndrome. J Child Neurol 20: 740-746.
3. Ellaway C, Peat J, Leonard H, Christodoulou J (2001) Sleep dysfunction in Rett syndrome: lack of age related decrease in sleep duration. Brain Dev 23 Suppl 1: S101-103.
4. Kerr AM, Julu PO (1999) Recent insights into hyperventilation from the study of Rett syndrome. Arch Dis Child 80: 384-387.
5. Southall DP, Kerr AM, Tirosh E, Amos P, Lang MH, et al. (1988) Hyperventilation in the awake state: potentially treatable component of Rett syndrome. Arch Dis Child 63: 1039-1048.
6. Campos-Castelló J, Peral Guerra M, Riviere Gómez A, Oliete García F, Herranz Tanarro J, et al. (1988) [Rett's syndrome: study of 15 cases]. An Esp Pediatr 28: 286-292.
7. Schlüter B, Aguigah G, Buschatz D, Trowitzsch E, Aksu F (1995) Polysomnographic recordings of respiratory disturbances in Rett syndrome. J Sleep Res 4: 203-207.
8. Marcus CL, Carroll JL, McColley SA, Loughlin GM, Curtis S, et al. (1994) Polysomnographic characteristics of patients with Rett syndrome. J Pediatr 125: 218-224.
9. Julu PO, Kerr AM, Apartopoulos F, Al-Rawas S, Engerström IW, et al. (2001) Characterisation of breathing and associated central autonomic dysfunction in the Rett disorder. Arch Dis Child 85: 29-37.
10. Rohdin M, Fernell E, Eriksson M, Albåge M, Lagercrantz H, et al. (2007) Disturbances in cardiorespiratory function during day and night in Rett syndrome. Pediatr Neurol 37: 338-344.
11. Weese-Mayer DE, Lieske SP, Boothby CM, Kenny AS, Bennett HL, et al. (2008) Autonomic dysregulation in young girls with Rett Syndrome during nighttime in-home recordings. Pediatr Pulmonol 43: 1045-1060.
12. d'Orsi G, Demaio V, Scarpelli F, Calvario T, Minervini MG (2009) Central sleep apnoea in Rett syndrome. Neurol Sci 30: 389-391.
13. Katz DM, Dutschmann M, Ramirez JM, Hilaire G (2009) Breathing disorders in Rett syndrome: progressive neurochemical dysfunction in the respiratory network after birth. Respir Physiol Neurobiol 168: 101-108.
14. Galetke W, Ghassemi BM, Priegnitz C, Stieglitz S, Anduleit N, et al. (2014) Anticyclic modulated ventilation versus continuous positive airway pressure in patients with coexisting obstructive sleep apnea and Cheyne-Stokes respiration: a randomized crossover trial. Sleep Med 15: 874-879.

Sleep Bruxism and Orthodontic Appliance among Children and Adolescents

Ivana Meyer Prado, Marcela Oliveira Brant, Sheyla Márcia Auad, Saul Martins Paiva, Isabela Almeida Pordeus and Junia M Serra-Negra*

Department of Pediatric Dentistry and Orthodontics, Federal University of Minas Gerais, Belo Horizonte, Brazil

***Corresponding author:** Junia Maria Serra-Negra, Department of Pediatric Dentistry and Orthodontics, Federal University of Minas Gerais, Belo Horizonte, Brazil, E-mail: juniaserranegra@hotmail.com

Abstract

Objective: The aim of this study was to evaluate the association between sleep bruxism and orthodontic treatment in children and adolescents.

Methods: Analysis was performed both before and during such treatment. A retrospective cross-sectional study was undertaken in two groups of seven to 15-year-old patients from the orthodontic clinic of a public university in Belo Horizonte, Brazil. The first group contained 22 patients with a mean age of ten years (SD = 2.058) who were awaiting orthodontic treatment.

The second group contained 44 patients with a mean age of nine years (SD = 1.79) undergoing orthodontic treatment. Data collection was performed using a questionnaire completed by parents/caregivers and data from the medical records of the clinic. Diagnosis of bruxism was determined in accordance with American Academy of Sleep Medicine criteria. Descriptive analysis and Chi-square test were used for statistical analysis.

Results: Sleep bruxism was observed in 27.3% of patients who were awaiting orthodontic treatment. Regarding the group undergoing treatment, 36.4% had sleep bruxism prior to the start of treatment and 25% continued to suffer from the Para function following placement of an orthodontic appliance.

Among those who had sleep bruxism before treatment, 75% reported that the Para function ceased after placement of the appliance. There was an association between the presence of sleep bruxism among parents/caregivers and among patients ($p = 0.035$). Interceptive orthodontics was associated in 77% of sleep bruxism stop during treatment ($p = 0.029$). The corrective orthodontics was in 22.8% patients with sleep bruxism only after fitting orthodontic appliance compared to 9% with interceptive orthodontic treatment ($p = 0.002$).

Conclusion: There was an association between sleep bruxism in parents/caregivers and the presence of the Para function among children/adolescents. The type of orthodontic treatment influenced the time that sleep bruxism appeared. The interceptive orthodontic treatment was associated with the cases which sleep bruxism stopped during treatment.

Keywords: Adolescents; Bruxism; Children; Para function; Corrective orthodontics; Interceptive orthodontics; Orthodontic treatment

Introduction

Sleep bruxism is a movement disorder characterized by the gnashing and/or grinding of teeth during sleep [1,2,3].

It manifests itself as rhythmic muscle contractions with a strength greater than that used in normal chewing [1,2,4].

An accurate etiology of sleep bruxism has not been clearly identified and the para function is considered multifactorial [3,5].

Some studies have highlighted an association with emotional factors [6-11], while one study highlighted the influence of genetics on sleep related problems during childhood and adolescence, and also the presence of the condition among parents [12].

Teeth grinding is a major concern for dentists because of its consequences, such as tooth wear, fracture of dental restorations, periodontal problems, exacerbation of temporomandibular disorders, stress induction leading to headaches, and grinding sounds, which may interfere with the sleep of family members or partners [1,3,4].

The prevalence of this nocturnal disorder in children is significant. Percentages vary depending on the diagnosis method used, and range from 8% to 38% [6,13,14].

The condition is usually diagnosed in children and adolescents from the reports of parents and caregivers [13,14].

Orthodontics is the area of dentistry that cares for preventing, intercepting and correcting dental irregularities and skeletal discrepancies [15-17].

The intercepted orthodontics is the treatment for preventing or reduces severe malocclusion installation, generally used to correct abnormal habits that can interfere with the growth pattern of the jaws and teeth position [16].

Usually the interceptive treatment is performed in younger patients with mixed dentition [16]. Corrective orthodontics is the treatment of malocclusions and growth patterns already installed, manly using fixed mechanisms, like orthodontic appliance [15,17].

Orthodontic treatment is sought by a large number of children and adolescents. Some authors have identified a relationship between the use of orthodontic appliances and its negative impact on oral health related quality of life [18], and have described the discomforts that come with the appliances, such as difficulty in speaking, difficulty in cleaning and dental mobility problems [19].

From these works it is unclear whether there is a relationship between sleep bruxism and emotional factors associated with the use of braces.

A search of the PubMed and Scopus databases in November 2015 using the key words: bruxism, orthodontic treatment and malocclusion did not reveal any published scientific studies of this subject.

Given the above, the aim of the present study was to analyze the prevalence of sleep bruxism among children and adolescents before and during orthodontic treatment and the possible association of this para function with the type of orthodontic treatment, corrective or interceptive.

Method and Material

A retrospective epidemiological survey was undertaken. The study was conducted at the Orthodontic Clinic of the Dental School of Federal University of Minas Gerais (FOUFMG) in Belo Horizonte, Brazil.

The parents/caregivers of patients yet to receive treatment and of those already being treated in the second half of 2014 were contacted. A total of 135 individuals were contacted.

Of these, 66 were included in the study, 44 of whom had children undergoing orthodontic treatment and 22 of whom had children who were waiting for treatment.

A convenience sample was used. The patients awaiting orthodontic treatment had been evaluated by clinical orthodontists and all had dental records.

All parents/caregivers and patients signed a Free and Informed Consent Form (FICF).

Parents responded to a questionnaire prepared in accordance with the criteria of the American Academy of Sleep Medicine (AASM) [13]. Thus, bruxism was diagnosed if parents/caregivers reported that their child had the habit of grinding or clenching his/her teeth during sleep and exhibited sounds associated with sleep bruxism [13].

The parent's questionnaire questions considered the development of children, sleep quality and characteristics, and the presence or absence of sleep bruxism before and after placement of an orthodontic appliance [20].

A single dentist who had undergone a training and calibration exercise with satisfactory kappa values conducted the clinical examinations. The participation of parents/caregivers was voluntary.

Data relating to the occlusal characteristics of patients undergoing treatment was collected from the documentation and orthodontic records of the clinics using a separate form.

Changes in anterior overlap, over jet and overbite were based on criteria described in literature: normal overbite was defined as when the upper incisors overlapped the lower incisors by no more than 3 mm, and normal over jet was defined as no more than 2 mm. Changes of more than 3 mm were considered altered over jet and overbite [21,22].

The methodology of the study was tested in a pilot study involving 20 parents/caregivers of patients undergoing orthodontic treatment at FOUFMG. These participants were not included in the main study.

This study was approved by the Human Research Ethics Committee of the Universidade Federal de Minas Gerais (COEP/UFMG) (protocol ETIC 03205).

All data was analyzed using the SPSS 21.0 software program. Descriptive data analysis and the chi-square test were used to analyze the correlations between the dependent variable "sleep bruxism" and the other variables collected, with a 5% significance level.

Results

A total of 135 parents/caregivers were contacted. Of these, 108 agreed to participate (80%), but only 66 (61.1%) were included in the study. The loss of 42 participants (39%) was the result of a failure to fully complete the questionnaire and/or incomplete information available in the medical records consulted.

Participants were divided into two groups. The first group consisted of 44 patients undergoing orthodontic treatment, which 29 were male (65.9%). The second group consisted of 22 patients awaiting orthodontic treatment, the majority were male (72.7%).

Patients undergoing orthodontic treatment

The participants in the study were patients aged from seven to 15 years (Table 1) with a mean age of 10.6 years (SD = 2.058). The age range of the parents/caregivers of the patients ranged from 18 to 69 years (Table 1), with a mean age of 42 years (SD = 9.77). Not all parents/caregivers responded to the item "age".

Among the 44 patients already undergoing orthodontic treatment, 36.4% suffered from sleep bruxism before orthodontic treatment (Table 1).

The other results referring to sleep bruxism before treatment among patients are at Table 1. The prevalence of sleep bruxism among parents/guardians was 15.9% (Table 1).

Most patients slept in various positions at night (31.8%), according to the reports of parents/caregivers (Table 1).

Some parents/caregivers reported that patients frequently slept in more than one position, and these were counted separately in statistical analysis.

There was no significant association between the presence of sleep bruxism, before and after treatment, and the type of malocclusion (Table 2).

Variables	Case Group		Control Group	
	N	%	N	%
Bruxism Before Treatment				
Yes	16	36.4	6	27.3
No	28	63.6	16	72.7
Bruxism Continued After Treatment				
Yes	4	25		
No	12	75	-	-
Bruxism Only After The Beginning Of Orthodontic Treatment				
Yes	4	9.1	-	-
No	40	90.9		
Parent/Caregiver Experienced Bruxism				
Yes	7	15.9	7	31.8
No	37	84.1	15	68.2
Hours of Sleep per Night				
>8 hours	38	86.4	18	81.8
<8 hours	6	13.6	4	18.2
***Patient's Sleep Position**				
On side	13	29.5	3	13.6
On back	13	29.5	9	40.9
On stomach	11	25	4	18.2
Various Positions	14	31.8	6	27.3
Age of Patients Undergoing Treatment				
07 to 10 years	22	50	15	68.2
11 to 15 years	22	50	7	31.8
Age of Parents/Caregivers of Patients Undergoing Treatment				
18 to 42 years	23	56.1	14	63.6
43 to 69 years	18	43.9	8	36.4
Patients That Drool During Sleep	17	38.6	13	59.1
Patients Complaining of Pain in TMJ	3	6.8	1	4.5
Patients Using Medication				
Yes	6	13.6	5	22.7
No	38	86.4	17	77.3
Type of Parent/Caregiver				
Father	3	20.5	7	31.8
Mother	31	10.5	13	59.1

Grandmother or Grandfather	9	6.8	1	4.5
Brother/Sister	1	2.3	-	-
Aunt/Uncle	-	-	1	4.5

Table 1: Descriptive analysis of studied variables in children and adolescents patients undergoing orthodontic treatment and patients yet to receive orthodontic treatment at the orthodontic clinic of a public university in Belo Horizonte, Brazil. *Parent/caregiver could describe more than one sleeping position.

	Bruxism before beginning of treatment		**P***	**Bruxism after beginning of treatment**		**P***
Malocclusion	**No**	**Yes**		**No**	**Yes**	
	n (%)	**n (%)**		**n (%)**	**n (%)**	
Crowding	3 (60%)	2 (40%)	0.962	5 (100%)	0 (0%)	0.433
Jaw Atresia	1 (100%)	0 (0%)	0.418	1 (100%)	0 (0%)	0.739
Class II canine	0 (0%)	1 (100%)	0.206	1 (100%)	0 (0%)	0.739
Class II	4 (100%)	0 (0%)	0.092	4 (100%)	0 (0%)	0.489
Altered overjet	5 (55.6%)	4 (44.4%)	0.706	9 (100%)	0 (0%)	0.264
Altered overbite	4 (57.1%)	3 (42.9%)	0.819	7 (100%)	0 (0%)	0.339
Class III	2 (66.7%)	1 (33.3%)	0.834	2 (66.7%)	1 (33.3%)	0.153
Midline Deviation	2 (100%)	0 (0%)	0.246	2 (100%)	0 (0%)	0.634
Anterior Open Bite	3 (75%)	1 (25%)	0.545	4 (100%)	0 (0%)	0.489
Diastema	1 (100%)	0 (0%)	0.418	1 (100%)	0 (0%)	0.739
Anterior Crossbite	9 (53%)	8 (47%)	0.375	14 (82.4%)	3 (17.6%)	0.152
Bilateral Posterior Crossbite	4 (66.7%)	2 (33.3%)	0.757	5 (83.3%)	1(16.7%)	0.537
Unilateral Posterior Crossbite	2 (50%)	2 (50%)	0.636	4 (100%)	0 (0%)	0.489

Table 2: Presence of bruxism compared to type of malocclusions presented by children and adolescents patients undergoing orthodontic treatment at an orthodontic clinic of a public university in Belo Horizonte, Brazil. *Chi-squared test; p = Probability value. Note: some patients suffered from more than one type of malocclusion.

There was no association between gender and sleep bruxism before starting treatment, but there was a higher percentage of the parafunction among women (46.7%, $p = 0.307$). A high percentage of patients with sleep bruxism (71.4%) had parents/caregivers that also suffered from the condition ($p = 0.035$) (Table 3).

When compared the type of treatment, interceptive or corrective, with the moment that sleep bruxism manifested in patients the result found was: interceptive orthodontic treatment was present in 77% of the cases that sleep bruxism stopped during treatment ($p = 0.029$); corrective orthodontic treatment was present in 22.8% of patients which sleep bruxism started only after the beginning of orthodontic treatment, comparing to 9% of patients having interceptive treatment ($p = 0.002$) (Table 3).

Patient awaiting orthodontic treatment

A total of 27.3% of the 22 patients awaiting orthodontic treatment had sleep bruxism (Table 1). The age of these patients ranged from seven to 14 years, with an average age of 9.1 years (SD = 1.79) (Table 1). The average age of parents/caregivers was 38.8 years (SD = 8.9), with the youngest aged 24 and the oldest 58 years old (Table 4).

According to information supplied by parents/caregivers, 40.9% of patients slept on their backs (Table 1), while only one patient (4.5%) complained of pain in the TMJ. The majority of the parents/caregivers (59.1%) reported that patients drooled during sleep (Table 1).

A total of 33.3% of parents/caregivers said that they ground their teeth at night. When parents/caregivers with sleep bruxism were compared with patients with the parafunction, the result found was 57.14% ($p = 0.035$) (Table 3). It was observed that 72.72% of patients had frequent headaches. Among these patients, 33.3% grinded their teeth at night ($p = 0.350$) (Table 3).

Anterior crossbite was the most prevalent malocclusion among patients undergoing orthodontic treatment (41.5%) (Table 4). Many patients had more than one type of malocclusion.

Variables	Case Group		P*	Control Group		P*
	Bruxism before beginning of treatment			Bruxism in patients before treatment		
	No (%)	Yes (%)		No (%)	Yes (%)	
Headache						
No	17 (73.9%)	06 (26.1%)	0.138	06 (85.7%)	01 (14.3%)	0.35
Yes	11 (52.4%)	10 (47.6%)		10 (66.7%)	06 (33.3%)	
Parent/Caregiver with Bruxism						
No	26 (70.3%)	11 (29.7%)	0.035	13 (86.7%)	02 (13.3%)	0.035
Yes	02 (28.6%)	05 (71.4%)		03 (42.9%)	04 (57.1%)	
Gender						
Female	08 (53.3%)	07 (46.7%)	0.307			
Male	20 (68.9%)	09 (31.1%)				
Type of Orthodontic Treatment						
Interceptive	19 (52.7)	17 (47.3)	0.097			
Corrective	21 (47.7)	23 (52.3)				
	Bruxism stop during treatment		p*			
	No (%)	**Yes (%)**				
Type of Orthodontic Treatment						
Interceptive	03 (23.0)	10 (77.0)	0.029			
Corrective	25 (92.5)	02 (7.5)				
	Bruxism only after beginning of orthodontic treatment		p*			
	No(%)	**Yes(%)**				
Type of Orthodontic Treatment						
Interceptive	20 (91.0)	02 (09.0)	0.002			
Corrective	17 (77.2)	05 (22.8)				

Table 3: Relationship between sleep bruxism before the start of orthodontic treatment and studied variables in chindren and adolescents patients undergoing orthodontic treatment and patients yet to receive treatment at an orthodontic clinic of a public university in Belo Horizonte, Brazil. *Chi-squared test; p = Probability value. Not all questions were answered in orthodonticrecords. Not all questions were answered by all parents.

Discussion

The true etiology of the bruxism remains controversial in literature [3,5], with the most likely cause of the parafunction being linked to emotional factors and genetics [6,11,12]. The prevalence of sleep bruxism in patients undergoing orthodontic treatment before starting the treatment (36.4%) in the present study were similar to those found in literature [14,20].

An association was found between parents/caregivers with bruxism and patients with sleep bruxism in both groups, which corroborates the findings of other studies [12,23]. The association found between patients with sleep bruxism and parents/caregivers also with the parafunction confirms potential familial relationship [23-25].

No genetic evaluations made between the groups. So, we can't call with word "heredity". However, as exits a strong influence of behavioral factors and the environment in which he lives the bruxer perhaps this explains the same behavior between parents and children [24]. This aspect deserves further study. An evaluation of the possible relationship between sleep bruxism and type of orthodontic treatment found a high percentage of participants for whom the parafunction ceased following treatment (75%).

Patients who continued to suffer from sleep bruxism following the beginning of orthodontic treatment (25%) are perhaps those whose quality of life was impacted most by the discomforts of the appliance, or who had a very high expectation of aesthetic change following orthodontic correction, which subsequently generated some emotional frustration [18,19].

These findings referring to an association of sleep bruxism and the type of orthodontic treatment, corrective or interceptive, is unprecedented in literature, showing the importance to dedicate in further investigation.

A comparison of the relationship between sleep bruxism both before and after the beginning of treatment and the type of malocclusion suffered by patients undergoing treatment showed that there was no statistical association between these factors, a finding which disagreed with another Brazilian study [26].

Malocclusion	n	%
Anterior Crossbite	17	41.5
Accentuated Overjet	9	22
Accentuated Overbite	7	17.1
Bilateral Posterior Crossbite	6	14.6
Crowding	5	12.2
Anterior Open Bite	4	9.8
Class II	4	9.8
Unilateral Posterior Crossbite	4	9.8
Class III	3	7.3
Midline deviation	2	4.9
Atresia	1	2.4
Class II Canine	1	2.4
Diastema	1	2.4

Table 4: Most frequent types of malocclusion in children and adolescents patients undergoing orthodontic treatment at an orthodontic clinic of a public university in Belo Horizonte, Brazil. Note: Some patients had more than one type of malocclusion.

This result may have been influenced by the small sample size of the present study and the fact that data regarding malocclusions was collected from medical records of patients. As the present study was undertaken in a university environment, many students record information in these files, with diagnostic criteria varying from student to student, even when under the supervision of a professor.

In addition, it was observed that a higher percentage of parents responded to the questionnaire in this other Brazilian study. The present study had a lower adhesion rate, with many blank questionnaires blank due to parents saying they had a lack of time to complete the questionnaire.

This behavior was different to that recorded in another study conducted at the same institution which evaluated the knowledge of parents/caregivers, and where mothers made up the largest group of parents/caregivers participating. Perhaps as a result, there was greater compliance and lower loss in said study [23].

The use of more accurate diagnosis, by electronic means or through the use of polysomnography and electromyography, may generate a more accurate diagnosis. However, this was an epidemiological study based on the AASM criteria [6]. Parents/caregivers responsible for caring for their children at night are often able to identify the noise made during the parafunction studied [14].

The main aim of the present study was to find a possible association between sleep bruxism and the type of orthodontic treatment. An association with the interceptive and corrective orthodontic treatment was proven in this study and in a 2011 study, Costa et al. found an association between the use of orthodontic appliances and their impact on the quality of life of children [18].

Other studies have sought to identify an association between malocclusion and oral health related quality of life [21,26]. These studies raise questions regarding the emotional influence attributed to the use of orthodontic appliances and the treatment itself, such as how a patient will react to the prospect of orthodontic treatment.

The association between quality of life and the use of orthodontic appliances can be something related to the prevalence of sleep bruxism among children and adolescents during orthodontic treatment since in our study we found that corrective orthodontic treatment was more related to beginning of sleep bruxism after placing the appliance (22.8%) when compared to interceptive treatment (9%).

The association between sleep bruxism and orthodontic treatment is something to be observed in other studies since this find can, with further investigation, influence the choice of orthodontic treatment in children and adolescents.

We need to be very careful when treating children and adolescents with emotional problems and distress once the orthodontic treatment can interfere negatively in their quality of life.

It's a preliminary study. For this hypothesis to be proven, longitudinal studies with larger sample groups and monitoring of the patient from the pre-treatment phase until the end of treatment will be required.

Acknowledgement

The present study received financial support from the following Brazilian funding agencies: Conselho Nacional de Pesquisa (CNPq), Fundação de Amparo à Pesquisa de Minas Gerais (FAPEMIG) and Pró-reitoria de Pesquisa da Universidade Federal de Minas Gerais (PRPq/UFMG).

Authors Contribution

Conceived and designed the experiments: IMP; SMA; JMSN. Performed the experiments: IMP; MOB. Analyzed the data: SMA; SMP; IAP; JMSN. Contributed reagents/materials/analysis tools: SMP IAP. Wrote the manuscript: IMP; MOB; JMSN. Final edition of the manuscript: JMSN; SMA; SMP; IAP.

References

1. Laat AD, Macaluso GM (2002) Sleep bruxism as a motor disorder. Mov Disord 17: 67-69.
2. Gonçalves LVP, Toledo AOD, Otero AS (2010) The relationship between bruxism, occlusal factors and oral habits. Dental Press J Orthod 15: 97-104.
3. Lavigne GL, Shoury S, Abe S, Yamaguchi T, Raphael K (2008) Bruxism physiology and pathology: an overview for clinicians. J Oral Rehabil 33: 476-494.
4. Nishigawa K, Bando E, Nakano M (2001) Quantitative study of bite force during sleep associated bruxism. J Oral Rehabil 28: 485-491.
5. Behr M, Hahnel S, Faltermeier A, Bürgers R, Kolbeck C, et al. (2012) The two main theories on dental bruxism. Ann Anat 194: 216-219.
6. Serra-Negra JM, Paiva SM, Seabra AP, Dorella C, Lemos BF, et al. (2010) Prevalence of sleep bruxism in a group of Brazilian schoolchildren. Eur Arch of Paediatr Dent 11: 192-195.
7. Ferreira-Bacci AV, Cardoso CL, Díaz-Serrano KV (2012) Behavioral Problems and emotional stress in children with bruxism. Braz Dent J 23: 245-251.
8. Manfredini D, Landi N, Romagnoli M, Bosco M (2004) Psychic and occlusal factors in bruxers. Aust Dent J 49: 84-89.
9. Clark GT, Rugh JD, Handelman SL (1980) Nocturnal masseter muscle activity and urinary catecholamine levels in bruxers. J Dent Res 59: 1571-1576.
10. Vanderas AP, Menenkuo M, Kouimtzis TH, Papagiannoulis L (2009) Urinary catecholamine levels and bruxism in children. J Oral Rehabil 26: 103-110.
11. Giraki M, Schneider C, Schäfer R, Singh P, Franz M, et al. (2010) Correlation between stress, stress-coping and current sleep bruxism. Head Face Med 6: 1-8.
12. Moore M, Slane J, Mindell JA, Burt AS, Klumb KL (2011) Genetic and enviromental influences on sleep problems: a study of preadolescent and adolescent twins. Child Care Health Dev 37: 638-641.
13. Castelo PM, Gavião MBD, Pereira LJ, Bonjardim LR (2005) Relationship between oral parafunctional/nutritive sucking habits and temporomandibular joint dysfunction in primary dentition. Int J Paediatr Dent 15: 29-36.
14. Cheifetz AT, Osganian SK, Allred EM, Needleman HL (2005) Prevalence of bruxism and associated correlates in children as reported by parents. J Dent Child 72: 67-73.
15. Guimarães CH, Henriques J, Janson G, Moura WS (2015) Stability of interceptive/corrective orthodontic treatment for tooth ankylosis and Class II mandibular deficiency: A case report with 10 years follow-up. Indian J Dent Res 3: 315-319.
16. Sandoval P, Bizcar B (2013) Benefits of Implementation of Orthodontics Interceptive in the Children's Clinic. Int J Odontostomat 7: 253-265.
17. Patel MP, Henriques JFC, Almeida RR, Pinzan A, Janson G, et al. (2013) Comparative cephalometric study of class II malocclusion treatment with Pendulum and Jones jig appliances followed by fixed corrective orthodontics. Dental Press J Orthod 6: 58-64.
18. Costa AA, Ferreira MC, Serra-Negra JM, Pordeus IA, Paiva SM (2011) Impact of wearing fixed orthodontic appliances on oral health-related quality of life among Brazilians children. J Orthod 38: 275-281.
19. Marques LS, Paiva SM, Vieira-Andrade RG, Pereira LJ, Ramos-Jorge ML (2014) Discomfort associated with fixed orthodontic appliances: determinant factors and influence on quality of life. Dental Press J Orthod 19: 102-107.
20. Serra-Negra JM, Paiva SM, Flores-Mendoza CE, Ramos-Jorge ML, Pordeus IA (2012) Association among stress, personality traits, and sleep bruxism in children. Pediatr Dent 34: 30-34.
21. Gois EGO, Ribeiro-Junior HC, Vale MPP, Paiva SM, Serra-Negra JMC, et al. (2008) Influence of nonnutritive sucking habits, breathing pattern and adenoid size on the development of malocclusion. Angle Orthod 78: 647-654.
22. Góis EG, Vale MP, Paiva SM, Abreu MH, Serra-Negra JM, et al. (2012) Incidence of malocclusion between primary and mixed dentitions among Brazilian children. A 5-year longitudinal study. Angle Orthod 82: 495-500.
23. Serra-Negra JM, Tirsa-Cosra D, Guimarãoes FH, Paiva SM, Pordeus IA (2013) Evaluation of parents/caregiver knowledge about the bruxism of their children: family knowledge of bruxism. J Indian Soc Pedod Prev Dent 31: 153-158.
24. Serra-Negra JM, Paiva SM, Auad SM, Ramos-Jorge ML, Pordeus IA (2012) Signs, symptoms, parafunctions and associated factors of parent-reported sleep bruxism in children: a case-control study. Braz Dent J 23: 746-752.
25. Serra-Negra JM, Paiva SM, Fulgêncio LB, Chavez BA, Lage CF, et al. (2014) Environmental factors, sleep duration, and sleep bruxism in Brazilian schoolchildren: a case-control study. Sleep Med 15: 236-239.
26. Sousa RVD, Ribeiro GL, Firmino RT, Martins CC, Granville-Garcia AF, et al. (2014) Prevalence and associated factors for the development of anterior open bite and posterior crossbite in the primary dentition. Braz Dent J 25: 336-342.

Sleeping through the Ages: An Examination of Sleep in Older Adults

Pennie S Seibert[1*], **Jennifer Valerio**[1,2], **Codieann Dehaas**[1,2], **Danielle Nebeker**[1,2], **Fred Grimsley**[1,2] **and Christian G Zimmerman**[1]

[1]*Physician Research Services at Saint Alphonsus Regional Medical Center, Boise, Idaho, USA*

[2]*Boise State University, Boise, Idaho, USA*

***Corresponding author:** Pennie S Seibert, Saint Alphonsus Regional Medical Center, 1055 North Curtis Road Boise, ID 83706, USA, E-mail: penseibert@msn.com

Abstract

It is widely recognized that sleep disorders (SD) are highly prevalent, despite being under diagnosed and under treated in practice. SDs occurs at all ages, although presentation and subsequent consequences for an individual's health varies throughout the lifespan. Currently, evaluation of SDs are inadequate across all age ranges, and for both sexes, as they are compromised by under reporting and relying on self-report, rather than professional sleep studies (i.e., nocturnal polysomnography (NPS) and multiple sleep latency tests (MSLT)). Moreover, there is a paucity of data specific to the elderly; many older individuals report dissatisfaction with quality of sleep. Indeed, literature has shown that geriatric populations spend less time in slow-wave sleep and rapid eye movement (REM) sleep and have more difficulties maintaining sleep. Their dissatisfaction may occur from changes in sleep architecture associated with the aging process; however, it has been suggested that it largely stems from comorbid illness, social problems, hormonal effects, altered circadian rhythms, or side effects of medications that are common in the elderly. Further, geriatric sleep is related to depression, impaired health and functioning, and weaker/ less synchronized circadian rhythms. In response, we utilized a 111-item questionnaire in conjunction with NPS, MSLT, the Epworth Sleepiness Scale (ESS) and medical chart reviews of individuals referred for SD evaluation to compare sleep in geriatrics with adults. Analysis revealed numerous differences between adult and geriatric groups, with the elderly experiencing more SDs, longer sleep latencies, and fewer sleep complaints. Based on the outcomes of this investigation, we posit further consideration to SDs across the age groups to achieve the best health care and quality of life for all.

Keywords: Geriatric, Sleep disorders, Sleep architecture, Quality of life, Circadian rhythms

Abbreviations:

SD: Sleep Disorder, NPS: Nocturnal Polysomnography, MSLT: Multiple Sleep Latency, ESS: Epworth Sleepiness Scale, REM: Rapid Eye Movement

Introduction

Sleep disorders (SDs) affect approximately one-third of the world's population and impact a multitude of physiological and psychological functions [1-3]. The presence of SDs occurs at all ages, though the presentation and subsequent consequences for an individual's health change in accordance with the natural aging process [4]. At any age, chronic sleep disturbances compromise response times, performance, and short-term memory. These disturbances can have serious consequences for the elderly in particular; geriatric sleep problems are associated with increased risk of falls, increased depressive/anxious feelings, impaired cognitive functioning and overall poorer quality of life [5].

It is commonplace for older individuals to complain that their sleep is not as good as it once was, as an estimated 50% of adults aged 65 and older experience sleep disturbances [6,7]. Indeed, aging is associated with numerous changes in average sleep; it becomes increasingly shallow and fragmented, less time spent in slow–wave and rapid eye movement (REM) sleep, and may result in difficulties maintaining sleep [4,5,8]. However, these changes in sleep architecture do not account for all sleep complaints reported by elderly adults. The majority of sleep complaints seen with increased age are more attributed to myriad medical and psychiatric illnesses, and the lifestyle challenges that present with these illnesses, rather than the aging process itself [5,8-11]. It is also plausible that the relationship shared by sleep disturbances and health status could be bi-directional; wherein chronic disease contributes to poor sleep and, poor sleep adversely affects the course of chronic disease [10].

SDs not attributed to illness or abnormal sleep architecture may also result from lack of stimulation, poor diet, or medications that lead to early onset of sleep [5]. It is not uncommon for the elderly to intake numerous medications, both prescription and over-the-counter, typically with one or more contributing to disrupted sleep [5,12]. Stimulating or alerting drugs that are often taken by older individuals affect and delay sleep onset at bedtime, and while sedative-type drugs can be useful for the relief of temporary insomnia, long-term use may result in habituation, loss of efficacy, drug-induced insomnia, and can gradually begin to imitate the dementia-like symptoms seen in individuals with Alzheimer's disease [4].

Though the aging process can affect one's ability to sleep, sex differences confound an already complex understanding of SDs in the elderly [10]. It has been postulated that sex differences explain the largest proportion of variance in measures of sleep architecture [13]. The factors that are most strongly related to sex differences in geriatric sleep disturbances are the use of medication, sleep apnea, and marital status [14].

It has been observed that women typically have longer sleep duration and higher sleep efficiency, yet are more likely to report sleep-related complaints, and to experience psychological effects such as depression and anxiety than their male counterparts [14]. These trends may be a reflection of gender based psychological and sociocultural factors, in addition to genetic and biologic factors [15].

In addition to psychological and sociocultural factors, hormonal effects may account for many of the sex differences in elderly sleep [14]. Coinciding with a decrease in estrogen and progesterone levels during menopause, postmenopausal women are more likely to suffer from sleep disturbances. Similarly, decreases in testosterone associated with male aging coincide with decreased sleep efficiency in men [13].

Our team constructed a 111-item questionnaire to help develop an understanding of how SDs in the elderly differ from those found in adults in conjunction with how they differ between the sexes through the process of data-driven, observational research utilizing both basic and applied designs. This study design's goal was to focus on sleep patterns revealed by naturally occurring phenomena (e.g. lifestyle, gender, age) to maximize knowledge advancement and applicability of sleep disorder treatment.

Materials and Methods

Currently, evaluations of SDs are inadequate across the ages and sexes, as they are compromised by under reporting and relying on self-reported data rather than professional sleep studies (i.e. nocturnal polysomnography (NPS) and multiple sleep latency tests (MSLT)). Moreover, there is a paucity of data specific to older adults. In response, we partnered with the sleep center at a regional medical center, and constructed a 111-item questionnaire to use in conjunction with NPS, MSLT, the Epworth Sleepiness Scale (ESS), and medical chart reviews of patients referred for evaluation of SDs. In this partnership, every individual referred for NPS at the regional medical hospital's sleep disorder center by his/her general care physician was given the opportunity to enroll in our study, regardless of proposed sleep disorder. Through this inclusive enrollment, our analysis is not limited to any particular SD; instead, patterns are revealed showing the disparities in which individuals are routinely referred to sleep centers, and which individuals do not receive treatment. Those who chose to participate in the study completed informed consent upon arrival at the sleep center for NPS.

Participants were asked, prior to their sleep study, to complete an extensive questionnaire. The 111-item questionnaire, developed over the course of 19 years by our team, collects a variety of behavioral, physiological, psychological, and medical data from each participant. Rather than being sleep-specific, this comprehensive approach allows for objective analysis of sleep effects and overall QoL, without bias to merely sleep disorder symptomatology. During the sleep study, baseline data regarding sleep patterns were collected utilizing NPS and MSLT. Following the study, our team collected impressions and diagnoses were given by trained sleep technicians. After collection of the baseline data, participants were then contacted six months post-sleep study for follow up questioning. These follow up questions collected data that is similar to the baseline questionnaire, geared towards comparing sleep pre-study to sleep experienced after diagnosis. . Following descriptive analysis comparing geriatric and adult sleep, we examined sex differences to further characterize geriatric sleep. The study population consisted of 568 adults (304 male and 264 female) and 151 geriatric participants (92 male and 59 female). Our investigation of sex differences looked at how sleep architecture, marital status, sleep diagnoses, and sleep associates varied between men and women (Tables 6-10). All participants in the study were independent adults not living in care facilities.

Results

We compared SDs and their associates by categorizing participants in two broad age groups: adult (ages 19-65, M=46.2) and geriatric (ages 66-90, M=71.6) to illuminate a characterization of the geriatric population. Chi-square analysis and t-tests revealed differences in the associated sleep disturbance symptoms reported between the adult and geriatric groups. BMI was significantly higher in the adult group (M=35.2) than the geriatric group (M=31.7, p<0.001). NPS revealed expected sleep architecture differences specific to the geriatric group spending significantly more time in N1 and less in N3 and REM (Table 1).

	Adult	Geriatric
N1***	12.6%	18.4%
N2	61.8%	60.3%
N3*	5.2%	3.6%
REM***	15.0%	11.58%
p*<0.05, p**<0.01, p***<0.001		

Table 1: NPS sleep architecture across sleep disorders.

Although the geriatric group had a higher prevalence of SD and physiological diagnoses (Tables 2 and 3), they experienced longer sleep latencies, spent significantly less time asleep, and reported fewer sleep related complaints than the adult group (Table 4).

	Adult	Geriatric
Nocturnal hypoxemia**	12.0%	21.5%
Periodic limb movement disorder**	6.1%	14.1%
Poor sleep efficiency***	26.8%	45.6%
Restless leg syndrome*	1.1%	3.4%
Hypersomnolence*	12.8%	6.0%
p*<0.05, p**<0.01, p***<0.001		

Table 2: Sleep diagnoses.

	Adult	**Geriatric**
Allergies*	63.7%	54.1%
Chronic Lung Disease***	12.2%	32.9%
Diabetes*	15.3%	22.4%
Headaches***	70.9%	41.7%
Heart Attack***	6.4%	16.4%
Heart Failure***	7.1%	20.7%
High Blood Pressure Treatment***	36.8%	66.7%

Nasal/Sinus Problems*	43.5%	33.8%
Stroke***	4.8%	13.0%
Thyroid Disease***	16.5%	28.4%
Anxiety***	56.8%	41.2%
Depression**	58.8%	45.6%
Irritability***	76.8%	53.3%
Stress***	83.8%	64.6%
p*<0.05, p**<0.01, p***<0.001		

Table 3: Physiological/Psychiatric symptoms across sleep disorders.

	Adult	Geriatric
NPS Sleep Duration (min)***	340.2	299.4
Wake rested***	14.9%	39.9%
NPS Sleep Latency (min)***	20.5	27.7
Concerned with well-being**	59.8%	41.0%
Bizarre dreams***	51.9%	34.1%
Choking sensation***	39.6%	23.2%
Feels paralyzed**	16.4%	6.5%
Grinds teeth***	29.7%	9.1%
Nightmares*	49.6%	36.1%
Restroom more than 3x/night***	41.5%	64.4%
Reported sleep latency*	27.6%	22.0%
p*<0.05, p**<0.01, p***<0.001		

Table 4: Sleep associated variants across sleep disorders.

The geriatric group reported fewer bizarre dreams, nightmares, and waking with choking sensations. Moreover, they reported waking rested more frequently than the adult group. Daytime detriments were also less frequent in the geriatric group in areas such as difficulty concentrating, sleep disturbances interfering with social life, and memory/ attention to detail (Table 5). Additionally, they experienced fewer headaches, less anxiety, depression, irritability and stress (Table 3).

	Adult	Geriatric
Difficulty concentrating***	66.8%	38.1%
ESS-passenger in car**	56.8%	45.3%
ESS-rest in afternoon**	87.4%	72.0%
Go to bed same time every night*	72.1%	87.7%
Like to sleep late***	65.8%	21.1%
Oxygen aid while sleeping***	7.5%	18.5%
Sleep interference with social life***	61.2%	30.4%
Take naps***	44.7%	64.1%
Wake at same time every day*	66.4	86.4%
Accident due to sleepiness***	22.5%	7.5%
Memory/attention to detail***	71.1%	56.6%
p*<0.05, p**<0.01, p***<0.001		

Table 5: Day time symptoms across sleep disorders.

When comparing sex differences in the geriatric group, we found that males spent more time in REM, experienced sleep problems longer before being diagnosed, and experienced more snoring, while females experienced longer sleep latency (Tables 6 and 7). Additionally, more elderly men were married and more geriatric women report living alone (Table 8).

	Male	Female
N1	19.6%	15.5%
N2	58.1%	60.8%
N3	2.7%	4.6%
REM*	12.8%	10.8%
p*<0.05, p**<0.01, p***<0.001		

Table 6: Sex differences: NPS sleep architecture across sleep disorders.

	Male	**Female**
NPS sleep latency (min)**	21.6	37
Sleep problem length (years)*	11.7	6.6
Snore**	86.2%	66.7%
Stop breathing***	77.4%	44.2%
Arm/leg jerk	51.8%	34.0%
ESS total***	11.7	9.2
Fall asleep while driving**	25.0%	10%
Sleep walking**	0%	4.3%
Enjoy sleep*	43.3%	55.7%
p*<0.05, p**<0.01, p***<0.001		

Table 7: Sex differences: Sleep associates across sleep disorders.

	Male	**Female**
Single	3.8%	7.1%
Married	80.8%	38.6%
Divorced	3.8%	24.3%
Widowed	7.7%	10.8%

p*<0.05, p**<0.01, p***<0.001

Table 8: Sex differences: Marital status*** across sleep disorders.

Despite significant differences in physiological comorbidities such as heart attack, body pain, high blood pressure, and thyroid disease; sleep diagnoses did not significantly differ between sexes (Tables 9 and 10). In our population, women more frequently reported body pain, high blood pressure, anxiety, and had concerns for their mental health. Conversely, men reported a higher incidence of breathing cessation, heart attack, and heart failure. We found this trend across age groups.

	Male	Female
OSA	88.5%	81.4%
Periodic leg movement	14.4%	15.7%
Poor sleep efficiency	51.9%	51.4%
Abnormal sleep architecture	75.0%	77.1%
Hypersomnolence	7.7%	2.9%
Nocturnal hypoventilation	1.0%	2.9%
Primary snoring	10.6%	7.1%
Restless leg syndrome	3.8%	2.9%
Normal sleep	5.8%	4.3%
Nocturnal hypoxemia	19.2%	28.6%
p*<0.05, p**<0.01, p***<0.001		

Table 9: Sex differences: Sleep diagnoses across sleep disorders.

	Male	Female
Allergies*	47.6%	64.8%
Anxiety*	33.7%	51.9%
Asthma**	7.7%	18.6%
Body Pain**	31.3%	81.8%
Heart Attack*	23.1%	6.9%
Heart burn/acid reflux*	32.6%	50.0%
Heart Failure*	25.6%	12.1%
High Blood Pressure**	57.6%	81.0%
Medication for mental health concerns**	26.0%	45.7%
Thyroid Disease***	11.8%	55.2%
p*<0.05, p**<0.01, p***<0.001		

Table 10: Sex differences: Physiological symptoms across sleep disorders.

Discussion

These findings indicate that comparison of SDs and their characterizations in the adult and geriatric groups result in similarities and differences between groups. The adult group had a significantly higher BMI than the geriatric group. Though it is widely accepted that increased BMI is associated with sleep disruptions, the difference in BMI skewed towards the adult group while the geriatric group reported the expected higher prevalence of chronic diseases. This suggests that circadian, social, and behavioral changes associated with aging may outweigh BMI as a predictor for sleep disturbances.

The most profound differences between adult and geriatric sleep exist in self-reported sleep adequacy. NPS revealed expected sleep architecture differences specific to the geriatric population spending significantly more time in N1 and less in N3 and REM. Yet, while the geriatric population experienced longer sleep latencies, spent significantly less time asleep, and had a higher prevalence of sleep disorder diagnoses and chronic disease, they reported fewer sleep-related symptomatology (including psychiatric symptoms). Moreover, the geriatric group reported waking rested more frequently than the adult group. As sleep quality is related to both psychological and physiological factors, future research would likely benefit from a thorough examination of which is more important for perceived sleep satisfaction. Further examining sex differences in elderly adults revealed some differences in perspective. Despite having similar sleep disorder diagnoses, these women reported fewer sleep complaints. Indeed, unlike men, women were more likely to accept sleep problems as a normal part of life. In this research, more geriatric men were married, whereas geriatric women were more likely to be single, divorced, or widowed. Women in the geriatric group were more likely to be diagnosed with physiological health problems and were more likely to be taking medication related to mental health.

These results could be a product of under reporting by the geriatric population or perhaps habituation to the challenges associated with sleep disturbances. It is plausible that the under reporting of geriatric sleep disturbances may be in part attributed to an 'ordering' of health issues. Wherein, perceived higher risk conditions/ chronic diseases such as heart disease, diabetes, or arthritis take precedence in the health concerns of elderly adults while their sleep issues fall to the wayside. It is also the case that our samples of adults versus geriatrics differed dramatically in size (i.e. 151 geriatric cases versus 568 adult cases) which suggests that significantly fewer older adults were referred for sleep studies. We ponder whether this is because sleep complaints by older adults are marginalized, disregarded, or regarded as simply part of the aging process. Given that we assessed all who presented for sleep study to a regional medical center; our sample may representative of referring patters specific to our particular region of the United States. This study is also limited by the fact that we did not seek or select participants according to sleep diagnosis and match the number of participants per diagnosis, we cannot address specific differences between specific sleep disorder diagnoses and the mechanisms therein. Instead, we simply report the outcomes from those referred to the regional medical center. Further, our investigation involved the physical health of participants. All participants were individuals living independently; not in a long-term care facility. Inclusions of elderly people living in dependent care may reveal different characteristics than found in the present study. We suggest that sleep disturbances across all age groups be given ample consideration to provide the best health care and quality of life for all.

References

1. Seibert PS, Valerio J, Rafla Y, Grimsely F, Writer S (2011) llluminating the relationship shared by cardiovascular disease and sleep. Presented at: 9th International Congress on Coronary Artery Disease (ICCAD).
2. Seibert PS1, Whitmore TA, Parker PD, Grimsley FP, Payne K, et al. (2006) The emerging role of telemedicine in diagnosing and treating sleep disorders. J Telemed Telecare 12: 379-381.
3. Seibert PS, Whitmore TA, Dufty BM, Whitener N, Grimsley FP, O'Donnell, JE. (2005) Sleep Disorders: Age Makes a Difference. Sleep Review.
4. Prinz PN, Vitello MV, Raskind MA, Thorpy MJ. (1990) Geriatrics: Sleep disorders and aging. New England Journal of Medicine 323: 520-526.
5. Ancoli-Israel A, Ayalon L, Salzman C (2008) Sleep in the elderly: Normal variations and common sleep disorders. Harv Rev Psychiatry 16:279-286.
6. Krishnan P1, Hawranik P (2008) Diagnosis and management of geriatric insomnia: a guide for nurse practitioners. J Am Acad Nurse Pract 20: 590-599.
7. Neikrug AB1, Ancoli-Israel S (2010) Sleep disorders in the older adult - a mini-review. Gerontology 56: 181-189.
8. Ohayon MM1, Carskadon MA, Guilleminault C, Vitiello MV (2004) Meta-analysis of quantitative sleep parameters from childhood to old age in healthy individuals: developing normative sleep values across the human lifespan. Sleep 27: 1255-1273.
9. Vitiello MV1, Moe KE, Prinz PN (2002) Sleep complaints cosegregate with illness in older adults: clinical research informed by and informing epidemiological studies of sleep. J Psychosom Res 53: 555-559.
10. Endeshaw Y (2012) Aging, subjective sleep quality, and health status: the global picture. Sleep 35: 1035-1036.
11. Subramanian S, Surani S. (2007) Sleep disorders in the elderly. Geriatrics 62:10-32.
12. Administration on Aging. (2012) Prescription medication misuse and abuse among older adults. Older Americans Behavioral Health 5:1-4.
13. Redline S, Kirchner HL, Quan SF, Gottlieb DJ, Kapur V, Newman A. (2004) The effects of age, sex, ethnicity, and sleep-disordered breathing on sleep architecture. Arch Intern Med 164:406-18.
14. van den Berg JF1, Miedema HM, Tulen JH, Hofman A, Neven AK, et al. (2009) Sex differences in subjective and actigraphic sleep measures: a population-based study of elderly persons. Sleep 32: 1367-1375.
15. Troxel WM, Buysse DJ, Hall M. (2009) Marital happiness and sleep disturbances in a multi-ethnic sample of middle-aged women. Behavioral Sleep Medicine 7:2-19.

22

Sleep Status and its Relationship with Other Coronary Artery Diseases Risk Factors

Najafipour Hamid[1], **Sabahi Abdolreza**[2,*], **Mirrashidi Fatemeasadat**[3], **Afshari Mahdi**[4] **and Haghdoost Ali Akbar**[5]

[1]*Physiology Research Center, Institute of Neuropharmacology, Kerman University of Medical Sciences, Kerman, Iran*

[2]*Religion and Medicine Research Center and the Department of Psychiatry, Kerman University of Medical Sciences, Kerman, Iran*

[3]*Cardiovascular Research Center, Institute of Basic and Clinical Physiology sciences, Kerman University of Medical Sciences, Kerman, Iran*

[4]*Department of Community Medicine, Zabol University of Medical Sciences, Zabol, Iran*

[5]*Research Center for Modeling in Health, Institute of Future Studies in Health, Kerman University of Medical Sciences, Kerman, Iran*

[*]**Corresponding author:** Sabahi Abdolreza, Religion and Medicine Research Center and the Department of Psychiatry, Kerman University of Medical Sciences, Kerman, Iran, E-mail: abdsaba@kmu.ac.ir

Abstract

Introduction: Coronary artery diseases (CADs) are one of the main causes of mortality and morbidity in Iran. Due to the shortage of information regarding sleep status in the area and also the close relation between CADs and sleep health, this study attempted to examine sleep status in a large urban area of southeast Iran in order to find its relation with CADs risk factors such as anxiety and depression, hypertension, blood glucose level, smoking, low physical activity, and obesity.

Method: A Single-stage cluster sampling cross-sectional study was carried out on 5900 people aged 15 to75 in Kerman city to examine the CAD risk factors (KERCADR study). Alongside, sleep screening and a physical activity (PA) questionnaire regarding their sleep quantity and PA level were also used. Beck Anxiety and Beck Depression Inventories (for anxiety and depression assessment), medical examination and fasting blood sample were taken to collect the participants' demographic and blood glucose data.

Findings: From 3238 (54.9%) women and 2662 (45.1%) men who participated in this study 30.5%suffered from abnormal sleep (11.5% from insomnia and 19% from hypersomnia). 39.3% of the men and 45.1% of the women had low physical activity. There was a significant relationship between smoking (p=0.02), anxiety and depression (p<0.001), hypertension (p=0.03) and low PA (p=0.01) with sleep disorders.

Conclusion: the results showed that nearly one-third of the adult population suffered from abnormal sleep. Also, the prevalence of hypersomnia was 1.65 times more than that of insomnia. This issue along with the high prevalence of low physical activity exposed the population to different diseases.

Keywords: Insomnia; Hypersomnia; Anxiety; Depression; Physical activity; Obesity; High blood pressure; Kerman

Introduction

Sleep is one of the circadian cycles and is a basic human need which is necessary to maintain energy, happiness and physical well-being [1]. Sleep is a process which the brain requires in order to function properly. It is not merely a passive process; in fact, it is related to high brain activity [2]. According to DSM-5 there are different forms of sleep disorders such as insomnia-hypersomnia, narcolepsy, breathing-related, circadian rhythm-related and somatic-related diseases or substance abuse related disorders.

Sleep disorders, in terms of pathology, are interconnected with other psychiatric disorders like depression-anxiety or other somatic diseases [3]. Hence, a smaller part of sleep disorders, which is primary as 25% of the patients who refer to sleep disorder clinics, suffer from a psychiatric disorder - half of whom have a mood disorder [4].

Sleep disorders are dangerous and costly as well. The direct cost per annum of sleep disorders in the United States is estimated at 16 billion dollars, with indirect costs ranging up to 100 billion dollars. Men over 30 years or older who slept less than 4 hours per night were 2.8 times more likely to die within 6 years than were those who slept 7 to 8 hours per night. Also, men who slept more than 10 hours per night had a higher death rate (1.8 times) than normal sleepers [5]. Studies show that there is a relation between obstructive sleep apnea and high blood pressure, heart failure, and heart attack (which are among the main causes of mortality and morbidity in developing countries such as Iran). Different factors can cause reduction in sleep. An anxiety-arousing experience or expecting a stressful event such as the loss of a dear one, can be associated with insomnia [2]. Poor sleepers commonly complain from daytime fatigue, disturbed mood, faulty memory, trouble in thinking and concentration, restlessness and irritability, stress intolerance and lack of energy in performing innovative and complex tasks [4]. Some studies consider sleep deprivation as a risk factor for depression, anxiety and substance abuse in the future; also, frequent absences from work and increased direct and indirect medical costs are also some of its negative effects [6].

Insomnia influences cognitive functioning, neuroendocrine, immune and inflammatory systems as well [7]. Recent studies show that sleep deprivation increases insulin resistance, compensatory hyper-insulinemia and the risk of diabetes among young adults with familial history of type 2 diabetes [8]. In a study doneby Gohansson et al. people with insomnia had increased variability in heart rate and blood pressure - which are risk factors for cardiovascular diseases. In addition, studies have shown that smokers suffer more from insomnia disorders [9]. Ohayon and Lemoine reported that the prevalence of insomnia was 20-40% in Western Europe and showed that it was more common among women and elderly people [10].

Another issue related to sleep disorder is hypersomnia. A longitudinal study carried out on 1200 men and women showed that people who slept more than 8.5 hours per night had 15%higher risk of death than those who slept 7 hours per night [6]. The lifetime prevalence of hypersomnia was found to be 8.2%. In a study done by Shirakawa and Takahashi, the rate of sleep disorder was reported to be 44% among the Japanese [11].

The studies devoted to sleep rate in Iran have been so far limited, and they are more frequently conducted to examine the sleep status in specific groups. In a study done in 2008 in Kashan-Iran, the prevalence of insomnia was reported to be 59% which had been more prevalent among women and middle-aged people [12]. In another study on students in Kurdistan University of Medical Sciences, the prevalence of insomnia was 57.4% [13]. This is why the sleep duration in the general population has been less investigated. Given the importance of sleep, its effects upon mental and general health, and its relation with cardiovascular diseases, the sleep status has not been investigated so far in southeast Iran according to the existing resources. As coronary artery diseases (CADs) are among main causes of mortality and morbidity in Iran and due to the shortage of information regarding the sleep status in the area, and also the close relation between CADs and sleep health, this study attempted to examine the prevalence of two main sleep disorders symptoms(insomnia and hypersomnia)in the general population of Kerman (the largest city in southeast Iran) and their relation with CADs risk factors such as anxiety and depression, hypertension, blood glucose level, smoking, low physical activity, and obesity. Also, in low and middle income countries, the sleep duration is affected by occupation as some people are obliged to have more than one job to manage their living expenses and the rate of unemployment is also high, the relation between sleep disorders and occupation was also investigated.

Methods

The present paper is a sub-analysis of data collected in a study which focused on the risk factors of coronary artery diseases (i.e. Kerman Coronary Artery Disease Risk Factor Study; KERCADRS). Four of these risk factors were the sleep status, the physical activity level, smoking, and obesity. The study was carried out on 5900 individuals ranging from 15 to 75 years old in 2010-2011on an urban population in South East of Iran. The study protocol was approved by the ethical committee of Kerman University of Medical Sciences, Iran (Permission No. 88/110KA).The unit of sampling was households who have been living in Kerman for at least one year prior to the interview. Using the zip code in the mail office as the sampling frame, we marked 250 post codes and approached the households in the area to recruit around 6000 individuals in the twelve strata of age and sex. The recruited people were invited to complete the informed consent and participate in the research. They were investigated in a clinical study site located in Kerman downtown where they went through several steps of in-person interview to disclose their demographic characteristics, occupation and CAD risk behaviors. They were also asked to report some possible factors influencing sleep such as their mental status (anxiety and depression), physical activity and smoking. A fasting blood sample was taken from each participant at the time of their attendance. The blood samples were then centrifuged and after 20 minutes of clotting time to separate the serum components, the glucose level was measured in a clinical laboratory by commerciallab kits. Details of this procedure are provided in another publication [14].

The blood pressure (BP) was measured by the physician using Rishter mercury BP manometer (RishterCo, Germany) after at least five minutes of rest, while the participant was required to hold his/her right arm in a sitting position. Also, participants with self-reported history of hypertension or anti-hypertensive drug used by participant were considered as hypertensive. More details are provided in another paper [15].

A sleep screening questionnaire was used by the interviewer to quantify the participants' sleep duration. Insomnia is defined to be the difficulty that one undergoes when initiating sleep or maintaining sleep, or having non-restorative sleep. Hypersomnia defined to be the excessive quantity of sleep, the deteriorated quality of wakefulness and sleep inertia [3]. Based on the American sleep association (A.S.A) an average of 7-8 hours of sleep is the best length of time for an adult [3]. In this study, cases with one hour less and one hour more than the normal range were placed in the following two groups respectively: insomnia and hypersomnia.

Beck Anxiety Inventory (BAI) and Beck Depression Inventory (BDI) [16], were translated and adapted for use in Iran. questionnaires were completed by trained interviewers. Beck Anxiety Inventory (BAI) is designed to quantify the anxiety level and contains 21 phrases (each phrase describes one of the symptoms of anxiety with severity ranged from 0 to 3). The total score of the inventory is 63. For depression, the Beck Depression Inventory (BDI) includes 21 groups of statements and each statement has 4 responses with severity ranged from 0 to 3. The total score of the inventory is 63. In the present study, based on the score of the inventories, the anxiety and depression level of the participants were divided into 3 levels: mild, moderate and severe. The score range for the different levels of anxiety was as follows: scores 0-7, normal; 8-15, mild anxiety; 16-25, moderate anxiety; and 26-63, severe anxiety.

The score range for the different levels of depression was as follows:

Scores 0-15, without symptom; 16-30, mild depression; 31-46, moderate depression and 47-63, severe depression.

Daily physical activities at home and workplace were recorded using WHO Global Physical Activity Questionnaire (GPAQ). To evaluate the intensity of the physical activities, metabolic equivalent (MET) was used. MET is the amount of energy an individual adult uses while s/he is sitting. Moderate physical activities are believed to consume four times the energy used while sitting, and intense physical activities consume eight times more. Low physical activities are believed to consume energy less than four times in proportion to the amount used while sitting.

About smoking, by use of an interview-assist questionnaire, we asked about the number of cigarettes that the participants smoked per day and those who smoked at least one cigarette per day were considered as cigarette smokers.

Body mass index (BMI) was calculated by dividing the participants' weight in kg to their height in meters squared (kg/m2) and based on the WHO definition, BMI was classified into three categories of normal [BMI 18.5-24.9 kg/m2], overweight [BMI 25-29.9 kg/m2], and obese [BMI ≥ 30 kg/m2].

The study Methodology has been explained more precisely in a previous publication [17].

Statistical analysis

The prevalence of Insomnia and hypersomnia were compared between the subjects with and without disorders using Chi square test. The prevalences were standardized according to Kerman's population distribution in 2006. We fitted univariate and multivariate (adjusted for age, gender, job and level of physical activity) Poisson regression models to show the crude and adjusted associations between the sleep disorders and other cardiovascular risk factors. Risk ratio (RR) is defined as the proportion of the existance of one risk factor in a case group to the existance of the same risk factor in the control group (crude RR). Adjusted RR is RR when the effect of the related confounding factors (such as the effect of aging on hypertension and diabetes) on the relationship/association was omitted by statistical methods (multivariate analysis). All the analyses were performed under survey data analysis considering the households as primary sampling units. Data analysis was conducted using STATA v.P value less than 0.05 was considered statistically significant.

Results

Out of 5900 participants in this study, 3238 (54.9%) and 2662 (45.1%) were men and women, respectively. Low physical activities were observed in 32.9% of the males (95% CI=37.9-40.6) and 45.1% of the females (95% CI=43.8-46.4). On the whole, 1800 (30.5%) had abnormal sleep. Accordingly, the prevalence of insomnia and hypersomnia were 11.5% and 19%, respectively; and their prevalence was more in the females than in males ($p<0.001$). In terms of occupation, the least prevalence of insomnia was related to employees (prevalence: 13.8%; 95% CI=8.3-21.9%) and the highest prevalence of hypersomnia was observed among the unemployed, retired individuals (prevalence: 43.2%; 95%Cl, 36.8-50.4%) and housewives. A significant relationship was found between smoking and sleep disorder ($p<0.02$), and the prevalence of hypersomnia was significantly higher in smokers (45.2%; 95%Cl: 38.3-52.4%) than in non-smokers (35.4%; 95%Cl: 33.5%-37.4%). In terms of physical activity, the prevalence of hypersomnia was significantly higher in those individuals who had low physical activity (37.9%) (95% CI: 34.9-40.9%) than in those with high physical activity (29.6%) (95% CI: 27.2-32.0%) (P=0.01). The prevalence of insomnia in anxious and depressed participants and the prevalence of hypersomnia in the participants having high blood pressure were significantly higher than in the people in good health (Table 1). The prevalence of insomnia and hypersomnia in the obese participants (BMI>30) was not significantly different from the others (p=0.09).

Disorders		Prevalence (95%Cl) of insomnia (<6 hours)	Prevalence (95%Cl) of hypersomnia (>9hours)	P-Value
Depression	Yes(BDI>15) (N=2283)	18%(15.8-20.4)	34.7%(31.4-38.3)	<0.0001
	no (N=3571)	7.7%(6.8-8.8)	37.1%(34.9-39.3)	
Anxiety	Yes(BAI>7) (N=4499)	12.8%(11.7-14)	35.6%(33.4-37.7)	0.0006
	no (N=1352)	6.7%(5.2-8.4)	38.5%(34.5-42.6)	
Hypertension	Yes(BP>140/80 or taking drug) (N=1321)	14.4%(9.4-21.6)	45.4%(37.4-53.7)	<0.0001
	no (N=4531)	11.4%(10.4-12.5)	35.7%(33.8-37.6)	
Obesity	Yes(BMI>30) (N=1043)	9.8%(7.6-12.4)	41.9%(35-49.2)	0.09
	no (N=4731)	11.6%(10.6-12.7)	35.3%(33.4-37.3)	

Table 1: The prevalence of different sleep disorders in relation to depression, anxiety, hypertension and obesity.

Sleep time	Disorders							
	Depression(BDI>15)		Anxiety(BAI>7)		Hypertension		Obesity (BMI>30)	
	Crude RR	Adjusted RR	Crude RR	Adjusted RR	Crude RR	Adjusted RR	Crude RR	Adjusted RR
	(p-value)	(p-value)	(p-value)	(p-value)	(p-value)	(p-value)	(p-value)	(p-value)
6-9hours (ref)	1	1	1	1	1	1	1	1

<6 hours	1.77 (<0.0001)	1.59 (<0.0001)	1.16 (<0.0001)	1.14 (<0.0001)	1.39 (<0.0001)	1.10 (0.1)	1.23(0.01)	1.05(0.5)
>9hours	1.06 (0.2)	0.99 (0.9)	1.01 (0.6)	0.99 (0.8)	1.01 (0.9)	1.14 (0.03)	1.13(0.1)	1.15(0.06)

Table 2: Crude and adjusted risk ratios (p-value) among sleeping time and other disorders BDI: Beck Depression Index; BAI: Beck Anxiety Index; Hypertension: (BP>140/80 or taking drug).

In a multivariate analysis carried out on people having insomnia, the risk of anxiety and depression increased up to 14% and 59% after adjusting the variables of age, gender, occupation and physical activity level (p<0.0001)(Table 2).

Also, the risk of hypersomnia was higher (12% more) in people with low physical activity (p=0.01) (Table 3). On the other hand, hypersomnia raised the risk of high blood pressure (above 140/80 mm Hg) up to 14% which was statistically significant (p<0.03). In addition, the risk ratio between obesity and insomnia and hypersomnia were 1.05(p=0.5) and 1.15 (p=0.06), respectively (Table 2).

In comparison with those having normal sleep, the mean of fasting blood glucose (FBG) in people having insomnia was 2.2 mg/dl more, and among people having hypersomnia it was 0.8 mg/dl lesser. However, none of these differences were significantly different (P=0.3 and P=0.5, respectively).

Sleep time	crude RR	p- value	Adjusted RR*	p-value
<6 hours	1.1	0.09	1.03	0.6
>9 hours	1.13	0.006	1.12	0.01

Table 3: Crude and adjusted associations between sleep disorder and low physical activity (*controlling demographic and clinical characteristics).

Discussion

The findings of this study showed that nearly one-third of the 5900 participants in this study had sleep disorders whose rate was higher among the females. The results corresponded to the results of Shirakawa and Takahashi's study which indicated that the prevalence of sleep disorders was 44% in Japan [11], and it was also in line with another study done in Kashan, Iran in 2008 with the prevalence of insomnia being 59% in which the highest rate was related to the women [12]. Ohayon et al. carried out a research on French individuals who were between 14-96 years of age. It was observed that the prevalence of sleep disorders was higher in the females than in the males. The overall prevalence of sleep disorders in the population was 36.2% [10]. A variety of factors influence females' sleep including stress, illness, changes in the level of female hormones, sleeping environment, and being overweight [18]. In another study conducted in Tabriz on people having mental disorders and on general population [19], it was concluded that the prevalence of sleep disorders was 35.2% in the general population which is a little higher than that of Kerman.

In this study, the prevalence of hypersomnia in smokers increased significantly which corresponded with the study done by Zarowski [20] and Wetter [21], in which smokers suffered from sleep disorders more than non-smokers. The risk of anxiety and depression increased significantly after the variables of age, gender, occupation and physical activity level were adjusted in the multivariate analysis. This confirmed the studies in which insomnia was recognized as a risk factor for depression and anxiety [5]. In their study, Saleh et al. found that there was a relationship between reduced sleep quality and abnormal anxiety [22]. Also, a significant and direct relation was found between the scores of sleep disorders and those of depression intensity in the participants. There were also serious disorders in all aspects of sleep quality and quantity in the patients suffering from depression [3]. It is important to note that it was not possible to determine whether insomnia caused anxiety and depression or it was the consequence of anxiety and depression since having sleep disorders can be the main symptom of depression [3]. In other words, it is possible that this problem occurs as a result of reverse causality, and this requires an independent research.

In this study, hypersomnia increased the risk of high blood pressure after the confounding factors were adjusted. In a study done by Gohansson et al. [9] in Finland the increased variability of heart beat and blood pressure among the patients having insomnia had been recognized as a risk factor for cardiovascular diseases. Both hypersomnia and insomnia may increase the blood pressure, however, with different mechanisms. Of course, lifestyle especially one's diet, level of physical activity and daily stresses are important factors influencing the blood pressure, and these factors vary in different countries. The overall 19% hypersomnia along with 18.4% prevalence of hypertension (HTN)and 35.5% prevalence of pre-HTN in the study population[15] while considering the fact that hypersomnia had a significant association with hypertension (Table 2) would render this population at a high risk of suffering from cardiovascular diseases in the future. Especially, when we found that smoking, anxiety, and obesity were the most significant predictors for HTN [15].

Although, insomnia and hypersomnia increased the risk of obesity more than 5% and 15% respectively, none of these associations were statistically significant. However, the P value of 0.06 regarding the association of hypersomnia with obesity (Table 2) is close to the significant level. The global prevalence of 9% diabetes and 18.7% pre-diabetes that we observed in our study population [14] in conjunction with 42.1% prevalence of low physical activity (unpublished observation), and significant association of hypersomnia with LPA (Table 2) are also important cautions for general health in the studied population. Compared with normal sleepers, fasting blood glucose was higher in insomnia sufferers and lower in hypersomnia sufferers (although not statistically significant). According to a previous study, sleep deprivation increases insulin resistance, compensatory hyper-insulinemia and also the risk of diabetes among young adults with familial risks for type 2 diabetes [23], or makes a significant relationship between one's overall sleep status and the disturbances in one's glucose metabolism and increased circulating insulin levels [23]. Also, a review of different studies shows a bidirectional relation between sleep status and diabetes, and it notes that the reduced sleep duration paves the way for diabetes type 2among females [24]. This relationship can be justified by referring to the fact that sleep reinforces neuro-hormonal receptors that control blood glucose [3]. Thus, pathophysiologic changes related to sleep disorders seem to lead to the development of type 2 diabetes. Keeping the results of the above mentioned studies at mind, the difference in the relation between insomnia and the risk of diabetes in the present study may be due to the higher susceptibility of the individuals with familial risk of having diabetes to fall sick when exposed to stress.

Regarding the significant association between insomnia and anxiety/depression (Table 2), it may note that it is required to have normal mental function in order for one to have normal sleep. And it is acceptable that individuals who are anxious or depressed may have shorter sleep durations. Due to the effect of stress hormones on other body functions, such as the effect of cortisol and sympathetic hormones on glucose metabolism, anxiety and depression, this may cause insomnia on one hand and lead to diabetes on the other hand. In this regard, we found that the maximum prevalence of co-morbidities among the patients with diabetes were anxiety (87.5%), depression (57.9%) and overweight/obesity (47.1%) [14].

One of the limitations of the present study is that it was cross-sectional. It also used simultaneous data collection concerning risk factors and their outcomes, which prevents an exact examination of the temporal transposition between them. In other words, we cannot be sure whether the higher prevalence of CAD risk factors leads to sleep disorders, or sleep disorders account for the increase of the prevalence of CAD risk factors. In order to find an answer to this, it is required to conduct a prospective longitudinal study on this issue. We have now commenced the second phase of KERCADR study as a longitudinal cohort to answer such important questions.

Conclusion

Given the high prevalence of abnormal sleep among nearly one-third of the population in this study and its relation with smoking, anxiety, depression, low physical activity and high blood pressure, (which are among the main risk factors of coronary artery diseases) and also by considering the fact that these diseases are currently the main causes of mortality and morbidity in Iran, it is suggested that necessary measurements should be considered to improve sleep health in the population. The prevalence of hypersomnia was concluded here to be 65% higher than the prevalence of insomnia. This along with high prevalence of low physical activity and body weight would render individuals exposed to various metabolic and cardiovascular diseases in the future.

Acknowledgements

We thank all who have participated in the KERCADR study. We are also deeply indebted to Medical Physicians: HesamiKh, YazdanpenahSh, Tajadini H, andAhmadiGohari N. Interviewers: Ebrahimian Z., Kalantari M., Shahabi Sh., Shahabi F. and Nazarieh S., Administration: Namjoo H., Sadeghi Z., andKhajooei S. Clinical Laboratory: DoostMohammadi M, Sheikholeslami Y. and KhajehHasani H.Community/Social Mobilizer: Nikvarz A., Nikvarz N., Iran-nejad H., Iran-nejad S., and Molaei F., Servants: Soltani M., Mohammadi Z., Ghanbari N., Bagheri M., Mortazapour M. and Iranmanesh M. We would like to thank Nadia Ghazanfari-Moghaddam for proof-reading this manuscript. Also, we send our best gratitude to Dr Maliheh Shadkam Farrokhi who contributed generously to the project and unfortunately passed away in the middle of the study (may she rest in peace).

Conflict of Interest

The authors declare that there is no conflict of interest in this study.

References

1. Hays RD, Martin SA, Sesti AM, Spritzer KL (2005) Psychometric properties of the Medical Outcomes Study Sleep measure. Sleep Med 6: 41-44.
2. Sadock BJ, Kaplan HI, Sadock VA (2007) Kaplan and Sadock's synopsis of psychiatry: behavioral sciences/clinical psychiatry (10thedn). Philadelphia: Wolter Kluwer, Lippincott Williams & Wilkins, 363-364.
3. American psychiatric association (2013) Sleep-wake disorder: In Diagnostic and stastical manual of mental disorders (5thedn).
4. Max H, Rhoda GS, Amir SH (2009) Sleep disorders. Comprehensive text book of psychiatry (9thedn). Lippincott, Williams & Wilkins, 2150-2178.
5. American Psychiatric Association, Insomnia: both symptom and syndrome. Clinical and Research News. Psychiatric News.
6. Breslau N, Roth T, Rosenthal L, Andreski P (1996) Sleep disturbance and psychiatric disorders: a longitudinal epidemiological study of young adults. Biol Psychiatry 39: 411-418.
7. Faraut B, Boudjeltia KZ, Vanhamme L, Kerkhofs M (2012) Immune, inflammatory and cardiovascular consequences of sleep restriction and recovery. Sleep Med Rev 16: 137-149.
8. Darukhanavala A, Booth JN 3rd, Bromley L, Whitmore H, Imperial J, et al. (2011) Changes in insulin secretion and action in adults with familial risk for type 2 diabetes who curtail their sleep. Diabetes Care 34: 2259-2264.
9. Johansson JK, Kronholm E, Jula AM (2011) Variability in home-measured blood pressure and heart rate: associations with self-reported insomnia and sleep duration. J Hypertens 29: 1897-1905.
10. Ohayon MM, Lemoine P (2004) [Sleep and insomnia markers in the general population]. Encephale 30: 135-140.
11. Shirakawa S, Takahashi K (1998) [Epidemiology of sleep disorders]. Nihon Rinsho 56: 475-481.
12. Ahmadvand A, Sepehrmanesh Z, Ghoreishi F, Mousavi GA (2010) Prevalence of insomnia among 18 years old people and over in Kashan city, Iran in 2008. Feyz, Journal of Kashan University of Medical Sciences; 13: 313-320
13. Arasteh, M (2007) Prevalence of insomnia in students of Kurdistan University of Medical Sciences. Scientific Journal of Kurdistan University of Medical Sciences; 12 autumn: 58-63.
14. Najafipour H, Sanjari M, Shokoohi M, Haghdoost AA, Afshari M, et al. (2014) Epidemiology of diabetes mellitus, pre-diabetes, undiagnosed and uncontrolled diabetes and its predictors in general population aged 15 to 75 years: A community-based study (KERCADRS) in southeastern Iran. J Diabetes 7: 613-621.
15. Najafipour H, Nasri HR, Afshari M, Moazenzadeh M, Shokoohi M, et al. Hypertension: diagnosis, control status and its predictors in general population aged between 15 and 75 years: a community-based study in southeastern Iran. Int J Public Health 59: 999-1009.
16. Beck, AT, Steer, RA, Garbin, MG (1988) Psychometric properties of the Beck Depression Inventory: Twenty-five years of evaluation. Clinical Psychology Review 8: 77-100.
17. Smith M, Robinson L, Segal R, Sleep Disorders and Sleeping Problems.
18. Pourafkari NA, Arfaee A, DadashZadeh H, GhaemMaghami SJ (2004) Prevalence of sleep disorders in patients with mental disorders and general population of Tabriz, Journal of Tabriz University of Medical Sciences, 64, winter: 28-33
19. Zarowski M, Mojs E, Kleka P, Steinborn B (2007) [The impact of smoking cigarettes on insomnia and excessive daytime sleepiness symptoms among teachers]. Przegl Lek 64: 645-648.
20. Wetter DW, Young TB (1994) The relation between cigarette smoking and sleep disturbance. Prev Med 23: 328-334.

23

Sleep Status in Male Wheelchair Basketball Players on a Japanese National Team

Kenji Tsunoda[1,2*], Kazushi Hotta[2], Hirotaka Mutsuzaki[3], Kaori Tachibana[4], Yukiyo Shimizu[5], Takashi Fukaya[6], Eiji Ikeda[7], Naruki Kitano[8] and Yasuyoshi Wadano[9]

[1]*Physical Fitness Research Institute, Meiji Yasuda Life Foundation of Health and Welfare, Tokyo, Japan*

[2]*Department of Occupational Therapy, School of Healthcare, Ibaraki Prefectural University of Health Sciences, Ibaraki, Japan*

[3]*Department of Orthopaedic Surgery, Ibaraki Prefectural University of Health Sciences, Ibaraki, Japan*

[4]*Department of Physical Therapy, School of Healthcare, Ibaraki Prefectural University of Health Sciences, Ibaraki, Japan*

[5]*Department of Rehabilitation Medicine, University of Tsukuba Hospital, Ibaraki, Japan*

[6]*Department of Physical Therapy, Faculty of Health Sciences, Tsukuba International University, Ibaraki, Japan*

[7]*Faculty of Education, Art and Science, Yamagata University, Yamagata, Japan*

[8]*Institute of Health and Sport Sciences, University of Tsukuba, Ibaraki, Japan*

[9]*Department of Rehabilitation Medicine, Ibaraki Prefectural University of Health Sciences, Ibaraki, Japan*

***Corresponding author:** Tsunoda K, PhD, Physical Fitness Research Institute, Meiji Yasuda Life Foundation of Health and Welfare, 150 Tobuki, Hachioji, Tokyo 192-0001, Japan, E-mail: tsunoda@my-zaidan.or.jp

Abstract

Background: Sufficient sleep is required for optimal performance in athletes; however, there is no published information regarding sleep status in top wheelchair basketball players. This study has two objectives: to compare sleep status between the general population of young Japanese males and male wheelchair basketball players, and to examine differences in sleep status by physical disordered conditions of wheelchair athletes.

Methods: Study participants included 14 male wheelchair basketball players on a Japanese national team. Sleep status was assessed by the Pittsburgh Sleep Quality Index (PSQI). A higher PSQI score indicates poor sleep quality. To compare sleep status between the general Japanese population and wheelchair athletes, we used data from a previous study that assessed PSQI in the former population. We divided athletes' disordered conditions into two categories: spinal cord injury (n=9) and skeletal system diseases (n=5).

Results: The mean PSQI score was 5.8 ± 3.0 points; six athletes (42.9%) were over the cutoff point (5.5) for insomnia. The wheelchair athletes had significantly higher scores for sleep quality, sleep efficiency, and total PSQI than the general population of young Japanese males. The PSQI score of athletes with skeletal system diseases was significantly higher than athletes with spinal cord injury. Additionally, athletes with skeletal system diseases were significantly more likely to score over the cutoff point for insomnia than those with spinal cord injury.

Conclusions: Top male wheelchair basketball players had poorer sleep than the general population of young Japanese men, and athletes with skeletal system diseases more frequently suffered from insomnia compared with athletes with spinal cord injury. Effective methods to improve sleep are needed to help top wheelchair basketball players to achieve optimal performance.

Keywords: Insomnia; Adapted sports; Disability; Top athlete; Wheelchair sports

Introduction

Sufficient sleep is required to bring about maximal performance in athletes. According to previous studies, sleep can affect both physical [1] and technical performance [2,3]. For example, Mougin et al. [1] reported that peak oxygen consumption dropped after partial sleep deprivation compared with normal sleep conditions. Similarly, in the study by Reyner and Horne [2], serving accuracy in tennis players was decreased in situations of sleep deprivation. In a study on the benefits of sleep extension for performance in basketball players [3], subjects were required to spend at least 10 hours in bed each night. Results of the extended sleep intervention showed that athletes' sprint time, reaction time, and three-point field goals were typically enhanced.

Since wheelchair basketball requires both physical and technical levels of performance that are similar to regular basketball [4], getting the best quality sleep is important to wheelchair athletes. However, no information has been reported on sleep status in wheelchair basketball players. People who have disorders of the spine and/or lower limbs frequently wake to change position, to prevent pressure ulcers [5] or because of pain [6-8]. Therefore, the sleep status of wheelchair basketball players could be poorer than that of healthy people. Additionally, disordered conditions in wheelchair basketball players are varied. For example, a healthy thermoregulation system is necessary to fall asleep smoothly [9]. Wheelchair athletes with spinal cord injury have a weaker thermoregulation system than other wheelchair athletes [10]. Such differences of disordered conditions may affect sleep. Revealing the sleep status of wheelchair basketball players could help in building sleep assistance strategies that could lead to optimal athlete performance.

This study has two objectives: to compare sleep status between young Japanese males in the general population and male wheelchair basketball players, and to examine differences in sleep status by physical disordered conditions in wheelchair athletes.

Methods

Study participants

Study participants included 14 male wheelchair basketball players who were members of a Japanese national team. The mean age was 29.5 ± 5.2 years (range: 22 to 39 years). Of the total 14 participants, 9 athletes (64.3%) had spinal cord injury and 5 (35.7%) had skeletal system diseases. The study examination was conducted on June 18, 2014 as a part of a health checkup before the World Wheelchair Basketball Championship on July 3–15, 2014.

The athletes played wheelchair basketball 2 to 5 days/week for 2 to 4 hours/day. The mean years of experience playing wheelchair basketball was 10.4 ± 4.7 years. All participants provided informed consent. The Human Ethics Review Committee of Ibaraki Prefectural University of Health Sciences (No. 485) approved this study.

Measurement variables

Sleep: We assessed sleep status during the past week using the Pittsburgh Sleep Quality Index (PSQI) [11]. The PSQI consists of seven domains: sleep latency, subjective sleep quality (very good, fairly good, fairly bad, and very bad), sleep duration, sleep efficiency (sleep duration per total time in bed), sleep disturbance, use of sleep medication, and daytime dysfunction. A higher PSQI score indicates poor sleep quality; a person with a PSQI score over 5.5 points is regarded as having insomnia.

Conditions of physical disorders

Orthopedists and physiatrists assessed the conditions of physical disorders. We divided the disordered conditions into two categories: spinal cord injury (n=9) including spinal injury (n=6) and spina bifida (n=3), and skeletal system diseases (n=5) including amputation (n=3), congenital lower limb loss (n=1), and arthropathy (n=1).

Statistical analysis

A previous epidemiological study [12] reported the PSQI of the general Japanese adult population. To examine differences in sleep status between young Japanese males in the general population and male wheelchair basketball players, we used data of that previous study.

We compared sleep status between young Japanese males and male wheelchair basketball players using the Student's t-test. To examine difference in sleep status between disordered conditions, the Student's t-test for continuous variables and chi-squared tests for categorical variables were also used. We used IBM SPSS Statistics package, Version 21.0 (IBM Corp., Armonk, NY, USA) for statistical analysis, with the level of significance set at $P<0.05$.

Results

Table 1 shows characteristics of the study participants. Mean sleep latency was 24.9 ± 21.5 minutes, sleep duration was 6.5 ± 0.9 hours, sleep efficiency was 87.8 ± 9.3%, and 6 athletes (42.9%) reported poor sleep quality. The mean PSQI score was 5.8 ± 3.0 points, and 6 athletes (42.9%) were over the cutoff point (5.5) for insomnia. With respect to the reasons for sleep disturbance, participants most frequently reported "wake up in the middle of the night or early morning" (42.9%), "feel too hot" (35.7%), and "cannot get to sleep within 30 minutes" (28.6%).

Age	29.5 ± 5.2
Spinal cord injury	9(64.3%)
Skeletal system diseases	5(35.7%)
Sleep latency (minutes)	24.9 ± 21.5
Sleep duration (hours)	6.5 ± 0.9
Sleep efficiency (%)	87.8 ± 9.3
Reasons for sleep disturbance (≥1 times/week)	
Cannot get to sleep within 30 minutes	4(28.6%)
Wake up in the middle of the night or early morning	6(42.9%)
Have to get up to use the bathroom	3(21.4%)
Cannot breathe comfortably	0(0.0%)
Cough or snore loudly	2(14.3%)
Feel too cold	0(0.0%)
Feel too hot	5(35.7%)
Have bad dreams	0(0.0%)
Have pain	2(14.3%)
Other reasons	0(0.0%)
Daytime dysfunction	
Daytime sleepiness (≥1 times/week)	2(14.3%)
Daytime enthusiasm (somewhat/very big problem)	3(21.4%)
Sleep medication usage	0(0.0%)
Sleep qualtiy (faily/very bad)	6(42.9%)
Total PSQI score (points)	5.8 ± 3.0
Insomnia (PSQI >5.5 points)	6(42.9%)

Table 1: Participant characteristics (PSQI: Pittsburgh Sleep Quality Index).

Table 2 shows differences in sleep status between young Japanese men in the general population and male wheelchair basketball players. The wheelchair athletes had significantly higher scores for sleep quality, sleep efficiency, and total PSQI than the general population of Japanese males.

Scores of PSQI domains	General Japanese men (aged 20-29 years)†	Male wheelchair basketball players	P
	(n=103)	(n=14)	
Sleep quality	1.05 ± 0.71	1.5 ± 0.65	0.027
Sleep latency	0.83 ± 0.85	1.07 ± 1.07	0.336
Sleep duration	0.99 ± 0.77	1.29 ± 0.99	0.196
Sleep efficiency	0.11 ± 0.31	0.36 ± 0.74	0.026
Sleep disturbance	0.62 ± 0.49	0.79 ± 0.43	0.231
Hypnotic medication use	0.04 ± 0.31	0 ± 0	–
Daytime dysfunction	0.84 ± 0.81	0.79 ± 0.89	0.817
Total PSQI score	4.51 ± 2.14	5.79 ± 3.02	0.049

Table 2: Differences in sleep status between general Japanese male population and wheelchair basketball players (PSQI: Pittsburgh Sleep Quality Index, A high score for each variable indicates poor sleep status, †Data were obtained from Doi et al. [12]).

Table 3 presents a comparison of sleep status by disordered conditions. Scores of sleep quality and PSQI of athletes with skeletal system diseases were significantly higher than that of athletes with spinal cord injury. Additionally, athletes with skeletal system diseases were significantly more likely to score above the cutoff for insomnia than those with spinal cord injury.

Scores of PSQI domains	Spinal cord injury	Skeletal system diseases	P
	(n=9)	(n=5)	
Sleep quality	1.22 ± 0.44	2 ± 0.71	0.025
Sleep latency	0.78 ± 1.09	1.6 ± 0.89	0.178
Sleep duration	1 ± 0.87	1.8 ± 1.1	0.156
Sleep efficiency	0.22 ± 0.67	0.6 ± 0.89	0.384
Sleep disturbance	0.67 ± 0.5	1 ± 0	0.169
Hypnotic medication use	0 ± 0	0 ± 0	–
Daytime dysfunction	0.67 ± 1	1 ± 0.71	0.525
Total PSQI score	4.56 ± 2.65	8 ± 2.45	0.034
Insomnia (PSQI > 5.5 points)	2(22.2%)	4(80.0%)	0.036
Reasons for sleep disturbance (≥1 times/week)			
Cannot get to sleep within 30 minutes	2(22.2%)	2(40.0%)	0.480
Wake up in the middle of the night or early morning	3(33.3%)	3(60.0%)	0.334
Have to get up to use the bathroom	1(11.1%)	2(40.0%)	0.207
Cannot breathe comfortably	0(0.0%)	0(0.0%)	–
Cough or snore loudly	2(22.2%	0(0.0%)	0.255
Feel too cold	0(0.0%)	0(0.0%)	–
Feel too hot	3(33.3%	2(40.0%)	0.803
Have bad dreams	0(0.0%)	0(0.0%)	–
Have pain	1(11.1%)	1(20.0%)	0.649
Other reasons	0(0.0%)	0(0.0%)	–

Table 3: Comparisons of sleep status by disordered conditions (PSQI: Pittsburgh Sleep Quality Index, A high score for each variable indicates poor sleep status).

Discussion

This study investigated the sleep status of male wheelchair basketball players on a Japanese national team. The sleep variables of the wheelchair athletes were significantly poorer than those of the general population of young Japanese men, and about half of wheelchair athletes suffered from insomnia.

The wheelchair athletes had poorer sleep quality and sleep efficiency than the general population, and they frequently cited nocturnal awakening as a reason for sleep disturbance. Amputees frequently suffer from phantom pain and restless legs syndrome during the night [6]. Additionally, to prevent pressure ulcers, people with physical disordered conditions wake frequently to change sleeping position [5]. Such nocturnal awakening may be unavoidable for athletes with such conditions, to protect their bodies.

The wheelchair athletes cited feeling hot as a reason for sleep disturbance. To obtain restful sleep, downregulation of core body temperature is important [9]. Although core body temperature is typically increased with vigorous physical training [13], wheelchair athletes cannot effectively downregulate their core body temperature compared with people who have no physical disability [14]. In particular, it is known that people with spinal cord injury have seriously impaired thermoregulatory control [10,15]. Edinger et al. [16] reported that people with elevated core body temperature after vigorous exercise had longer sleep latency than those whose core temperature did not rise substantially. Susceptibility to such overheating could be a reason for poor sleep in wheelchair athletes. Additionally, nearly all study participants worked during the daytime so they typically trained at night. Vigorous exercise before sleep can interfere with falling asleep owing to enhanced physiologic excitement [13]. To moderate core body temperature and physical arousal level, it is important that vigorous physical training finish as early as possible before bedtime.

Although the sleep status of wheelchair basketball players was generally poor, athletes with skeletal system diseases suffered more frequently from insomnia than athletes with spinal cord injury. Compared with the latter, athletes with skeletal system diseases are assigned to higher ability classes [17], so they are required to perform more vigorously and precisely; therefore, excessive physical and mental stress may negatively affect sleep in these athletes. Additionally, vigorous performance in the athletes with higher ability classes could increase core body temperature extremely. It is also possible that people with spinal cord injury are frequently prescribed muscle relaxant [18] and analgesic [19] drugs, which can assist with sleep as a side effect [18,20]. However, in the current study, we did not have a determinant reason for the higher ratio of insomnia among athletes with skeletal system diseases. Future studies should investigate these reasons with more detailed assessment of sleep and disordered conditions.

This study had some limitations. First, the sample size was small. With a more adequate sample size, greater statistical differences in sleep status between disordered conditions might be observed. Second, sleep variables were assessed by a self-reported questionnaire that may induce recall/reporting bias. Third, the study examination was conducted before the World Wheelchair Basketball Championship 2014. Athletes are more likely to have nervousness and insomnia before an important competition [21], and the study time may affect results. To build sound evidence, further studies with various seasons are needed. Forth, although this study reported poor sleep status among top wheelchair basketball players, generalizability to other wheelchair athletes is uncertain. Finally, we did not assess actual performance in wheelchair basketball among athletes included in the study. Although a previous study revealed the effect of sleep on basketball performance [3], to clarify the importance of sleep in wheelchair basketball, future studies should examine the association between sleep and wheelchair basketball performance.

Conclusion

Top male wheelchair basketball players had poorer sleep than young Japanese males in the general population. Additionally, athletes with skeletal system diseases more frequently suffered from insomnia compared with athletes with spinal cord injury. To promote optimal performance, sleep assistance strategies should be developed for top wheelchair basketball players.

Acknowledgement

The authors thank the members of the Japan Wheelchair Basketball Federation (JWBF), Tokyo, Japan, for their support. This work was supported by a Grant-in-Aid for Project Research (1248-3) from the Ibaraki Prefectural University of Health Sciences. The authors declare that there are no conflicts of interest.

References

1. Mougin F, Simon-Rigaud ML, Davenne D, Renaud A, Garnier A, et al. (1991) Effects of sleep disturbances on subsequent physical performance. Eur J Appl Physiol Occup Physiol 63: 77-82.
2. Reyner LA, Horne JA (2013) Sleep restriction and serving accuracy in performance tennis players, and effects of caffeine. Physiol Behav 120: 93-96.
3. Mah CD, Mah KE, Kezirian EJ, Dement WC (2011) The effects of sleep extension on the athletic performance of collegiate basketball players. Sleep 34: 943-950.
4. International Wheelchair Basketballand Federation (2014) Official Wheelchair Basketball Rules 2014.
5. Evans JM, Andrews KL, Chutka DS, Fleming KC, Garness SL (1995) Pressure ulcers: prevention and management. Mayo Clin Proc 70: 789-799.
6. Giummarra MJ, Bradshaw JL (2010) The phantom of the night: restless legs syndrome in amputees. Med Hypotheses 74: 968-972.
7. Norrbrink Budh C, Hultling C, Lundeberg T (2005) Quality of sleep in individuals with spinal cord injury: a comparison between patients with and without pain. Spinal Cord 43: 85-95.
8. Widerström-Noga EG, Felipe-Cuervo E, Yezierski RP (2001) Chronic pain after spinal injury: interference with sleep and daily activities. Arch Phys Med Rehabil 82: 1571-1577.
9. Lack LC, Gradisar M, Van Someren EJ, Wright HR, Lushington K (2008) The relationship between insomnia and body temperatures. Sleep Med Rev 12: 307-317.
10. Veltmeijer MT, Pluim B, Thijssen DH, Hopman MT, Eijsvogels TM (2014) Thermoregulatory responses in wheelchair tennis players: a pilot study. Spinal Cord 52: 373-377.
11. Buysse DJ, Reynolds CF 3rd, Monk TH, Berman SR, Kupfer DJ (1989) The Pittsburgh Sleep Quality Index: a new instrument for psychiatric practice and research. Psychiatry Res 28: 193-213.
12. Doi Y, Minowa M, Uchiyama M, Okawa M (2001) Subjective sleep quality and sleep problems in the general Japanese adult population. Psychiatry Clin Neurosci 55: 213-215.
13. Oda S, Shirakawa K (2014) Sleep onset is disrupted following pre-sleep exercise that causes large physiological excitement at bedtime. Eur J Appl Physiol 114: 1789-1799.
14. Bhambhani Y (2002) Physiology of wheelchair racing in athletes with spinal cord injury. Sports Med 32: 23-51.
15. Webborn A (1996) Heat-related problems for the Paralympic Games, Atlanta 1996. Br J Ther Rehabil 3: 429-436.
16. Edinger JD, Morey MC, Sullivan RJ, Higginbotham MB, Marsh GR, et al. (1993) Aerobic fitness, acute exercise and sleep in older men. Sleep 16: 351-359.
17. International Wheelchair Basketballand Federation (2014) International Wheelchair Basketball Federation Official Player Classification Manual.
18. Taricco M, Adone R, Pagliacci C, Telaro E (2000) Pharmacological interventions for spasticity following spinal cord injury. Cochrane Database Syst Rev : CD001131.
19. Felix ER (2014) Chronic neuropathic pain in SCI: evaluation and treatment. Phys Med Rehabil Clin N Am 25: 545-57, viii.
20. Furlan AD, Sandoval JA, Mailis-Gagnon A, Tunks E (2006) Opioids for chronic noncancer pain: a meta-analysis of effectiveness and side effects. CMAJ 174: 1589-1594.
21. Erlacher D, Ehrlenspiel F, Adegbesan OA, El-Din HG (2011) Sleep habits in German athletes before important competitions or games. J Sports Sci 29: 859-866.

Does CPAP Use in the First 15 Days Predict its Use after 4 Months?

Thibaut Gentina[1], Elodie Gentina[2,*], Catherine Lamblin[1], François Jouniaux[1], François Codron[1] and Aiman Tulaimat[3]
[1]*Hôpital Privé La Louvière, Générale de Santé, Lille, France*
[2]*Skema Business School – Université de Lille, MERCUR Research, France*
[3]*Cook County Health and Hospital Systems, Division of Pulmonary, Critial Care, and Sleep Medicine, USA*

Abstract

Objective: Early prediction of which patients with obstructive sleep apnea will not adhere with CPAP can trigger physicians to correct possible causes or offer alternative therapies. This study aims to determine the ability of early CPAP use to predict long-term adherence with CPAP independent from its definition and to test previously described predictors of adherence.

Method: This is a prospective, observational cohort study that was performed in nine sleep disorder centers in France. Patients were newly diagnosed with obstructive sleep apnea and a CPAP was prescribed for the first time. We collected socioeconomic, medical, sleep, and psychological variables to be associated with adherence with CPAP. The patients were evaluated 15 days after CPAP set up and monthly for 4 months until they were adherent. We assessed potential predictors of CPAP adherence at 4 months with emphasis on CPAP use at 15 days. CPAP adherence was defined as an average daily use of at least 3, 4, 5, and 6 hours.

Results: We enrolled 420 patients. Early CPAP use and CPAP use at 4 months were similar. At 4 months, 94% of patients used a CPAP ≥3 hours and 49% of patients used it ≥6 hours. The area under the ROC curve for early CPAP use predicting adherence at 4 months was ≥0.85 for all adherence definitions. The optimal threshold for early CPAP use to predict adherence increased from 3.2 to 6.4 hours as the definition of CPAP adherence increased from 3 to 6 hours. CPAP use at 4 months was higher in older patients.

Conclusions: Early CPAP use was the single best predictor of CPAP adherence and was independent of how adherence was defined. Physicians must assess CPAP use no later than 2 weeks to address its causes or prescribe an alternative therapy.

Keywords: Obstructive sleep apnea (OSA); Continuous positive airway pressure (CPAP); Adherence; predictors

Introduction

Treatment of obstructive sleep apnea (OSA) with continuous positive airway pressure (CPAP) improves sleep quality, reduces sleepiness, enhances quality of life and reduces cardiovascular morbidities [1-3]. As in most medical conditions, the benefits of therapy are reaped only by adherent patients. Unfortunately, and as in other conditions, adherence to the use of a CPAP is suboptimal. In one study which defined adherence arbitrarily as using a CPAP ≥3 hours on 70% of nights, found that 54% of patients were non-adherent [4]. Understanding the barriers to and predictors of CPAP treatment uptake and long-term adherence is therefore critical for successfully establishing and maintaining patients on effective CPAP treatment [5]. It allows physicians to apply interventions that improve adherence early because waiting until patients declare themselves after few months of treatment to be non-adherent might be too late. It also allows physicians to select the patients that need these interventions instead of applying these interventions to all patients at a much higher cost. Knowing which patients are unlikely to adhere to the use of CPAP also prompts physicians to discuss alternative treatments early [6,7].

Socio-economic factors, disease severity, health problems, psychological variables, social variables, testing methods, side effects, and behavioural traits have been associated with adherence to the use of a CPAP. This large number of variables suggests that adherence is a complex process (Appendix 1).

This complexity underscores some of the limitations of published reports. First, the reports focus on one variable or a limited number of variables to predict CPAP adherence. Second, the samples of many of these studies are small. This not only reduces the generalizability of the findings, but also reduces the number of variables that can be reliably tested. Lastly, the sometimes vaguely described follow-up process of the patients reduces the reproducibility of the findings.

Furthermore, the definitions of adherence are arbitrary. The most frequently used definition is 4 hours per night and it is based on the improvement in consequences of OSA in patients that use CPAP for at least 4 hours. There is, however, growing interest in setting CPAP targets based on a patient needs [8-10].

Therefore, we conducted this study to validate a large number of variables as predictors of the adherence to CPAP use in a large sample of patients that were followed meticulously for 4 months. We focused on early use of CPAP and we defined adherence at 4 months in various ways.

***Corresponding author:** Elodie Gentina, 2SKEMA Business School – Université de Lille, MERCUR Research, France; E-mail: elodie. gentina@skema.edu

Materials and Methods

Study design

This prospective cohort study was performed in nine medical centers in the north of France. The protocol was approved by the French Research Ethics Board of The Patient Protection Committee. All patients provided written informed consent before participation.

Study sample

Adult patients (18-75 years old) were recruited from nine centers in France. Each center utilized the same method to recruit and follow their patients in order to avoid any differences between centers (Table 1).

All consecutive patients for whom CPAP had been prescribed for the first time for the treatment of OSA between March 2013 and June 2013 were eligible for the present study. We excluded patients that were cognitively deficient and unable to fill in the questionnaires, patients unable (or refused) to give their informed consent, patients unable to read and/or speak French, and patients with neuromuscular diseases.

Diagnosis of obstructive sleep apnea

The diagnosis was based on a full in-laboratory polysomnogram (PSG) or home sleep test (HST). The PSG was performed with the Alice 5 (Philips, Eindhoven, Netherlands) that included 6 EEG channels, 2 EOG channels, chin EMG, bilateral anterior tibialis EMG, nasal/oral thermister, nasal pressure transducer, chest and abdominal wall movements, EKG, and pulse oximetry. The PSG scoring was standardized across centers. HST was performed with Embletta polygraph (Resmed, San Diego, CA) that included nasal/oral thermister, nasal pressure transducer, chest and abdominal wall movements, heart rate, and pulse oximetry.

Sleep was scored with the Rechtschaffen and Kales criteria. Apneas, hypopneas, and arousals were scored according to the American Academy of Sleep Medicine 2007. The apnea hypopnea index that was calculated by dividing the number of apneas and hypopnea by the total sleep time (recording time for HST) in hours.

Prescription of CPAP

CPAP was prescribed if a patient met 1 of 2 conditions: 1) the apnea-hypopnea index (AHI) ≥30 events per hour, or 2) the AHI index was between 15 and 30 events per hour with respiratory arousal >10 per hour and at least 2 symptoms of OSA symptoms (snoring, choking or gasping during sleep, unrefreshing sleep, daytime fatigue, impaired concentration, or nocturia).

CPAP initiation and monitoring

Patients were seen by sleep physicians in consultation and then referred for a sleep study [11-13]. Because knowledge is a pre-condition for health behavior or a change in health behavior, patient were subjected to a specific educational intervention [14]. Before starting CPAP, each patient was educated by a physician and a technician about the health risk of OSA and about the use of the CPAP machine. Patients also watched a 10-min video about the definition of OSA, symptoms of OSA, CPAP machine, the sensation of wearing CPAP, and benefits of using CPAP [15]. The delay between seeing the physician and the sleep study was 15 days and between the sleep study and starting CPAP was less than 48 hours.

The CPAP devices include counters that measure machine-on time using a microprocessor. Patient adherence data was obtained on day 15 and at the end of the first month. Patients with CPAP use ≥3 hours at the end of the first month were evaluated at the end of fourth months. Patients with CPAP use <3 hours at the end of the first month were visited monthly until they became adherent. During each visit, the average nightly use CPAP hours over the last month was recorded (Table 1).

Data collected

Independent variables: The socio-economic variables were age, gender, marital status (married or living as a couple versus living alone), employment status (fulltime, part-time, or unemployed), type of health insurance (government or government insurance with private health insurance). The health variables were infarction, or arrhythmia. The psychological variables were assessed with two scales: The Pichot scale16 and the Epworth Sleepiness Scale (ESS17). The Pichot scale is divided in 2 subscales: depression (13 items) and fatigue (8 items). The ESS measures the level of sleepiness (8 items). OSA related variables were method of diagnosing OSA (PSG or HST), the apnea-hypopnea index (AHI), average nightly use of CPAP in the first 15 days (early CPAP use).

Dependent variable: Adherence was monitored using the smart card technology embedded in the CPAP machines and was defined as the average nightly use of CPAP at the set pressure.

Statistical analysis

To determine the ability of early CPAP use in predicting adherence with CPAP at 4 months, we calculated the area under the receiver operator characteristic curve (AU-ROC) for 4 adherence definitions (3, 4, 5, 6 hours).We determined the optimal thresholds of early CPAP use to predict adherence based on the Youden Index and calculated the sensitivity (Sn) and specificity (Sp) for these thresholds. We also determined, at each definition of adherence, the thresholds of early CPAP use that had a sensitivity of 90% (Sn90) or a specificity of 90% (Sp90). Bias-corrected bootstrapping of 1000 iterations was used to determine these thresholds and their confidence intervals.

The French government reimburses patients for CPAP if they use it for more than 3 hours per night. Therefore, we used the 3-hour definition for the rest of the analysis, with patients using CPAP ≥ 3 hours per day considered as adherent, patients using CPAP <3 hours considered as non-adherent.

We compared between adherent and non-adherent patients all other variables available for the physician before initiating CPAP (pre-CPAP predictors). We used the t-test or chi-squared as indicated by the data type. Differences were significant if the p value is ≤0.05. We tested the significant pre-CPAP predictors with early CPAP use in a multiple regression analysis to determine the smallest number of independent predictors of adherence.

Results

Patients

We give the study questionnaire to 465 patients: 429 patients responded, 9 were lost during the follow-up, and 420 patients were included in the final analysis (useable response rate of 92%). Most patients were men, obese, and had severe sleep apnea. The majority of patients had private insurance in addition to government insurance (Table 2).

Adherence CPAP use: early CPAP use (5.6 ± 2.0 hours) and CPAP use at 4 months (5.7 ± 1.7 hours) were similar, p=0.09. The correlation

Visit	Patients	Where	Personnel	What was done	Education
CPAP set up	All patients	Clinic	Physician	Questionnaire	A 15-min video about the definition of OSA, symptoms of OSA, CPAP machine, the sensation of wearing CPAP, and benefits of using CPAP. Discussion and demonstration
Visit 15 days	All patients	Home	Technician	Early CPAP use	Individualized and face to face education and specific information about OSA, performance, treatment relevance, symptom change with CPAP, troubleshooting advice… A written document on CPAP was provided Demonstration of the Website "Elia Medical Education http://eliamedical-education.com/
First month	All patients	Clinic	Physician	CPAP use	Discussion, demonstration and support
Second month	Non-adherent first month	Home	Technician	CPAP use	Discussion, demonstration and support
Third month	Non-adherent second month	Home	Technician	CPAP use	Discussion, demonstration and support
Fourth month	All patients	Clinic	Physician	CPAP use	Discussion, demonstration and support

Table 1: Visit types during the 1-4 month study.

between early CPAP use and CPAP use at 4 months was high (r=0.71, p<0.001). The linear regression equation for CPAP was use at 4 months (hours)=2.2 + 0.6 × early use of CPAP (hours).

Early CPAP use was equally predictive of use of CPAP at 4 months no matter what the threshold was (Table 3 and Figure 1). The accuracy of early CPAP in predicting adherence changed with the type of insurance. The AU-ROC was higher when patients had only government insurance than when they had additional private insurance (4-hours: 0.95 ± 0.04 versus 0.86 ± 0.02, p=0.04; 5-hours: 0.92 ± 0.06 versus 0.85 ± 0.02, p=0.2; 6-hours: 0.96 ± 0.03 versus 0.83 ± 0.02, p=0.002). We did not evaluate the 3 hours adherence because the sample was two small. The accuracy of early CPAP use in predicting adherence at 4 months was not affected by ESS, age, gender, employment, or marital status.

As the threshold to define CPAP adherence increased from 3 hours to 4 hours, the optimal threshold of early CPAP use increased, then was stable for adherence defined as 4 or 5 hours, and then increased again for adherence define as 6 hours. The ranges of thresholds for Sn90 (3.3-4.6 hours) and for Sp90 (5.5-6.5 hours) were narrow.

When the definition of adherence changes, the distribution of adherence status (remained adherent, became non-adherent, remained non-adherent, became adherent) at 4 months changes. When we used the same threshold to define adherence at 15 days and at 4 months, increasing the threshold for adherence from 3 to 6 hours increased the percentage of patients that remain non-adherent at 4 months and decreased the percentage remained adherent over the 4 month (Figure 2).

Pre-CPAP predictors of adherence at 4 months

Adherent patients were older than non-adherent patients (57 ± 12 versus 49 ± 11, p=0.002). The AU-ROC curve for age as a predictor of adherence was 0.67 and the optimal threshold was 53 years with a sensitivity of 0.62 and a specificity of 0.67. The threshold for a specificity of 90% was 67.

We divided patients into 2 groups: older patients>53 years (252 patients), and younger patients ≤ 53 years (168 patients). In comparison to the older patients, the younger patients had a higher BMI (34 ± 7 versus 31 ± 6), had a higher Pichot fatigue score (15 ± 8 versus 14 ± 8, p=0.01), and a higher ESS score (11, IQR 8-15 versus 10, IQR 6-14, p=0.03), and they used CPAP slightly less in the first 15 days (0.5 ± 0.2 hours). There was also a weak but significant correlation between the Pichot fatigue score and the drop in CPAP use from 15 days to 4 months (r=0.1, p=0.036).

When age and early use of CPAP were entered in a logistic regression, age became non-significant and early use of CPAP was the only predictor of adherence at 4 months. The odds ratio associated with every hour of early CPAP use for predicting CPAP adherence at 4 months was 2.1 (95% CI: 1.6-2.7, p<0.001). On the other hand, in a linear regression model with the hours of CPAP use as the dependent variable, age and early CPAP use were significant and the regression equation was CPAP use at 4 months=1.5+ [early CPAP use in hours × 0.62] + [age in years×0.01].

There was no correlation between CPAP use at 4 months and ESS (r=-0.05, p=0.3) or between CPAP use and AHI (r=0.09, p=0.06). Similarly, none of the other pre-CPAP variables (including the methods of diagnosing OSA) was associated with CPAP use at 4 months.

Discussion

In this relatively large sample of patient with OSA that was followed closely for 4 months, we found that early CPAP use was the strongest predictor of adherence at 4 months independent of its definition. Of the variables available for the physician before starting CPAP, age was the only variable associated, though weakly, with CPAP adherence at 4 months.

Our results complement the results reported by others that long-term CPAP adherence patterns are often established within the first weeks of therapy [15-18]. Budhiraj et al. [12] reported that CPAP use by the third day was predictive of CPAP use at 30 days. Popescu et al. [13] reported that CPAP use in the first 2 weeks predicts CPAP adherence at 1 year. Chai-Coetzer et al. [19] reported that adherence at one month predicted CPAP adherence at 1 year. McArdle et al. [5] reported that CPAP use at 3 months predicts adherence after 2 years. This composite of evidence suggests that adherence to CPAP use must be evaluated early and continuously after initiating therapy.

A novel and interesting finding of our study was the relationship between the area under the ROC curve for early CPAP use and the insurance type. It has been shown in the past that socioeconomic status (especially poverty) is associated with CPAP use (see appendix). In our study, early CPAP use was more predictive of long-term use in patients with government only (suggestive lower income). The type of insurance was not, however, associated the adherence itself. This finding deserves

Socio-economic variables	
Men, %	70
Age, years	56 ± 12
Married, %	78
Fully employed, %	59
Government insurance with private health insurance,%	94
Health variables	
Body mass index, kg/m^2	32 ± 6
Treated Hypertension, %	49
Heart disease (arrhythmia or congestive heart failure),%	12
Stroke,%	12
Myocardial infarction, %	11
Loss of libido, %	32
OSA related variables	
AHI	46 ± 19
Diagnosis made with HST, %	38
Daily CPAP use in the first 15 days	5.6±2
Psychological Variables	
Epworth Sleepiness Scale	10.7 ± 5
Pichot Fatigue Scale	14.2 ± 7
Pichot Depression Scale	4.7 ± 4

Table 2: Baseline characteristics of the patients at the onset of CPAP therapy (n=420).

Definition of adherence at 4 months	Adherence at 4 month based on definition	Threshold at 15 days	Sn	Sp	Sn_{90}	Sp_{90}
3 hours	94%	3.2 (2.2-3.9)	91%	70%	3.3	6.0
4 hours	81%	5.4 (3.3-5.6)	72%	86%	3.8	5.5
5 hours	69%	5.5 (5.1-5.5)	77%	83%	4.2	6.2
6 hours	49%	6.4 (5.7-6.8)	66%	89%	4.6	6.5

Table 3: The percentage of adherent patients at various definitions at four months, the optimal threshold of early use (15 days) to predict adherence based on bootstrap analysis, its sensitivity and specificity, and the threshold of early CPAP use with sensitivity of 90% (Sn_{90}) and specificity of 90% (Sp_{90}).

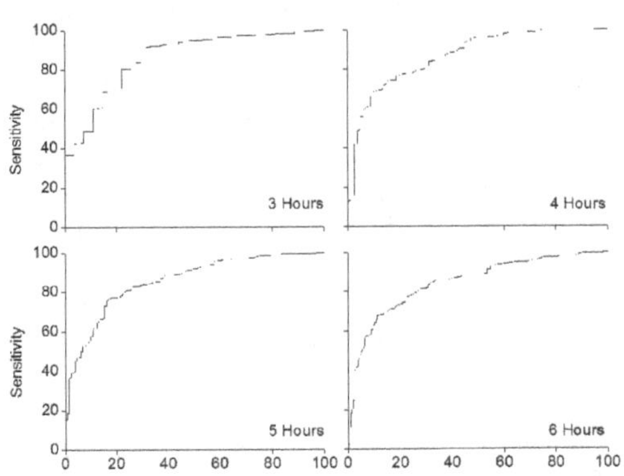

Figure 1: ROC curves for early CPAP use predicting adherence at the 4 thresholds at 4 months. The area was 0.86 (0.82-0.89) for 3 hours, 0.87 (0.83-0.89) for 4 hours, 0.86 (0.82-0.88) for 5 hours, and 0.85 (0.81-0.88) for 6 hours.

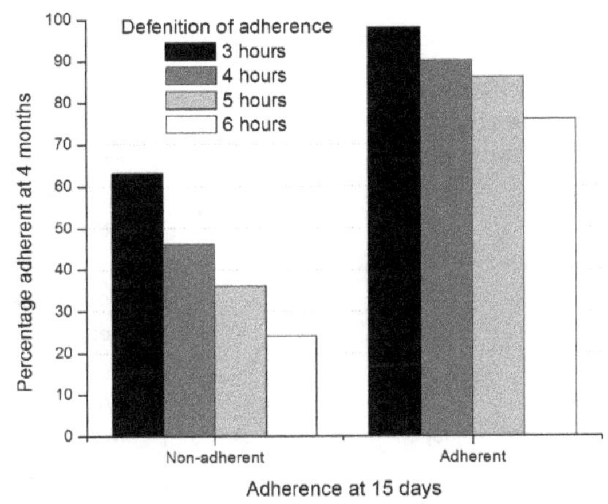

Figure 2: The relation between adherence on day 15 (x-axis) and adherence at 4 months defined with the same hours of CPAP use. When patients were non-adherent at 15 days, they are unlikely to be adherent at 4 months with a decreasing chance of adherence as the threshold for adherence increases. When patients were adherent at 15 days, the were likely to be adherent at 4 month but with a decreasing likelihood as the threshold for adherence increased; but, the lowest adherence rate, which was with a threshold of 6 hours, was still >70%.

further evaluation because it might reflect a motive behind the use of CPAP such as employment for drivers or just to avoid monetary penalty for not using CPAP.

Because the definition of CPAP adherence is arbitrary and studies have used definitions varying between 2 and 6 hours, we tested 3, 4, 5, and 6 hour thresholds. The AU- ROC curve for early CPAP use predicting later adherence was similar between all definitions of adherence. Therefore, our conclusions can be extended to settings where the criterion of adherence is different from that used in France, especially since Chai-Coetzer and colleagues have shown that the relation between early use and long-term adherence is independent from country [19].

Currently most clinicians rely on a single definition to identify patients not adherent to CPAP use. In the United States, patients are considered adherent if they use a CPAP for more than 4 hours most night of the week. This definition of adherence is required by Medicare to pay for CPAP. Nevertheless, to achieve maximal alertness and cognitive functioning, a reduction in carbon dioxide in patients with obesity hypoventilation syndrome, or a reduction in blood pressure, a patient must use a CPAP for more than 6 hours a day [20-22]. The thresholds we identified can help physicians predict if a patient will meet the required CPAP use. Therefore, for example, if a patient was a commercial driver that required maximal cognitive functioning, early CPAP use of less than 6.5 hours would be concerning and less than 4.5 hours would be very concerning.

Predicting non-adherent patients early helps physicians select patients that need attention and intensive follow-up. Of thc patients that were using CPAP ≥3 hours in the first two weeks, 98% were using it ≥3 hours at 4 months. On the other hand, 37% of the patients that were using CPAP < 3 hours at 15 days were still using it <3 hours at 4 months. Thus, when the desired dose of CPAP use is low, only patients with very low early use should probably be followed closely for the first few months.

Variable	This study
Socio-economic variables	
Age [12,13]	Confirmed
Gender [30]	Not confirmed
Marital status [26,30]	Not confirmed
Employment status [26,31]	Not confirmed
Type of health insurance [32]	Not confirmed
Race [33]	Not tested
Life events [34]	Not tested
Health variables	
Treated Hypertension [35]	Not confirmed
Heart disorders [4]	Not confirmed
BMI [13,36]	Not confirmed
Stroke [37]	Not confirmed
Myocardial infarction [38]	Not confirmed
Nasal anatomy [39]	Not tested
Psychological or behavioural variables	
Epworth Sleepiness [17]	Not confirmed
Pichot Fatigue Scale [40]	Not confirmed
Pichot Depression scale [16]	Not confirmed
Self-efficacy [27,28]	Not tested
Coping-styles [41]	Not tested
Locus of control [29]	Not tested
Initial CPAP exposure variables	
CPAP use in the first 15 days [4,13]	Confirmed
Diagnosed with HST [42]	Not confirmed
AHI [43]	Not confirmed
Social variables	
Spousal involvement [27,44]	Not tested
Bed partner sleep quality [45,46]	Not tested
Technical variable	
Mask-interface [47]	Not tested
Heated vs. cold pass-over humidity [48]	Not tested
Flexible pressure on CPAP (C-Flex vs continuous positive airway pressure) [49]	Not tested
Claustrophobia [50]	Not tested
Side effect [19]	Not tested

Table 4: Summary of variables from prior studies on significant predictors of CPAP.

In contrast, 76% of patients using a CPAP more than 6 hours at 15 days were still doing so at 4 months and only 24% of patients using a CPAP less than 6 hours increased above this threshold. Therefore, when the desired dose of CPAP is high, as in drivers and patients with obesity hypoventilation, all patient should be followed closely.

Age was the only pre-CPAP variable predictor of adherence: older patients were more likely to use a CPAP than younger patients. Sin et al. [23] reported a similar relation between age and CPAP adherence. In fact they reported that CPAP use increased by 0.24 hours per decade, while in our study it was 0.34 hours in a univariate regression and 0.1 hours after adjustment for early CPAP use. Similarly, Budhiraja et al. [12] showed that adherent (defined as >4 hours) patients were on average 3 years older than non-adherent patients. If we use the 4 hour definition, adherent patients were 8 years older.

Although they were more fatigued and sleepy, younger patients used a CPAP less than older ones. This profile is similar to that report by Pepin et al. [24] as a predictor of residual sleepiness after treatment with a CPAP. Because of the correlation between the Pichot fatigue score and the drop in CPAP use from 15 days to 4 months, it is plausible that these young, fatigued patients gradually reduced their CPAP use because they did not feel better with it. This observation is also concerning because younger patients will live longer than older ones, and if they remain non-adherent, they are likely to suffer cardiovascular complications at a younger age, further leading to a larger societal impact of OSA.

Many investigators have reported that AHI [4,13] and the ESS4, [25] predicted adherence. We did not find such a relationship. This is not due to spectrum bias because the distribution of both AHI and ESS were wide. A larger sample size might have resulted in a weak correlation between AHI and adherence, but it would have been too weak to be useful predictor. Yet, patients with high AHI and ESS should receive special attention from physicians because they are more likely to benefit when they adhere to CPAP use than patients with lower AHI or ESS.

This study has two particular strengths. First, the sample is relatively large (only 5 other studies included more than 500 patients) and the patients were recruited from multiple centers. This allowed us to simultaneously test a large number of variables previously tested by other investigators (Table 4). Second, the patients were followed monthly if they remained non-adherent and at 4 months. In comparison, the study by Gagnadoux et al. [26] included more than 1000 patients that were followed at the end of the first week, and then at the end of the third month. The follow-up was not regular or based on adherence. Another study from Sin et al. [23] provided a very detailed follow-up of the patients but the sample was small.

Follow-up and adherence in this study was higher than what is reported by others. Two reasons might explain this observation. First, the study had a dedicated physician who was specifically involved in the coordination of data collection to monitor the quality of the collection processing. Second, the French government reimbursed patients for CPAP use if they used it for more than 3 hours per night, which encouraged the patients to use the CPAP. This is slightly different from reimbursement in the United States where Medicare purchases the CPAP machine once the patients is deemed adherent. In fact, the relationship between the accuracy of early CPAP use in predicting adherence and the type of insurance suggests that the reimbursement mechanism might play a role in the change in adherence between the first 15 days and 4 months.

There are several limitations in this study. The first limitation is that we did not test side effects. Early complaints of side effects have previously been associated with long-term non-adherence with CPAP [19]. We assume that they were addressed with the patients during the frequent visits and should have been resolved by the fourth months of follow-up. The second limitation is that we did not test coping, locus of control, and self-efficacy, which have previously been shown to predict adherence [19,20,21,26-29]. They are probably mechanisms that lead to early non-adherence that ultimately continues long-term. Once a patient is identified early on to be at risk of non-adherence, the clinician must evaluate that patient's coping and self-efficacy. Lastly, our follow-up was 4 months only. The longer the follow-up, the more events that can affect adherence: seasonal allergy, mask failure, change work hours, etc. The 4 four month follow-up is probably optimal to reduce external events that can affect adherence.

In conclusion, CPAP use in the first 15 days is the best predictor of adherence to the use of a CPAP at 4 months and it was more accurate in patients than in government only insured patients. The threshold of early CPAP use should be adjusted based on the desired long term adherence. These observations might assist physicians identify early the patients that will not meets their target of CPAP use and these patients will be suitable for intensive follow-up or alternative therapy.

Contributions

Study conception and design: Thibaut Gentina. Thibaut Gentina designed the research plan and organized the study.

Acquisition of data: François Jounieaux, Catherine Lamblin and François Codron developed the methodology, participated in the collection of data and coordinated the data-analysis.

Analysis and interpretation of data: Elodie Dancoine and Aiman Tulaimat performed the analyses.

Drafting of manuscript: Thibaut Gentina, Elodie Dancoine and Aiman Tulaimat contributed to the writing of the manuscript.

Critical revision: Elodie Dancoine and Aiman Tulaimat.

Acknowledgment

1. Elia Medical (Manufacture and Installation of Medical-Surgical EquipmentaAnd Instruments) by supporting financially this research.

Elia Medical, 11 Avenue Léon Blum, 59370 Mons-en-Barœul, France.

2. Bernard DOUAY by supporting his help in the coordination of the mouse work.

3. Doctors by supporting their help in collecting data: François FORTIN, Lille (59), Jean Marc DERNIS, Lille (59), Marc BURE, Lille (59), Arnaud PRIGENT, Rennes (35), Christophe VERKINDRE, Béthune (62), Pierre Marie BROUSSIER, Bois Guillaume (76), Jean-Jacques GRES, Havre (76), Dominique GUFFROY, Maubeuge (59), Jamal KABBANI, Chelles (77), Laurent KEDZIORA, Denain (59).

Conflict of Interest

There is not conflict of interest in this research.

References

1. McArdle N, Devereux G, Heidarnejad H, Engleman HM, Mackay TW, et al. (1999) Long-term use of CPAP therapy for sleep apnea/hypopnea syndrome. Am J Respir Crit Care Med 159: 1108-1114.
2. Krieger J, Kurtz D, Petiau C, Sforza E, Trautmann D (1996) Long-term compliance with CPAP therapy in obstructive sleep apnea patients and in snorers. Sleep 19: S136-143.
3. Budhiraja R, Parthasarathy S, Drake CL, Roth T, Sharief I, et al. (2007) Early CPAP use identifies subsequent adherence to CPAP therapy. Sleep 30: 320-324.
4. Olsen S, Smith S, Oei T, Douglas J (2008) Health belief model predicts adherence to CPAP before experience with CPAP. Eur Respir J 32: 710-717.
5. Popescu G, Latham M, Allgar V, Elliott MW (2001) Continuous positive airway pressure for sleep apnoea/hypopnoea syndrome: usefulness of a 2 week trial to identify factors associated with long term use. Thorax 56: 727-733.
6. Sin DD, Mayers I, Man GC, Pawluk L (2002) Long-term compliance rates to continuous positive airway pressure in obstructive sleep apnea: a population-based study. Chest 121: 430-435.
7. Simon-Tuval T, Reuveni H, Greenberg-Dotan S, Oksenberg A, Tal A, et al. (2009) Low socioeconomic status is a risk factor for CPAP acceptance among adult OSAS patients requiring treatment. Sleep 32: 545-552.
8. Young T, Palta M, Dempsey J, Skatrud J, Weber S, et al. (1993) The occurrence of sleep-disordered breathing among middle-aged adults. N Engl J Med 328: 1230-1235.
9. Pelletier-Fleury N, Rakatonanahary D, Fleury B (2001) The age and other factors in the evaluation of compliance with nasal continuous positive airway pressure for obstructive sleep apnoea syndrome. Acox proportional hazars analysis. Sleep Medicine 2: 225-232.
10. Lewis KE, Seale L, Bartle IE, Watkins AJ, Ebden P (2004) Early predictors of CPAP use for the treatment of obstructive sleep apnea. Sleep 27: 134-138.
11. Ye L, Pien GW, Ratcliffe SJ, Weaver TE (2009) Gender differences in obstructive sleep apnea and treatment response to continuous positive airway pressure. J Clin Sleep Med 5: 512-518.
12. Bakker JP, O'Keeffe KM, Neill AM, Campbell AJ (2011) Ethnic disparities in CPAP adherence in New Zealand: Effects of socioeconomic status, health literacy and self-efficacy. Sleep 1: 1595-1603.
13. Ye L, Pack A, Maislin G, Dinges D, Hurley S, et al. (2012) Predictors of continuous positive airway pressure use during the first week of treatment. J Sleep Res 21: 419-426.
14. Gagnadoux F, Le Vaillant M, Goupil F, Pigeanne T, Chollet S, et al. (2011) Influence of marital status and employment status on long-term adherence with continuous positive airway pressure in sleep apnea patients. PLoS One 6: e22503.
15. Scharf SM, Seiden L, DeMore J, Carter-Pokras O (2004) Racial differences in clinical presentation of patients with sleep-disordered breathing. Sleep Breath 8: 173-183.
16. Billings ME, Auckley D, Benca R, Foldvary-Schaefer N, Iber C, et al. (2011) Race and residential socioeconomics as predictors of CPAP adherence. Sleep 34: 1653-1658.
17. Platt AB, Field SH, Asch DA, Chen Z, Patel NP, et al. (2009) Neighborhood of residence is associated with daily adherence to CPAP therapy. Sleep 32: 799-806.
18. Hoffstein V, Viner S, Mateika S, Conway J (1992). Treatment of obstructive sleep apnea with nasal continuous positive airway pressure. Patient compliance, perception of benefits, and side effects. American Review of Respiratory Disease 145: 841-745.
19. Loredo JS, Berry C, Nelesen RA, Dimsdale JE (2007) Prediction of continuous positive airway pressure in obstructive sleep apnea. Sleep Breath 11: 45-51.
20. Wild MR, Engleman HM, Douglas NJ, Espie CA (2004) Can psychological factors help us to determine adherence to CPAP? A prospective study. Eur Respir J 24: 461-465.
21. Redenius R, Murphy C, O'Neill E, Al-Hamwi M, Zallek SN (2008) Does CPAP lead to change in BMI? J Clin Sleep Med 4: 205-209.
22. Sugiura T, Noda A, Nakata S, Yasuda Y, Soga T, et al. (2007) Influence of nasal resistance on initial acceptance of continuous positive airway pressure in treatment for obstructive sleep apnea syndrome. Respiration 74(1): 56–60.
23. Reishtein JL, Maislin G, Weaver TE; Multisite Study group (2010) Outcome of CPAP treatment on intimate and sexual relationships in men with obstructive sleep apnea. J Clin Sleep Med 6: 221-226.
24. Margel D, Tal R, Livne PM, Pillar G (2005) Predictors of erectile function improvement in obstructive sleep apnea patients with long-term CPAP treatment. Int J Impot Res 17: 186-190.
25. Hung J, Whitford EG, Parsons RW, Hillman DR (1990) Association of sleep apnoea with myocardial infarction in men. Lancet 336: 261-264.
26. Phillips B, Shafazand S (2013) CPAP and hypertension in nonsleepy patients. J Clin Sleep Med 9: 181-182.
27. Palombini L, Guilleminault C (2006) Stroke and treatment with nasal CPAP. Eur J Ncurol 13: 198 200.
28. Martínez-García MA, Campos-Rodríguez F, Soler-Cataluña JJ, Catalán-Serra P, Román-Sánchez P, et al. (2012) Increased incidence of nonfatal cardiovascular events in stroke patients with sleep apnoea: effect of CPAP treatment. Eur Respir J 39: 906-912.
29. Hui DS, Choy DK, Li TS, Ko FW, Wong KK, et al. (2001) Determinants of continuous positive airway pressure compliance in a group of Chinese

patients with obstructive sleep apnea. Chest 120: 170-176.

30. Krieger J (1992) Long-term compliance with nasal continuous positive airway pressure (CPAP) in obstructive sleep apnea patients and nonapneic snorers. Sleep 15: S42-46.
31. Meurice JC, Dore P, Paquereau J, Neau JP, Ingrand P, et al. (1994) Predictive factors of long-term compliance with nasal continuous positive airway pressure treatment in sleep apnea syndrome. Chest 105: 429-433.
32. Bollig SM (2010) Encouraging CPAP adherence: it is everyone's job. Respir Care 55: 1230-1239.
33. Baron KG, Berg CA, Czajkowski LA, Smith TW, Gunn HE, et al. (2011) Self-efficacy contributes to individual differences in subjective improvements using CPAP. Sleep Breath 15: 599-606.
34. Morris LG, Setlur J, Burschtin OE, Steward DL, Jacobs JB, et al. (2006) Acoustic rhinometry predicts tolerance of nasal continuous positive airway pressure: a pilot study. Am J Rhinol 20: 133-137.
35. Fletcher E, Luckett R (1991) The effect of positive reinforcement on hourly compliance in nasal continuous positive airway pressure users with obstructive sleep apnea. American Review of Respiratory Disease 143(5): 936-41.
36. Engleman HM, Martin SE, Deary IJ, Douglas NJ (1993) Effect of continuous positive airway pressure treatment on daytime function in sleep apnoea/hypopnoea syndrome. Lancet 343(8897): 572–575.
37. Waldhorn RE1, Herrick TW, Nguyen MC, O'Donnell AE, Sodero J, et al. (1990) Long-term compliance with nasal continuous positive airway pressure therapy of obstructive sleep apnea. Chest 97: 33-38.
38. Yinghui L, Preud'homme X, Harold W, Goforth MD, Omonua T, et al. (2011) The association of fatigue with depression and insomnia in HIV-seropositive patients: A pilot study. Sleep 34(12): 1723-1726.
39. Sawyer AM, Canamucio A, Moriarty H, Weaver TE, Richards KC, et al. (2011) Do cognitive perceptions influence CPAP use? Patient Educ Couns 85: 85-91.
40. Stepnowsky CJ Jr, Bardwell WA, Moore PJ, Ancoli-Israel S, Dimsdale JE (2002) Psychologic correlates of compliance with continuous positive airway pressure. Sleep 25: 758-762.
41. de Zeeuw J, Baberg HT, Duchna HW, Kempkens DJ, Walther JW, et al. (2007) Locus of control belief is a predictor of CPAP-compliance in patients with obstructive sleep apnea syndrome. Pneumologie 61(5): 283-290.
42. Tyrrell J, Poulet C, Pe Pin JL, Veale D (2006) A preliminary study of psychological factors affecting patients' acceptance of CPAP therapy for sleep apnoea syndrome. Sleep medicine 7(4): 375-379.
43. Balachandran JS, Yu X, Wroblewski K, Mokhlesi B (2013) A brief survey of patients' first impression after CPAP titration predicts future CPAP adherence: a pilot study. Journal of Clinical Sleep Medicine 9(3): 199-205.
44. Rosen CL , Auckley D , Benca R., Foldvary-Schaefer N, Iber C, et al (2012) A multisite randomized trial of portable sleep studies and positive airway pressure autotitration versus laboratory-based polysomnography for the diagnosis and treatment of obstructive sleep apnea: the HomePAP study . Sleep 35(6): 757-767.
45. Lettieri CF, Lettieri CJ, Carter K (2011) Does home sleep testing impair continuous positive airway pressure adherence in patients with obstructive sleep apnea? Chest 139: 849-854.
46. Parish JM, Lyng PJ (2003) Quality of life in bed partners of patients with obstructive sleep apnea or hypopnea after treatment with continuous positive airway pressure. Chest 124: 942-947.
47. McArdle N, Kingshott R, Engleman HM, Mackay TW, Douglas NJ (2001) Partners of patients with sleep apnoea/hypopnoea syndrome: effect of CPAP treatment on sleep quality and quality of life. Thorax 56: 513-518.
48. Cartwright R (2008) Sleeping together: a pilot study of the effects of shared sleeping on adherence to CPAP treatment in obstructive sleep apnea. J Clin Sleep Med 4: 123-127.

Appendix 1

Reference	Factors associated with compliance	Country	Sample (n)	threshold value to be adherent (/ night)
	Socio-economic variables			
Mc Ardle et al. (1999)[1]	Age	U.K.	1211	2 hours
Krieger et al. (1996)[2]	Age	France	728	4 hours
Budhiraja et al. (2007)[3]	Age, race	U.S.	100	4 hours
Olsen et al. (2008)[4]	Age	Australia	77	2 hours
Popescu et al. (2001)[5]	Age, gender	England	209	
Sin et al. (2002)[6]	Age, gender	Canada	296	4 hours
Simon-Tuval et al. (2009)[7]	Age, monthly income	Israel	162	Not indicated
Young et al. (1993)[8]	Gender	U.S.	602	4 hours
Pelletier et al. (2001)[9]	Gender	France	163	3 hours
Lewis et al. (2004)[10]	Gender, marital status, life event	United Kingdom	82	4 hours
Ye et al. (2009)[11]	Gender	7 sleep centers in the U.S. and Canada	176	4 hours
Bakker et al.[12]	Age, gender, ethnicity, education, employment, annual income, type of health insurance, health literacy	New Zealand	126	4 hours
Ye et al. (2012)[13]	Marital status, race	U.S.	91	4 hours
Gagnadoux et al. (2011)[14]	Marital status, employment status	France	1141	4 hours
Scharf et al. (2004)[15]	Race	U.S.	128	Not indicated
Billings et al. (2011)[16]	Race	U.S.	191	2 hours
Platt et al. (2009)[17]	Race, employment status, Neighborhood of residence	U.S.	266	4hours
Hoffstein et al. (1992)[18]	Type of health insurance	U.S.	96	4 hours

Reference	Factors associated with compliance	Country	Sample (n)	threshold value to be adherent (/ night)
	health variables			
Popescu et al. (2001)[5]	BMI	England	209	2 hours
Krieger et al. (1996)[2]	BMI	France	728	4 hours
Young et al. (1993)[8]	BMI	U.S.	602	4 hours
Pelletier et al. (2001)[9]	BMI	France	163	3 hours
Gagnadoux et al. (2011)[14]	BMI	France	1141	4 hours
Loredo et al. (2007)[19]	BMI, heart disorder	U.S.	76	6 hours
Wild et al. (2004)[20]	BMI	United Kingdom	119	3 hours
Olsen et al. (2008)[4]	BMI	Australia	77	4 hours
Redenius et al. (2008)[21]	BMI	U.S.	309	4 hours
Sugiera et al. (2007)[22]	BMI	Japan	77	5 hours
Reishten et al. (2010)[23]	Erectile dysfunction	U.S. and Canada	123	Not indicated
Margel et al. (2005)[24]	Erectile dysfunction	Israel	60	Not indicated
Mc Ardle et al. (1999)[1]	Treated Hypertension, heart disorder	U.K.	1211	2 hours
Hung et al. (1990)[25]	Treated Hypertension, myocardial infarction	Australia	101	Not indicated
Philips et al. (2013)[26]	Treated Hypertension	Spain	725	4 hours
Palombini et al. (2006)[27]	Stroke	Italy	50	4 hours
Martínez-García et al. (2012)[28]	Stroke, myocardial infarction	Italy	223	4 hours

Reference	Factors associated with compliance	Country	Sample (n)	threshold value to be adherent (/night)
	osa related variables			
Mc Ardle et al. (1999)[1]	AHI	U.K.	1211	2 hours
Popescu et al. (2001)[5]	AHI	England	209	2 hours
Krieger et al. (1996)[2]	AHI	France	728	4 hours
Pelletier et al. (2001)[9]	AHI	France	163	3 hours
Gagnadoux et al. (2011)[14]	AHI	France	1141	4 hours
Wild et al. (2004)[20]	AHI	United Kingdom	119	3 hours
Palombini et al. (2006)[27]	AHI	Italy	50	4 hours
Hui et al. (2001)[29]	AHI	China	112	4 hours
Krieger (1992)[30]	AHI	France	233	Not indicated
Meurice et al. (1994)[31]	AHI	France	44	5 hours
Bollig (2010)[32]	AHI	Synthetical article		
Baron et al. (2011)[33]	AHI	U.S.	31	Not indicated
Hoffstein et al. (1992)[18]	Minimum nasal cross-sectional area + reduced volume	U.S.	96	4 hours
Sugiera et al. (2007)[22]	AHI, Minimum nasal cross-sectional area + reduced volume	Japan	77	5 hours
Morris et al. (2006)[34]	Minimum nasal cross-sectional area + reduced volume	U.S.	34	Not indicated
Fletcher et al. (1991)[35]	Minimum nasal cross-sectional area + reduced volume	U.S.	Not indicated	Not indicated
Bakker et al. (2011)[12]	AHI	USA	126	4 hours
Simon-Tuval et al. (2009)[7]	AHI	Israel	162	Not indicated

Reference	Factors associated with compliance	Country	Sample (n)	threshold value to be adherent (/ night)
	psychological/ behavioral variables			
Mc Ardle et al. (1999)[1]	Epworth Sleepiness, Pichot Fatigue Scale	U.K.	1211	2 hours
Krieger et al. (1996)[2]	Epworth Sleepiness	France	728	4 hours
Pelletier et al. (2001)[9]	Epworth Sleepiness	France	163	3 hours
Lewis et al. (2004)[10]	Epworth Sleepiness	United Kingdom	82	4 hours
Ye et al. (2012)[11]	Epworth Sleepiness	U.S.	91	4 hours
Sin et al. (2002)[6]	Epworth Sleepiness, self-efficacy	Canada	296	4 hours

Loredo et al. (2007) [19]	Epworth Sleepiness	U.S.	76	6 hours
Wild et al. (2004)[20]	Epworth Sleepiness, self-efficacy	United Kingdom	119	3 hours
Meurice et al. (1994)[31]	Epworth Sleepiness	France	44	5 hours
Engleman et al. (1994)[36]	Epworth Sleepiness	U.K.	16	3.2 hours
Waldhorn et al. (1990)[37]	Epworth Sleepiness	U.S.	125	2 hours
Olsen et al. (2008)[4]	Pichot Fatigue Scale, Pichot Depression scale	Australia	77	4 hours
Yinghui et al. (2011)[38]	Pichot Fatigue Scale, Pichot Depression scale	U.S.	57	Not indicated
Bakker et al. (2011) [12]	Epworth Sleepiness, self-efficacy	USA	126	4 hours
Baron et al. (2011)[33]	Self-efficacy	U.S.	31	Not indicated
Sawyer et al. (2011)[39]	Self-efficacy	U.S.	66	20 minutes at effective pressure
Stepnowsky et al. (2002)[40]	Coping-styles	U.S.	23	Not indicated
de Zeeuw et al. (2007)[41]	Locus of control	Germany	85	Not indicated
Tyrrell et al. (2006)[42]	Locus of control	France	9	Not indicated

Reference	**Factors associated with compliance**	**Country**	**Sample (n)**	**Minimum threshold value to be adherent (/night)**
	initial cpap exposure variables			
Mc Ardle et al. (1999)[1]	CPAP use (in the first 15 days stage <3 hours)	U.K.	1211	2 hours
Popescu et al. (2001)[5]	CPAP use (in the first 15 days stage <3 hours)	England	209	2 hours
Lewis et al. (2001)[10]	Initial problems with CPAP use (in the first night)	United Kingdom	82	4 hours
Balachandran et al.(2013)[43]	CPAP perception questionnaire over the first 30 days of therapy	U.S.	1226	4 hours
Rosen et al. (2012)[44]	Diagnosed with HST	U.S.	373	4 hours
Lettieri et al. (2011)[45]	Diagnosed with HST	U.S.	210	4 hours

Reference	**Factors associated with compliance**	**Country**	**Sample (n)**	**Minimum threshold value to be adherent (/night)**
	social variables			
Baron et al. (2011)[33]	Spousal involvement	U.S.	31	Not indicated
Mc Ardle et al. (1999)[1]	Bed partner's sleep quality and overall quality of life	U.K.	1211	2 hours
Parish et al. (2003)[46]	Bed partner's sleep quality and overall quality of life	U.S.	51	6 hours (mean)
McArdle et al. (2001)[47]	Bed partner's sleep quality and overall quality of life	U.K.	49	Not indicated
Simon-Tuval et al. (2009)[7]	Partners sleeps separately and family and/or friends with positive experience of CPAP	Israel	162	Not indicated
Cartwright. (2008)[48]	Shared sleeping		20	
Ye et al. (2009)[49]	Spousal involvement	Synthetical article		

Reference	Factors associated with compliance	Country	Sample (n)	Minimum threshold value to be adherent (/night)
technical variables				
Anderson et al. (2003)[50]	Mask-interface (types of nasal vs face mask innovations)	New Zealand	11	Not indicated
Khanna et al. (2003)[51]	Mask-interface (types of nasal vs face mask innovations)	U.S.	38	4 hours
Massie et al. (2003)[52]	Mask-interface (types of nasal vs face mask innovations)	U.S.	39	4 hours
Mortimore et al. (1998)[53]	Mask-interface (types of nasal vs face mask innovations)	U.K.	30	Not indicated
Massie et al. (1999)[54]	Heated vs cold pass-over humidity	U.S.	38	1 hour
Aloia et al. (2005)[55]	Flexible pressure on CPAP adherence	U.S.	89	Not indicated
Pepin et al. (2009)[56]	Flexible pressure on CPAP adherence	France	218	4 hours
Chasen et al. (2005)[57]	Claustrophobia	U.S.	153	2 and 5 hours
Chai et al. (2013)[58]	Side effect	China, Australia, and New Zealand	275	3 hours

Study on the Current Situation of College Students' Sleep Quality

Anqiong Ji[1] and Rufang Wang[1,2*]

[1]Department of Management, Chengdu University of Traditional Chinese Medicine, Chengdu, P.R. China

[2]Department of Psychiatry & Health Behavior, Medical College of Georgia, Augusta University, Augusta, GA, USA

*Corresponding author: Wang R, Department of Management, Chengdu University of Traditional Chinese Medicine, Chengdu, P. R. China, E-mail: RUFWANG@augusta.edu

Abstract

In order to understand the current status of sleep quality of students in Chengdu University of Traditional Chinese Medicine, and to propose countermeasures. A simple random sampling method was used to select 255 university students as the survey subjects, and Pittsburgh Sleep Quality Index (PSQI) scale was used as a tool to evaluate the quality of college students' sleep. The survey found that the average score of PSQI was about 7.6 points. There were 128 people above 7 points, which accounted for 50.2% of the total number of students. This indicated that the overall quality of sleep of the undergraduates was poorer; the quality of sleep for boys was better than that of girls, and the quality of sleep among rural college students was better than that of girls. Urban college students, seniors and undergraduates have worse sleep than sophomores and juniors. The sleep quality of students in Chengdu University of Traditional Chinese Medicine is generally poor, and it is necessary to implement measures that target different populations for different demographic differences to achieve proper treatment and improve sleep quality.

Keywords: College students; Sleep quality; Influencing factors

Introduction

Sleep is necessary in people's life, work and study. Sleep quality affects health status [1]. At the same time, research from the World Health Organization (WHO) shows that about 27% of people worldwide suffer from sleep problems, and sleep problems need to be solved urgently. Sleep disorders are one of the most common health problems for late adolescents and young adults. Students report lack of sleep, difficulty sleeping or difficulty sleeping [2]. Studies have shown that sleep problems are common among college students [3-5] among them; about 20% of college students have sleep problems [6]. Despite this, many studies only examined total sleep rather than specific sleep components, highlighting the significance of further analysis of college students' sleep problems [7-11]. This article aims to investigate the current status of college students' sleep quality and their existing problems, so as to take appropriate measures to improve the quality of sleep for college students in order to promote their physical and mental health.

Research Objects and Methods

Research objects

A simple random sample was taken of students from Chengdu University of Traditional Chinese Medicine. During the survey, 300 questionnaires were actually sent out. A total of 262 questionnaires were returned, and 255 valid questionnaires were sent. Freshman students accounted for 20.0% (51/255), sophomores accounted for 44.7% (114/255), juniors accounted for 22.4% (57/255), and seniors accounted for 12.9% (33/255). Among them are 128 male students and 127 female students. Urban students accounted for 34.9% (89/255), rural students accounted for 65.1% (166/255).

Research methods

Questionnaire method, using the PSQI scale compiled by Liu et al. with the help of classmates from Chengdu University of Traditional Chinese Medicine, 255 university students were selected to conduct a questionnaire survey. The questionnaire used an anonymous method.

Survey tool

Analysis using the PSQI Scale [12], the scale has a total of 7 dimensions, which are sleep quality, fall-sleep time, sleep time, sleep disorders, and sleep efficiency, the application of sleep medicine and impact on daytime function. Each dimension score is divided into four levels, which are 0 -3 points, the scores of each component add up to the PSQI score, the total score is between 0-21. The high or low PSQI score indicates the quality of sleep. The higher the total score, the worse the quality of sleep. In this study, PSQI score of 7 was used as the standard for the classification of sleep disorders so as to understand the quality of sleep in the subjects in the past 1 month. According to this method, the quality of sleep can be demonstrated objectively and scientifically [13].

Confidence test

The reliability test of the questionnaire showed that the Cronbach alpha coefficient was 0.832, which had a high level of credibility and could be used as a tool for investigating the quality of sleep quality of college students.

Statistical Results

Different sex and sleep quality

The average score of boys (7.50 ± 1.97) is less than the average score of women (7.61 ± 2.37), and the difference is statistically significant ($P=0.000<0.05$) (Table 1). Taking the score criterion PSQI>7 as the critical value of sleep quality, there were 128 people with sleep disorders in college students, accounting for 50.2% of the total number of people. The average score of PSQI score was about 7.6 points. Slightly more than the study. About one-third of subjects had sleep problems (Table 1) [14].

Factors	Male (n=128)	Female (n=127)	T value	P-value
Total score	7.50 ± 1.97	7.61 ± 2.37	-1.514	0.004
Sleep time	1.94 ± 0.54	2.22 ± 0.57	-6.757	<0.001
Sleep efficiency	2.21 ± 0.47	2.97 ± 0.39	4.709	<0.001
Sleep quality	0.94 ± 0.68	0.88 ± 0.70	-3.241	<0.001
Hypnotic	0.09 ± 0.39	0.09 ± 0.31	-1.25	0.213
Fall-sleep time	1.13 ± 0.85	1.00 ± 0.79	1.751	0.08
Sleep disorder	0.85 ± 0.42	0.79 ± 0.43	5.143	<0.001
Day function	1.13 ± 0.79	1.16 ± 0.85	-2.727	0.786

Table 1: The influence of gender on sleep quality ($\bar{x} \pm s$).

Different grades and sleep quality

The differences in PSQI scores of different grades were statistically significant (P=0.000<0.05), the mean from the largest to the youngest is senior, freshman, sophomore and junior (Table 2).

Factors	Freshman (n=51)	Sophomore (n=114)	Junior (n=57)	Senior (n=33)	P-value
Total score	7.98 ± 2.19	7.37 ± 1.91	6.82 ± 2.06	8.78 ± 2.63	<0.001
Sleep time	0.63 ± 0.77	0.57 ± 0.76	0.37 ± 0.72	0.52 ± 0.91	0.109
Sleep efficiency	1.23 ± 0.25	2.34 ± 0.95	2.93 ± 0.53	1.38 ± 0.84	<0.001
Sleep quality	1.10 ± 0.88	0.84 ± 0.54	0.81 ± 0.70	1.06 ± 0.75	0.049
Hypnotic	0.04 ± 0.20	0.11 ± 0.35	0.05 ± 0.30	0.15 ± 0.57	<0.001
Fall-sleep time	1.22 ± 0.90	1.02 ± 0.75	0.81 ± 0.77	1.42 ± 0.90	<0.001
Sleep disorder	0.92 ± 0.39	0.73 ± 0.44	0.81 ± 0.44	0.97 ± 0.30	<0.001
Day function	1.08 ± 0.77	1.08 ± 0.75	1.05 ± 0.91	1.67 ± 0.78	<0.001

Table 2: Comparison of different grades of sleep quality ($\bar{x} \pm s$).

Different places of origin and quality of sleep

The detection rates of poor and relatively poor sleep quality in urban and rural areas were 55.06% and 47.59%, respectively, the difference was statistically significant (P<0.05) as shown in Table 3.

Source of origin	Number of people examined	Poor or relatively poor (%)
Urban	89	4955.06
Rural	166	7947.59
Total	255	12850.20

Table 3: Comparison of sleep quality in different habitats.

Discussion

The study found that the reporting rate of sleep quality problems among college students reached 50.2%, which was higher than that of and higher than that of poor quality of sleep, it is still not clear whether it is a downward trend. The reported rate of sleep quality problems among girls is higher than that of boys, and coincides. However, with some domestic surveys, the prevalence of sleep quality among boys is inconsistent with that of girls. Male and female students receive the same education at school and live in the same general environment. However, girls are more meticulous and sensitive, and their emotions fluctuate. As a result, anxiety and tension occur, which affects sleep quality. The unique physiological characteristics of women (menstrual period) can also affect Sleep quality. The difference in sleep quality at different grades was statistically significant, which is consistent with some domestic reports. The quality of the freshman's sleep is poor. Freshmen have just entered school and need to adapt to the new environment. The process of adapting to the new environment is accompanied by insomnia. This transition period is usually associated with an increase in stress levels, which in turn has a profound and lasting effect on sleep. The sleep quality of sophomores was gradually reduced from the second year to the fourth year, which is consistent with the related research. Seniors are facing the pressure of examinations or employment and are prone to sleep disorders. Studies show that there is a negative relationship between stress and emotion Schools, family, friends, etc. should pay attention to these problems and find practical solutions. This survey of college students in rural and urban areas found that the quality of sleep among urban students was worse than that in rural areas. This is contrary to the conclusion. Some domestic reports indicate that the difference between rural and urban areas is not statistically significant. However, this study did not find it. Urban students lived in a colorful world from childhood. They were tempted by the outside world, and their nightlife was abundant. This affected the quality of sleep. This is a manifestation of the simple quality of rural students. Early in the morning and early evening, there is less nightlife.

Conclusion

To resolve the existing problems, schools should pay attention to strengthening dormitory management, creating a good sleeping atmosphere, and paying attention to noise management to alleviate anxiety and depression caused by various reasons. Girls are more sensitive and must pay more attention to the psychological activities of girls. Visits to students from rural areas allow students to adapt to college new life as soon as possible, and reduce the negative emotions brought about by various pressures [15-22].

References

1. Zhu ZH, Zhang YL, Wang J (2016) An analysis of the status quo of sleep quality of military academy students. Chinese J Health Psychol 24: 1568-1570.
2. Yang CM, Wu CH, Hsieh MH, Liu MH, Lu FH (2003) Coping with sleep disturbances among young adults: A survey of first-year college students in Taiwan. Behav Med 29: 133-138.
3. Becker SP, Jarrett MA, Luebbe AM, Garner AA, Burns GL, et al. (2018) Sleep in a large, multi-university sample of college students: Sleep problem prevalence, sex differences, and mental health correlates. Sleep Health 4: 174-181.
4. Lund HG, Reider BD, Whiting AB, Prichard JR (2010) Sleep patterns and predictors of disturbed sleep in a large population of college students. J Adolesc Health 46: 124-132.
5. Orzech KM, Salafsky DB, Hamilton LA (2011) The state of sleep among college students at a large public university. J Am Coll Health 59: 612-619.
6. Xia CC, Geng LG, Sun GR (2015) Investigation on the correlation between Sleep Quality and Personality Traits of college students. Chinese Health Education 31: 20-23.
7. Brown FC, Buboltz WC Jr, Soper B (2002) Relationship of sleep hygiene awareness, sleep hygiene practices and sleep quality in university students. Behav Med 28: 33-38.
8. Gilbert SP, Weaver CC (2010) Sleep quality and academic performance in university students: A wake-up call for college psychologists. J Coll Stud Psychother 24: 295-306.
9. Lemma S, Gelaye B, Berhane Y, Worku A, Williams MA (2012) Sleep quality and its psychological correlates among university students in Ethiopia: A cross-sectional study. BMC Psychiatry 12: 237.
10. Adams SK, Kisler TS (2013) Sleep quality as a mediator between technology-related sleep quality, depression and anxiety. Cyberpsychol Behav Soc Netw 16: 25-30.
11. Cheng SH, Shih CC, Lee IH, Hou YW, Chen KC, et al. (2012) A study on the sleep quality of incoming university students. Psychiatry Res 197: 270-274.
12. Wang XD, Wang XL, Ma H (1999) Mental health assessment scale manual (updated version). Chinese Mental Health Magazine 375-378.
13. Xiao DM, Cai LB, Huang Y (2016) The relationship between college students' sleep quality and eating habits. Chinese School Health 37: 1424-1426.
14. Liu MW, Liu H, Rui B (2016) An Investigation on the Sleep Quality of University Students in Anhui Medical College. J Qiqihar Med College 37: 4566-4568.
15. Xu CY, Liu C, Hao LJ (2017) Study on Sleep Quality and Relationship among College Students. Prevent Med 29: 142-145.
16. Wu X, Liu C, Hao LJ (2008) Sleep quality and its influencing factors in medical students. Modern Prevent Med 35: 98-100.
17. Becker SP, Jarrett MA, Luebbe AM, Garner AA, Burns GL, et al. (2018) Sleep in a large, multi-university sample of college students: sleep problem prevalence, sex differences, and mental health correlates. Sleep Health 2: 174-181.
18. Åkerstedt T (2006) Psychosocial stress and impaired sleep. Scand J Work Environ Health 32: 493-501.
19. Nyer M, Farabaugh A, Fehling K, Soskin D, Holt G, et al. (2013) Relationship between sleep disturbance and depression, anxiety, and functioning in college students. Depress. Anxiety 30: 873-880.
20. Folkman S (2013) Stress: Appraisal and coping. Gellman, J.R. Turner (Eds.), Encyclopedia of Behavioral Medicine, Springer, New York.
21. Wei CQ, Lan QL, Liang HQ (2009) Sleep status and influencing factors of college students at a medical college. Chinese School Health 30: 941-942.
22. Qiao Y (2017) Sleep quality and its influencing factors among students in a medical school in Hebei. Mental Health 42: 106-110.

The Development of Posttraumatic Stress Disorder after Mild Traumatic Brain Injury in Civilian Populations

Xi Han[1], Ping Sheng[2,3]*, Chengguang Huang[2], Mingkun Yu[2], Lijun Hou[2] and Yan Dong[2,3]*

[1]*Department of Neurosurgery, Huashan Hospital, Fudan University, China*
[2]*Department of Neurosurgery, Second Military Medical University, China*
[3]*Neuroscience center, Second Military Medical University, China*

Abstract

Background: Posttraumatic stress disorder (PTSD) is an anxiety disorder following exposure to a traumatic event. Recent studies demonstrate that mild traumatic brain injury (mTBI) is strongly associated with PTSD among soldiers returning from Iraq. However, the effect of mTBI on development of PTSD in civilian populations is quite controversial. The study is aimed at identifying whether mTBI contributes to an increased risk of PTSD in civilian populations as it happens in the service members.

Methods: A comprehensive search of literature was undertaken in order to identify published studies on PTSD associated with mTBI. mTBI was defined according to the American Congress of Rehabilitation Medicine (ACRM). PTSD was operationalized as the presence of symptoms consistent with those defined by the *Diagnostic and Statistical Manual of Mental Disorders*. The effect of mTBI on the development of PTSD was assessed with odds ratio (OR) with 95% confidence intervals (CIs).

Results: The pooled data consisted of 1222 mTBI patients and 1468 general trauma participants. 14% of mTBI patients reported PTSD, and 9% of general trauma patients developed PTSD. Or of the pooled studies indicates a 61% increase in the prevalence of PTSD, suggesting that mTBI might increase the risk of development of PTSD in civilian settings (or 1.61, 95% CI 1.25-2.06. p=0.0002, I^2=0%). The occurrence of PTSD was not significantly different among 3-months, 6-months and 12-months follow up subgroups (p=0.28). A sensitivity analysis shows the results are affected by sequential exclusion of study reported by Bryant et al. (2010). When Bryant et al. data were removed, OR of the other six studies demonstrates that the prevalence of PTSD in mTBI and general trauma groups doesn't significantly differ (OR 1.30, 95% CI 0.88-1.93. p=0.19, I^2=0%). The study from Bryant et al contributed 57% of patients to overall data, which was derived from four levels I trauma centers across three states in Australia.

Conclusion: Our data indicate that mTBI patients are more prone to develop PTSD than general trauma patients without mTBI in civilian settings.

Keywords: Mild traumatic brain injury; Minor brain injury; Posttraumatic stress disorder; Anxiety.

Introduction

Traumatic brain injury (TBI) is a major public health problem. In the United States, more than 1.5 million individuals sustain TBI every year [1]. It is estimated that almost 320,000 deployed American personnel may have suffered varying degrees of TBI [2]. Mild TBI (mTBI) is the most frequent type of TBI among both veteran and civilian populations. In the civilian sector, the majority of cases with mTBI are associated with early symptoms that typically resolve within a few days to a few months post injury [3-6]. However, a minority of individuals continue to complain of ongoing post concussive somatic, cognitive, and/or behavioral symptoms that may lead to long-term functional limitation [7-10].

Posttraumatic stress disorder (PTSD) is an anxiety disorder characterized by reexperiencing, avoidance, and hyper arousal symptoms following exposure to a traumatic event. Historically, it was argued that trauma survivors with mTBI have no painful traumatic memories and, therefore cannot develop core PTSD symptoms characterized by intrusive re-experiencing of the event. However, evidence has accrued showing that PTSD symptoms can develop after mTBI [11-16]. Recent studies demonstrate that mTBI are strongly associated with PTSD among soldiers returning from Iraq [17]. On examination of multiple potential predictors of PTSD including non-TBI-related injuries, only combat intensity and mTBI with loss of consciousness (LOC) were significantly associated with PTSD once other variables were controlled. These findings suggest that mTBI might increase the likelihood of developing PTSD in service members. There has been extensive debate in the literature regarding whether mTBI has a strong effect on the development of PTSD in civilian populations [18-28]. So far, the published data investigating the incidence of PTSD after mTBI in civilian populations are difficult to interpret due to variations in the methodology and conflicting results. As indicated in a recent study by the World Health Organization Collaborating Centre Task Force on mTBI, different criteria used to define mTBI and lack of control groups or comparison of inappropriate control groups have been often found in the existing literature [29].

The current study employed meta-analysis to integrate the available literature on the incidence of PTSD associated with mTBI and bring

***Corresponding author:** Yan Dong, Department of Neurosurgery, Shanghai Institute of Neurosurgery, Military Institute of Neurosurgery, Changzheng Hospital, Second Military Medical University, 415 Fengyang Road, Shanghai 200003, China; E-mail: smmudongyan@163.com or li_hou@hotmail.com

a more clear evidence for the question whether PTSD can confer the risk of PTSD development after mTBI in civilian populations with a rigorous methodological quality assessment.

Materials and Methods

Selection of studies

A comprehensive search of Pubmed and PSYCHInfo databases was undertaken in order to identify published studies on PTSD associated with mTBI. Key search terms included "mild traumatic brain injury", "minor traumatic brain injury", "mild brain injury", "minor brain injury", "mild head injury", "minor head injury", "mild closed head injury", "minor closed head injury", "mild head trauma" and "minor head trauma". These search terms were paired with "posttraumatic stress", "posttraumatic stress disorder" and "anxiety disorder". The search was limited to English language published in peer-reviewed journals from January 1980 to December 2013 that involved human subjects and presented primary data. Reference lists from the relevant studies were searched for additional references.

Inclusion criteria

Original studies were considered for inclusion in the meta-analysis if they met with the following criteria: (1) adult civilians were studied; (2) mTBI was defined according to the American Congress of Rehabilitation Medicine (ACRM) [30]; (3) PTSD was operationalized as the presence of symptoms consistent with those defined by the *Diagnostic and Statistical Manual of Mental Disorders (DSM-III, SDM-III-R, DSM IV, or DSM-IV-TR)* [31-33], which were assessed through clinical diagnoses or interviews or "probable PTSD" based on indicated cutoff scores using self-report inventories or screening measures in not less than 3 months after injury. (4) Results were sufficient to allow calculation of effect sizes. (5) Results were not reported elsewhere.

Data collection

Titles and abstracts from all references identified in the literature search process were reviewed by two independent study investigators. For each study included in the meta-analysis, the author, date of publication, country and assessment tools for PTSD were summarized in Table 1. Several sample characteristics were also noted, including sample size, mean age, mean education, sex, CT examination, and severity of injury as measured by Injury Severity Score (ISS) for patients and control samples when available. Results were reviewed with another member of the research team. Studies included in the meta-analysis were assessed for risk of bias using Newcastle-Ottawa score (NOS) [34]. The score assigns a study a maximum of 9 points, with higher scores indicating a lower risk of bias.

Statistical analysis

The effect of mTBI on the development of PTSD was assessed with odds ratio (or) with 95% confidence intervals (CIs). A subgroup analysis was carried out based on education, mean age, NOS, follow-up, ISS and country. Egger's test was applied to check the potential publication bias. The statistical estimates of effect were derived using a random-effects model with Mantel-Haenszel statistics. Heterogeneity of mTBI effect on the development of PTSD between studies was investigated visually by scatter plot analysis and statistically by the heterogeneity I^2 statistic. I^2 statistic of 0%-40% indicates unimportant heterogeneity, 30%-60% indicates moderate heterogeneity, 50-90% indicates substantial heterogeneity, and 75%-100% indicates considerable heterogeneity. P values were calculated by χ^2 tests. All the reported P values are two-sided and value of P less than 0.05 was regarded as statistically significant for all included studies. All analyses were calculated using STATA (version 10.0).

Results

We identified 853 potentially relevant studies from our combined database, of which 734 were excluded after a preliminary review. The remaining 75 studies were retrieved for detailed assessment. Ultimately, 7 prospective cohort studies met the inclusion criteria (Figure 1). For the study from Bryant et al. [26], outcomes at 3-months and 12-months follow up were both included for analyses. A total of 1222 mTBI patients and 1468 general trauma participants were included. There was no evidence of publication bias for the development of PTSD after mild traumatic brain injury (P value for Egger's test, 0.38). Five high quality studies were judged by a NOS score of 7 or above. The baseline characteristics of the participants and the design of the studies were summarized in the Table 1.

The pooled data consisted of 2690 individuals with 304 PTSD patients. 14 % of mTBI patients reported PTSD, and 9% of general trauma patients developed PTSD. As shown in Figure 2, OR of the pooled studies indicates a 61% increase in the prevalence of PTSD in mTBI patients when compared with general trauma participants, suggesting that mTBI might increase the risk of development of PTSD in civilian settings (OR 1.61, 95% CI 1.25-2.06, p=0.0002, I^2=0%) (Figure 2). In order to evaluate the effect of time after injury on development of PTSD in mTBI populations, the pooled data were classified into 3 subgroups (3-months, 6-months and 12-months follow up groups). There was no significant difference among subgroups (p=0.28) (Figure 2). A sensitivity analysis shows the results are affected by sequential exclusion of study reported by Bryant et al. [26] When Bryant's research was removed, OR of the other six studies demonstrates that

Source	mTBI group		control group		follow up (month)	sex (male)	mean age (year)	ISS	education (year)	CT examination	Newcastle-Ottawa score	country	diagnosis of TBI	screening tools for PTSD
	PTSD	total	PTSD	total										
Levin HS [21] (2001)	8	60	6	52	3	71%	36	5.13	10.84	-/+	6	USA	ACRM	SCID
Jones C [23] (2005)	10	58	11	61	3	40%	37	3.22	N/A	N/A	4	UK	ACRM	PSS
Bryant RA [24] (2010)	48	377	43	555	3	73%	38	10.42	N/A	N/A	7	Australia	ACRM	CAPS
Ponford J [26] (2011)	7	90	3	80	3	70%	35	ND	13.87	-	7	Australia	ACRM	PCL-C
Bryant RA[19] (1999)	15	63	18	71	6	68%	32	6.82	N/A	N/A	7	Australia	ACRM	CIDI
Friedland JF [20] (2001)	17	64	7	35	7	64%	33	20.06	N/A	N/A	7	Canada	ACRM	IES+GHQ
Creamer M [22] (2005)	24	189	8	118	12	76%	37	13.67	N/A	N/A	7	Australia	ACRM	CAPS
Bryant RA [24] (2010)	43	321	36	496	12	73%	38	10.42	N/A	N/A	7	Australia	ACRM	CAPS

N/A, not available; ACRM, American Congress of Rehabilitation Medicine; CIDI, Composite International Diagnostic Interview; PCL-C, PTSD Checklist-civilian version; CAPS, Clinician-Administered PTSD Scale; SCID, structured clinical interview for DSM-IV; PSS, PTSD symptom scale; -/+, negative/positive; IES, Impact of Event Scale; GHQ, General Health Questionaire; CT, computed tomography.

Table 1: Design and patient characteristics for studies included in the meta analysis.

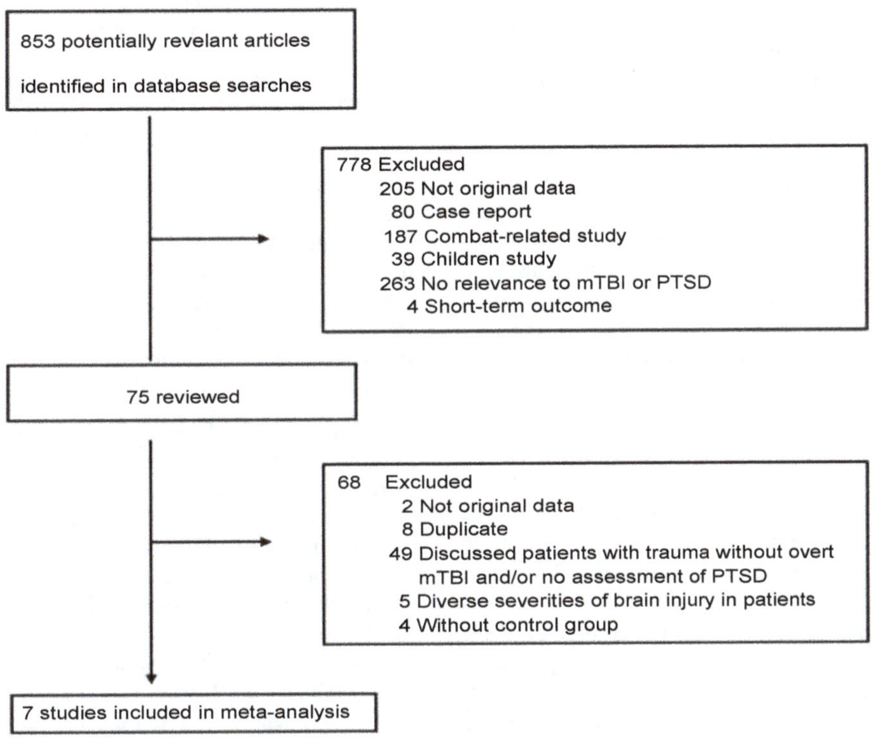

Figure 1: Flow diagram of the literature search and studies selection process.

Study or Subgroup	mTBI Events	mTBI Total	Control Events	Control Total	Weight	Odds Ratio M-H, Random, 95% CI
4.1.1 3 months follow up						
Bryant RA 2010	48	337	43	555	32.4%	1.74 [1.13, 2.68]
Jones C 2005	10	58	11	61	6.9%	0.95 [0.37, 2.43]
Levin HS 2001	8	60	6	52	4.8%	1.18 [0.38, 3.65]
Ponford J 2011	7	90	3	80	3.2%	2.16 [0.54, 8.67]
Subtotal (95% CI)		585		748	47.3%	1.55 [1.08, 2.22]
Total events	73		63			
Heterogeneity: Tau² = 0.00: Chi² = 1.76, df = 3 (P = 0.62); I² = 0%						
Test for overall effect: Z = 2.40 (P = 0.02)						
4.1.2 6 months follow up						
Bryant RA 1999	15	63	18	71	9.8%	0.92 [0.42, 2.02]
Friedland JF 2001	17	64	7	35	6.2%	1.45 [0.53, 3.92]
Subtotal (95% CI)		127		106	16.0%	1.10 [0.59, 2.03]
Total events	32		25			
Heterogeneity: Tau² = 0.00: Chi² = 0.49, df = 1 (P = 0.49); I² = 0%						
Test for overall effect: Z = 0.29 (P = 0.77)						
4.1.3 12 months follow up						
Bryant RA* 2010	43	321	36	496	28.0%	1.98 [1.24, 3.15]
Creamer M 2005	24	189	8	118	8.8%	2.00 [0.87, 4.61]
Subtotal (95% CI)		510		614	36.8%	1.98 [1.32, 2.98]
Total events	67		44			
Heterogeneity: Tau² = 0.00: Chi² = 0.00, df = 1 (P = 0.98); I² = 0%						
Test for overall effect: Z = 3.29 (P = 0.001)						
Total (95% CI)		1222		1468	100.0%	1.61 [1.25, 2.06]
Total events	172		132			
Heterogeneity: Tau² = 0.00: Chi² = 4.77, df = 7 (P = 0.69); I² = 0%						
Test for overall effect: Z = 3.76 (P = 0.0002)						
Test for subgroup differences: Chi² = 2.53. df = 2 (P = 0.28). I² = 20.9%						

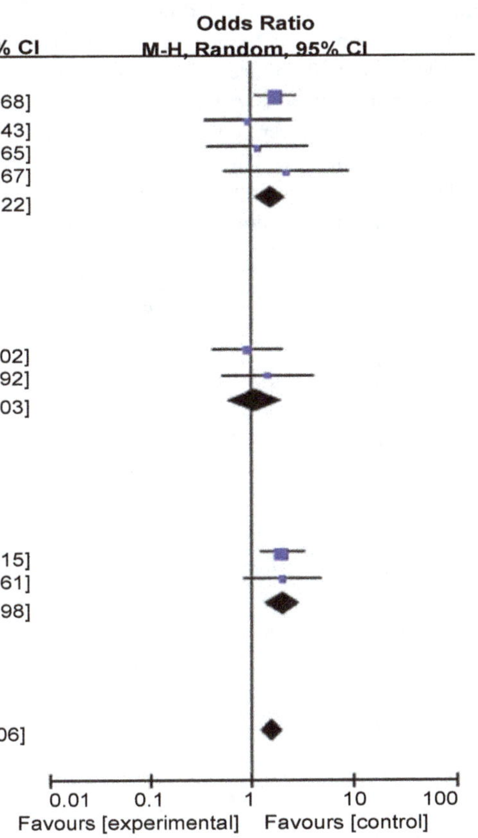

Figure 2: Effect of mTBI on the risk of development of PTSD in civilian populations. * Outcomes at 3-months and 12-months follow up were both included for analyses.

the prevalence of PTSD in mTBI and general trauma groups doesn't significantly differ (OR 1.30, 95% CI 0.88-1.93, p=0.19, I^2=0%). The study from Bryant et al. [26] contributed 57% of patients to overall data, which was derived from four levels I trauma centers across three states in Australia.

Subgroup analyses were carried out based on education, mean age, NOS, follow-up, ISS and country (Table 2). Outcomes at 12-months follow up were included for subgroup analyses in the study from Bryant et al. [26], with the exception of education, mTBI attributed to an increase in the prevalence of PTSD in the other five subgroup analyses, where Bryant's study contributed an overwhelming portion to overall data due to its huge sample size. It is possible that statistical significant difference might come out of contribution of specific study rather than subset factors.

Discussion

Our study is aimed at identifying whether mTBI contributes to a increased risk of PTSD in civilian populations as it happens in the service members. In this review, we surveyed 804 publications related to mTBI and PTSD and 7 studies were finally included in our meta-analysis. The overall incidence of PTSD is 14% in the mTBI patients in a civilian sample. The military or veteran studies reported probable PTSD in 33% to 39% of respondents who endorsed having experienced a probable mTBI [17,35,36]. Since a substantial number of mTBI survivors in the military is the result of non-combat-related injuries (i.e., sports injuries, assaults, motor vehicle accidents), comparison between civilian studies and military studies helps assess how often PTSD is due to the stress of combat/military life. The meta-analysis demonstrates that patients suffering mTBI are at higher risk of PTSD development compared to general trauma patients in the civilian populations. Some literature on PTSD following TBI has shown that PTSD symptoms decrease significantly over time within a year post injury [37-38]. However, quite a quantity of studies disputes the opinion because of the fact that the rates of PTSD don't drop over a year after TBI [26,39,40] Our stratified analyses showed that the prevalence of PTSD at 3-months, 6-months and 12-months follow up didn't differ, supporting the idea that the occurrence of PTSD may be maintained or even increase over time after injury.

Hesdorffer *et al.* [20] reported their systematic review on the long-term psychiatric outcomes following traumatic brain injury in 2009. They concluded, on the basis of their evaluation, that there is inadequate/insufficient evidence to determine whether an association exists between mTBI and PTSD in civilian populations [20]. Of note, they drew their conclusion mainly depending on the study reported by Creame, which was derived from one trauma center in Australia including 189 mTBI patients and 118 general trauma patients. In the present review, we included 2690 individuals in 7 studies with a broad range of baseline characteristics. We argue that the insufficient data might lead to the uncertainty about the relationship between PTSD and mTBI in Hesdorffer *et al.* [20] research.

There are several important limitations in the review. The major limitation is the quality of studies involved. Of the 7 studies, 71% (n=5) were from centers in Australia. Although all the studies are prospective investigation, only the study reported by Bryant, *et al.* [26] is a multisite design with a big sample size of more than 300 mTBI participants. The numbers of mTBI patients vary across the other six studies from 58 to 189. The meta-analysis demonstrates that patients suffering mTBI are at higher risk of PTSD development compared to general trauma patients in the civilian populations, which is in accordance with findings from Bryant *et al.* [26]. However, when the data were removed, a meta-analysis of the other six small studies does not predict the effect of mTBI on the development of PTSD. In some cases, a meta-analysis of several small studies may fail to predict the results of a single large study although it is now widely used to provide evidence to support clinical strategies [41]. The heterogeneity of sample sizes may partially account for the divergence in our study. When divergences are seen between meta-analysis and a large study, few will disagree that the value of the large and well designed studies is of more guidance to clinical practice than meta-analyses. Thus, more large researches of high quality will help us come to a consistent conclusion in the future.

Another limitation is the inconsistent assessment tools of PTSD applied in the studies, consisting of clinical interview and self-reported

Group	PTSD event/total patients		Odds Ratios (OR) and 95%CI	P value	heterogeneity	P value for heterogeneity
	mTBI	GT				
Education (years)						
≥ 12	7/90	3/80	2.16 [0.54, 8.67]	0.28	-	-
<12	8/60	6/52	1.18 [0.38, 3.65]	0.77	-	-
Mean age						
≥ 35	92/718	64/807	1.72 [1.22, 2.43]	0.002	0	0.64
<35	32/127	25/106	1.10 [0.59, 2.03]	0.77	0	0.49
NOS						
≥ 7	106/727	72/800	1.68 [1.21, 2.34]	0.002	0	0.54
<7	18/118	17/113	1.04 [0.50, 2.14]	0.92	0	0.77
Follow-up						
≥ 6	99/637	69/720	1.66 [1.18, 2.33]	0.004	0	0.40
<6	28/208	20/193	1.21 [0.64, 2.31]	0.55	0	0.63
ISS						
>10	60/385	43/531	1.87 [1.22, 2.85]	0.004	0	0.58
<10	33/181	35/184	0.98 [0.58, 1.67]	0.95	0	0.94
Country						
Australia	89/663	65/765	1.71 [1.21, 2.43]	0.003	0	0.39
Other	35/182	24/148	1.16 [0.65, 2.09]	0.61	0	0.83
Overall	124/845	89/913	1.55 [1.15, 2.09]	0.004	0	0.60

Table 2: Subgroup analyses based on education, mean age, NOS, follow-up, ISS and country.

questionnaires. Clinician-Administered PTSD Scale-IV (CAPS), a structured clinical interview with good sensitivity and specificity relative to the Structured Clinical Interview for DSM-IV (SCID), as well as sound test-retest reliability, was utilized to assess PTSD in the studies of Bryant and Creamer Compared to CAPS, self-reported questionnaires could interfere with the ascertainment of PTSD in the studies. Three of the studies used self-reported questionnaires to diagnose probable PTSD. The inclusion of such articles could elevate the estimated incidence of PTSD in the participants.

An additional limitation of the review is the classification of mTBI. All the studies categorized TBI patients according to Glasgow Coma Scale (GCS), widely used to assess the level of consciousness after TBI. GCS score ranges from 3 (most severely impaired) to 15 (no neurologic impairment). GCS 13-15 is often employed as one of criteria to define mTBI. However, GCS score doesn't accord with severity of brain damage all the time. Mild traumatic brain injury can be classified into two categories-complicated and uncomplicated mTBI, in which complicated mTBI means presence of an intracranial abnormality on neuroimaging. Almost all the studies included in our meta-analysis didn't discriminate complicated mTBI from uncomplicated mTBI. Data by Smits *et al.* [42] indicated that complicated mTBI was significantly associated with worse outcome [42]. Grouping all mTBI participants into a single category may oversimplify the complex characteristics of brain injury and obscure important differences related to mTBI severity [43]. In future study, it is necessary to clarify whether injury in the specific sites of brain tissue might confer the risk of development of PTSD following mTBI.

mTBI patients develop post concussion symptoms (PCS), a constellation of physical, cognitive and emotional symptoms. The presence of persistent PCS complicates the diagnosis of PTSD after mTBI because many of the complaints are similar, including irritability, depressive symptoms, sleep disturbance and cognitive difficulties. The issue that PCS are a result of organic or psychological factors, or an interaction between the two has been long debated. The facts that PCS is frequently encountered among healthy adults [44-45] and clinical groups without a history of mTBI [46] indicate that PCS might be nonspecific to mTBI. Recent studies show that PCS complaints after mTBI are more likely to be ascribed to psychological factors, such as anxiety, depression or PTSD rather than mTBI [47-50]. Apart from PTSD, mTBI could be associated with other psychiatric disorders, such as depression, generalized anxiety disorder, obsessive-compulsive disorder and substance abuse. It is a well-studied fact that PTSD patients have high rates of psychiatric comorbidity. Apparently, public health concerns are needed to address the huge health burden caused by the psychiatric effects of mTBI. New approaches that ease early identification of psychiatric disorders and prompt early interventions to prevent psychiatric condition might facilitate optimal recovery from mTBI.

Conclusion

This meta-analysis represents synthesis of the available data on the development of PTSD after mTBI in civilian populations. The overall incidence of PTSD is 14% in mTBI patients and 9% in general trauma patients among the civilian populations. Our data indicate that mTBI patients are more prone to develop PTSD than general trauma patients without mTBI in civilian settings.

References

1. Beauchamp K, Mutlak H, Smith WR, Shohami E, Stahel PF (2008) Pharmacology of traumatic brain injury: where is the "golden bullet"? Mol Med 14: 731-740.
2. Ling G, Bandak F, Armonda R, Grant G, Ecklund J (2009) Explosive blast neurotrauma. J Neurotrauma 26: 815-825.
3. Dikmen S, Machamer J, Temkin N (2001) Mild head injury: facts and artifacts. J Clin Exp Neuropsychol 23: 729-738.
4. Ryan LM, Warden DL (2003) Post concussion syndrome. Int Rev Psychiatry 15: 310-316.
5. Powell TJ, Collin C, Sutton K (1996) A follow-up study of patients hospitalized after minor head injury. Disabil Rehabil 18: 231-237.
6. Carroll LJ, Cassidy JD, Peloso PM, Borg J, von Holst H, et al. (2004) Prognosis for mild traumatic brain injury: results of the WHO Collaborating Centre Task Force on Mild Traumatic Brain Injury. J Rehabil Med 43: 84-105.
7. Hartlage LC, Durant-Wilson D, Patch PC (2001) Persistent neurobehavioral problems following mild traumatic brain injury. Arch Clin Neuropsychol 16: 561-570.
8. Vanderploeg RD, Curtiss G, Luis CA, Salazar AM (2007) Long-term morbidities following self-reported mild traumatic brain injury. J Clin Exp Neuropsychol 29: 585-598.
9. Deb S, Lyons I, Koutzoukis C (1999) Neurobehavioural symptoms one year after a head injury. Br J Psychiatry 174: 360-365.
10. van der Naalt J, van Zomeren AH, Sluiter WJ, Minderhoud JM (1999) One year outcome in mild to moderate head injury: the predictive value of acute injury characteristics related to complaints and return to work. J Neurol Neurosurg Psychiatry 66: 207-213.
11. Harvey AG, Bryant RA (1999) The relationship between acute stress disorder and posttraumatic stress disorder: a 2-year prospective evaluation. J Consult Clin Psychol 67: 985-988.
12. Hickling EJ, Gillen R, Blanchard EB, Buckley T, Taylor A (1998) Traumatic brain injury and posttraumatic stress disorder: a preliminary investigation of neuropsychological test results in PTSD secondary to motor vehicle accidents. Brain Inj 12: 265-274.
13. Mayou RA, Black J, Bryant B (2000) Unconsciousness, amnesia and psychiatric symptoms following road traffic accident injury. Br J Psychiatry 177: 540-545.
14. Gil S, Caspi Y, Ben-Ari IZ, Koren D, Klein E (2005) Does memory of a traumatic event increase the risk for posttraumatic stress disorder in patients with traumatic brain injury? A prospective study. Am J Psychiatry 162: 963-969.
15. Bombardier CH, Fann JR, Temkin N, Esselman PC, Pelzer E, et al. (2006) Posttraumatic stress disorder symptoms during the first six months after traumatic brain injury. J Neuropsychiatry Clin Neurosci 18: 501-508.
16. Yurgil KA, Barkauskas DA2, Vasterling JJ3, Nievergelt CM4, Larson GE5, et al. (2014) Association between traumatic brain injury and risk of posttraumatic stress disorder in active-duty Marines. JAMA Psychiatry 71: 149-157.
17. Hoge CW, McGurk D, Thomas JL, Cox AL, Engel CC, et al. (2008) Mild traumatic brain injury in U.S. Soldiers returning from Iraq. N Engl J Med 358: 453-463.
18. Bryant RA, O'Donnell ML, Creamer M, McFarlane AC, Silove D (2013) A multisite analysis of the fluctuating course of posttraumatic stress disorder. JAMA Psychiatry 70: 839-846.
19. Sbordone RJ, Liter JC (1995) Mild traumatic brain injury does not produce post-traumatic stress disorder. Brain Inj 9: 405-412.
20. Hesdorffer DC, Rauch SL, Tamminga CA (2009) Long-term psychiatric outcomes following traumatic brain injury: a review of the literature. J Head Trauma Rehabil 24: 452-459.

21. Bryant RA, Harvey AG (1999) The influence of traumatic brain injury on acute stress disorder and post-traumatic stress disorder following motor vehicle accidents. Brain Inj 13: 15-22.

22. Friedland JF, Dawson DR (2001) Function after motor vehicle accidents: a prospective study of mild head injury and posttraumatic stress. J Nerv Ment Dis 189: 426-434.

23. Levin HS, Brown SA, Song JX, McCauley SR, Boake C, et al. (2001) Depression and posttraumatic stress disorder at three months after mild to moderate traumatic brain injury. J Clin Exp Neuropsychol 23: 754-769.

24. Creamer M, O'Donnell ML, Pattison P (2005) Amnesia, traumatic brain injury, and posttraumatic stress disorder: a methodological inquiry. Behav Res Ther 43: 1383-1389.

25. Jones C, Harvey AG, Brewin CR (2005) Traumatic brain injury, dissociation, and posttraumatic stress disorder in road traffic accident survivors. J Trauma Stress 18: 181-191.

26. Bryant RA, O'Donnell ML, Creamer M, McFarlane AC, Clark CR, et al. (2010) The psychiatric sequelae of traumatic injury. Am J Psychiatry 167: 312-320.

27. Zatzick DF, Rivara FP, Jurkovich GJ, Hoge CW, Wang J, et al. (2010) Multisite investigation of traumatic brain injuries, posttraumatic stress disorder, and self-reported health and cognitive impairments. Arch Gen Psychiatry 67: 1291-1300.

28. Ponsford J, Cameron P, Fitzgerald M, Grant M, Mikocka-Walus A (2011) Long-term outcomes after uncomplicated mild traumatic brain injury: a comparison with trauma controls. J Neurotrauma 28: 937-946.

29. Carroll LJ, Cassidy JD, Holm L, Kraus J, Coronado VG, et al. (2004) Methodological issues and research recommendations for mild traumatic brain injury: J Rehabil Med 43: 113-125.

30. The Mild Traumatic Brain Injury Committee of the Head Injury Interdisciplinary Special Interest Group of the American Congress of Rehabilitation Medicine (1993) Definition of mild traumatic brain injury. J Head Trauma Rehabil 8: 86-87.

31. Arntz A (1999) Do personality disorders exist? On the validity of the concept and its cognitive-behavioral formulation and treatment. Behav Res Ther 37 Suppl 1: S97-134.

32. Diagnostic and Statistical Manual of Mental Disorders. 3rd ed. Washington, DC, American Psychiatric Association.

33. Diagnostic and Statistical Manual of Mental Disorders. 4th ed. Washington, DC,American Psychiatric Association.

34. Wells GA, Shea B, O'Connell D, Peterson J, Welch V, et al. The Newcastle-Ottawa Scale (NOS) for assessing the quality of nonrandomised studies in meta-analyses.

35. Schneiderman AI, Braver ER, Kang HK (2008) Understanding sequelae of injury mechanisms and mild traumatic brain injury incurred during the conflicts in Iraq and Afghanistan: persistent postconcussive symptoms and posttraumatic stress disorder. Am J Epidemiol 167: 1446-1452.

36. Center for Military Health Policy Research (2008) Invisible Wounds of War: Psychological and Cognitive Injuries, Their Consequences, and Services to Assist Recovery. Rand Corporation.

37. Blanchard EB1, Hickling EJ, Barton KA, Taylor AE, Loos WR, et al. (1996) One-year prospective follow-up of motor vehicle accident victims. Behav Res Ther 34: 775-786.

38. Shalev AY1, Freedman S, Peri T, Brandes D, Sahar T, et al. (1998) Prospective study of posttraumatic stress disorder and depression following trauma. Am J Psychiatry 155: 630-637.

39. Mayou R1, Bryant B, Duthie R (1993) Psychiatric consequences of road traffic accidents. BMJ 307: 647-651.

40. O'Donnell ML1, Creamer M, Pattison P, Atkin C (2004) Psychiatric morbidity following injury. Am J Psychiatry 161: 507-514.

41. LeLorier J1, Grégoire G, Benhaddad A, Lapierre J, Derderian F (1997) Discrepancies between meta-analyses and subsequent large randomized, controlled trials. N Engl J Med 337: 536-542.

42. Smits M1, Hunink MG, van Rijssel DA, Dekker HM, Vos PE, et al. (2008) Outcome after complicated minor head injury. AJNR Am J Neuroradiol 29: 506-513.

43. Pertab JL1, James KM, Bigler ED (2009) Limitations of mild traumatic brain injury meta-analyses. Brain Inj 23: 498-508.

44. Paniak C1, Reynolds S, Phillips K, Toller-Lobe G, Melnyk A, et al. (2002) Patient complaints within 1 month of mild traumatic brain injury: a controlled study. Arch Clin Neuropsychol 17: 319-334.

45. Iverson GL1, Lange RT (2003) Examination of "postconcussion-like" symptoms in a healthy sample. Appl Neuropsychol 10: 137-144.

46. Meares S1, Shores EA, Taylor AJ, Batchelor J, Bryant RA, et al. (2011) The prospective course of postconcussion syndrome: the role of mild traumatic brain injury. Neuropsychology 25: 454-465.

47. Lippa SM1, Pastorek NJ, Benge JF, Thornton GM (2010) Postconcussive symptoms after blast and nonblast-related mild traumatic brain injuries in Afghanistan and Iraq war veterans. J Int Neuropsychol Soc 16: 856-866.

48. Meares S1, Shores EA, Taylor AJ, Batchelor J, Bryant RA, et al. (2011) The prospective course of postconcussion syndrome: the role of mild traumatic brain injury. Neuropsychology 25: 454-465.

49. Ponsford J1, Cameron P, Fitzgerald M, Grant M, Mikocka-Walus A, et al. (2012) Predictors of postconcussive symptoms 3 months after mild traumatic brain injury. Neuropsychology 26: 304-313.

50. Wilk JE1, Thomas JL, McGurk DM, Riviere LA, Castro CA, et al. (2010) Mild traumatic brain injury (concussion) during combat: lack of association of blast mechanism with persistent postconcussive symptoms. J Head Trauma Rehabil 25: 9-14.

The Effects of a Self-Administered, Two-Session, Cognitive-Behavioral Intervention for Insomnia

Diana Maier[1], **Jonathan Savelle**[2], **Valerie Vidana**[3] **and Richard Shane**[4*]

[1]*Independent Researcher and Quality and Performance Improvement Consultant, Denver, United States*

[2]*Independent Researcher and Statistical Consultant, Cheyenne, United States*

[3]*Independent Researcher and Data Organization Specialist, Boulder, United States*

[4]*Founder and Manager, Sleep Easily LLC, Boulder, United States*

[*]**Corresponding author:** Richard Shane, Founder and Manager, Sleep Easily LLC, Boulder, United States, E-mail: drshane@sleepeasily.com

Abstract

Background: It is estimated that 1-in-3 (84M) adults in the US suffer from one or more symptoms of insomnia. This has a damaging effect on almost every area of life. Pharmacologic treatment carries dangers of addiction and side effects. Behavioral treatment is expensive and there are not enough therapists who offer such treatment. To meet this need, the present study explored the effectiveness of a two-session, self-administered cognitive-behavioral intervention.

Participants: Police personnel, firefighters, commercial airline pilots, veterans, patients of physicians and members of the general public.

Design: Data were collected on-line, with a within-subject, pre-post design.

Data source: Primary outcomes were the Insomnia Severity Index total score and two factor scores.

Data analysis: T-tests and chi-square/contingency statistics, as appropriate.

Results: The Baseline ISI was 13.8+/-4.1(range = 0-28). Factor scores: 5.2+/-1.8 (sleep continuity [SC]) and 8.5+/-3.1 (daytime effects [DE]). The Post treatment ISI was: 9.8+/-4.7 and factor scores were 3.7+/-2.1 (SC), and 6.1+/-3.0 (DE). Observed changes were significant ($p < 0.0001$) and had corresponding large effect sizes (Total ISI = 0.89, SC = 0.76, and daytime effects = 0.81). 40 of 49 participants (81.6%) had a Post-Treatment Summary Score that was lower (i.e., associated with improved sleep quality) than their Pre-treatment Summary Score.

On the post-treatment assessment, 71.4% reported their sleep began to improve within the first five nights. 65.3% reported the method was easy to use. 55.1% reported feeling better during the day and 36.7% reported reduced anxiety and/or stress during the day. 64% of subjects using sleep medications reported reduced dose or frequency of such substances.

Conclusions: The intervention produced significant change and large effects within a short time frame. Results suggest the Sleep Easily method may be ideal as a "first step" in a stepped care approach to the management of insomnia.

Future studies should assess this method within the context of a larger scale 1) controlled study and/or 2) dismantling study where the component parts of this method are assessed for their unique contribution to treatment outcome.

Keywords: Insomnia; Cognitive-behavioral Therapy; Stress; Anxiety; Depression; Trauma; Hypervigilance; Nonpharmacologic; Mind-body medicine

Introduction

Despite the evidence of the effectiveness of Cognitive-Behavioral Treatment for Insomnia (CBT- I) [1-21], most patients will not receive this form of treatment.

This is likely true for a variety of reasons including the ease and acceptability of pharmacotherapy and the lack of public awareness about CBT-I.

Additional considerations include the time commitment and cost involved, and the stigma of psychotherapy. Even if these factors were fully addressed, there would remain at least one profound barrier to treatment access: there are very few therapists who have been trained in, and provide, CBT-I.

Given these daunting considerations, it has been suggested that a stepped-care approach is required [22,23]; the first step of which might be a brief self-administered intervention.

The purpose of the present study was to explore the feasibility and effectiveness of a two-session, two-week, self-administered cognitive behavioral intervention referred to as "Sleep Easily" (hereinafter referred to as SE).

Method and Material

Overview

This study was designed as a within subject repeated measures design used in conjunction with the two session intervention that was self-administered over the course of two weeks.

Recruitment of subjects

The target sample for the study was people who reported difficulty falling or staying asleep, drawn from the following groups: Police personnel, firefighters, commercial airline pilots, and veterans, patients of physicians and members of the general public. No additional inclusionary or exclusionary criteria were applied. In order to acquire this sample, subjects were recruited from United Airlines, the Denver Police Department, the Boulder Fire Department, groups supporting veterans who have Post Traumatic Stress Disorder (PTSD), patients of physicians from the American College of Lifestyle Medicine (ACLM), and the general public.

1. Detailed information about the study was sent to the United Airlines Quality Control Manager, Denver Police Department Manager of Wellness Unit, Boulder Fire Department Fire Chief, the Director of American College of Lifestyle Medicine and the Director of Veterans Helping Veterans Now. These managers were asked to review the proposal and, if they approved, would they be willing to disseminate the information to staff and employees in their organizations.

2. The above directors and managers spoke with the Corresponding Author by phone or in person.

3. All of the above directors and managers approved of the study (the Denver Police Department manager submitted the study proposal to top chain of command and received approval) and circulated a request for participation email that disclosed the intent of the study, the study requirements, and stated that participation was purely voluntary and that all acquired information would be kept confidential.

To accurately reflect the population, no one was excluded from the study. Subjects were not paid for participating in the study.

Intervention and subject flow

Because the insomnia intervention is self-administered, there was no face-to-face or phone call contact with the participants. All interactions were through email or through the survey website.

Prospective study participants learned of the study through email received from the above-listed directors and managers. That announcement contained instructions that people interested in participating in the study should email their request to one of the independent investigators who emailed the participant a link to the on-line pre-treatment questionnaire conducted via Survey Monkey. Subjects requesting to participate were provided contact information for one of the independent investigators.

Participants filled out the online pre-treatment questionnaire.

Those who completed the survey were mailed a package containing a welcome to the study cover letter and study materials.

All participating subjects were mailed a package containing a booklet, two training CDs, two sleep CDs, two summary cards, and a set of specialized earplugs, and two summary cards. The booklet and training CDs provided the rationale for the elements and use of the method, plus basic instructions of the steps they should follow to use the method.

The booklet also provided instructions for 1) Sleep hygiene (habits and practices that are conducive to sleeping well on a regular basis) 2) Stimulus control (steps designed to associate the bed with sleeping and limit its association with stimulating behavior, i.e., go to bed only when tired, limit activities in bed to sleep and sex) and 3) Information to help people restructure dysfunctional thought patterns regarding sleep.

Sleep hygiene, stimulus control and cognitive restructuring were implemented through the participant reading and implementing the recommendations. The sleep CDs verbally guided the participant through the steps of the basic and advanced versions of the SE method. Earplugs were used to amplify the internal sound of sleep breathing, making it easier to hear. The summary cards enabled participants to use the method without the recording.

The self-administered intervention was structured to include two informational/training sessions and nightly use of stimulus control and the SE intervention. The SE component of the intervention was comprised of a sequence of steps that promotes an enhanced awareness of four body sensations (tongue, throat, heart and abdomen) and the breathing sound and sensation that seem to naturally occur during the transition from wake to sleep.

Awareness of these body sensations, in combination, is intended to create a subjective experience of safety that helps calm mind, emotions, and body and this is thought to help to transition the individual into sleep. The ear plugs were provided to help the individual hear the sound of the sleep breathing pattern.

The intervention was delivered over two informational/training session CDs that each involved approximately 45 minutes to review. The booklet of information about sleep hygiene, stimulus control and cognitive restructuring could be read in about one hour. The nightly use of the SE method-with or without the sleep CDs–was structured to take 20-30 minutes.

Ten days after participants received materials, they were emailed a reminder to fill out online post-treatment questionnaire #1. This first post treatment questionnaire was brief. It included a question asking if their sleep had improved at all and if so, when did they first notice that improvement (followed by multiple choice answers of 1st night, 2nd, etc.).

Many people using this sleep method (prior to this study) reported their sleep began to improve within the first few nights of use. Therefore, we sent this first post-treatment questionnaire early to capture that information while still fresh in memory. This sleep method does not ask people to use sleep diaries because over more than 20 years of working with insomnia patients, the developer of the method (and sponsor of the study) received feedback from many patients that sleep diaries made them more hypervigilant about their sleep, increasing their sleep difficulty.

Seven days after the first email reminder, any participants who did not fill out online post-treatment questionnaire #1, were sent a second reminder.

Three weeks after participants received their materials, they were emailed a reminder to fill out online post-treatment questionnaire #2. This time period was chosen because the method required two weeks to use and three weeks was deemed sufficient time to incorporate any delay in beginning to use the method.

Seven days after the reminder to fill out online post-treatment questionnaire #2, any participants who had not done so was sent a second reminder.

If they did not respond to that, the investigators decided that sending them a fourth email asking them why they had not responded to the previous three emails, could have annoyed the subjects, which would have skewed their reply and given us inaccurate information.

Data acquisition, analysis, and summary

This study was undertaken as contract between the developer of the SE method (and sponsor of the study) and three independent investigators who collected, analyzed, and summarized the data. No one associated with Sleep easily, Inc. interacted with the subjects or had access to the data acquisition or analysis.

All data were collected on-line via a web based survey that was comprised of several questionnaires including the ISI. Study subjects were assessed twice: once when joining the study and two weeks later. The analysis was conducted in two phases. The first phase of the analyses was descriptive.

The sample was characterized with regard to demographic variables. Categorical variables were summarized by frequencies, while continuous variables were summarized by the calculation of means, medians, standard deviations and ranges. The second phase of the analysis consisted of the analysis of continuous (e.g., ISI total score and "Factor" Scores) and categorical outcomes (e.g., response and remitter rates) by way of paired t-tests for pre-post means and chi-square/contingency statistics for percent and rate measures.

The initial treatment outcome report was written by the independent investigators. The present summary was written by the Senior Author in consultation with a specialist in Behavioral Sleep Medicine. The present summary was reviewed and approved by the three independent investigators.

Outcomes

The primary outcomes were assessed with the Insomnia Severity Index (ISI) (used with permission) [2]. The ISI has been validated in comparison with sleep diary and polysomnographic measurement and has been shown to be sensitive in measuring treatment response in patients. In the current study, the ISI was assessed in terms three scores: total score, and two factor scores. The first factor score was comprised of the first 3 items (sleep continuity disturbance) and the second factor score was comprised of the last 4 items (day time effects of insomnia). The ISI data were also used to type subjects in terms of response and remission.

Treatment outcome was assessed via pre and post-treatment replies to the ISI. Secondary outcomes were evaluated post hoc with single item questions from a brief end of study survey which included items regarding latency to response, ease of use re: the method, and change in medication use (Table 1).

Variable		Freq	%
Sex	M	29	59.18
	F	20	40.82
Age	20-30	3	6.12
	30-40	9	18.37
	40-50	17	34.69
	50-60	15	30.61
	60-70	4	8.16
	70-80	1	2.04

Table 1: Demographics of the study sample. Age and sex study sample.

Results

Subjects

Forty-nine of 73 subjects completed the study. Of the 67% subjects that completed the study, approximately 60% were male. Age was assessed categorically by decade: Approximately 90% of the samples were between the age of 20 and 60. Table 1 contains summary data regarding the demographics of the study cohort. Figure 1 provides the study consort data (Figure 1).

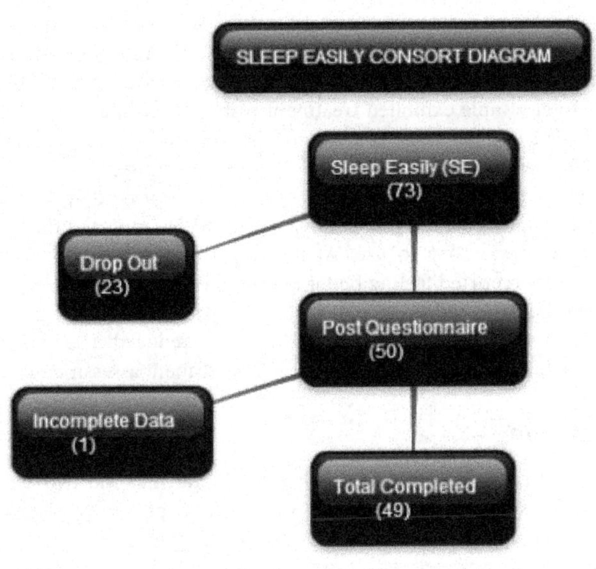

Figure 1: Sleep easily consort diagram.

Treatment outcome

As can be seen in Table 2 and Figure 2, the baseline score for the total ISI was 13.8+/-4.1 (range = 0-28) and the baseline scores for the factor scores were 5.2+/-1.8 (sleep continuity [range 0-12]) and 8.5+/-3.1 (daytime effects [range 0-16]). Following the Two Session two-week intervention, the post-treatment scores for the ISI were 9.8+/-4.7 (full scale score), 3.7+/-2.1 (sleep continuity factor), and 6.1+/-3.0 (daytime effects factor). The observed effects were significant ($p < 0.0001$ for all the pre-post comparisons) and had corresponding large effect sizes (total ISI = 0.89, sleep continuity = 0.76, and daytime effects = 0.81). The effects on sleep continuity factor and daytime effects were comparable (not significantly different) (Table 2 and Figure 2).

Variable	Pre Mean(SD)	Post Mean(SD)	Mean Change(SD)	Mean % Change (SD)	Cohen's d
ISI total score	13.76(4.11)	9.82(4.71)	3.94(3.84)	-28.64%	0.891
ISI factor 1	5.22(1.84)	3.73(2.09)	1.49(1.75)	-28.52%	0.757
ISI factor 2	8.53(3.05)	6.08(3.04)	6.08(3.04)	-28.71%	0.805

Table 2: Insomnia severity index scores measuring treatment outcome.

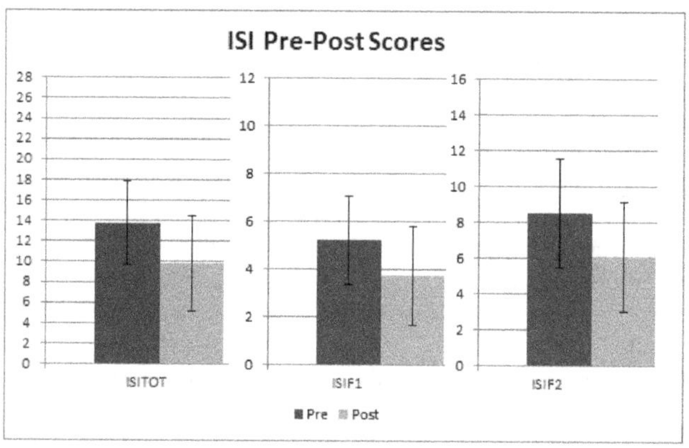

Figure 2: Insomnia severity index pre-post scores.

In terms of responder-remitter rates: 16% of the sample exhibited treatment responses, with the change in the total scale score of >8; 26% of the total sample exhibited treatment responses with a change in the total scale score of >50%; and 20% of the total sample met criteria for remission, with total scale scores of <7. These outcomes were not found to vary by sex or age. 71.4% of the completers reported that their sleep began to improve within the first five nights, 65.3% reported that use of the method was easy to use. After using the SE method, 55.1% of participants reported feeling better during the day and 36.7% reported reduced anxiety and/or stress during the day. Finally, 64% of the subjects using sleep medications reported reduced use (dose or frequency) of such substances on the post treatment assessment.

Discussion

The present study provides preliminary data that the two-session, two-week, self-administered SE intervention produces significant outcomes for people with insomnia. While the average outcome is less than might be expected with 8-week in person CBT-I (e.g., responder rates from 70-80% and remission rates at approximately 40%), this may be due to the modest level of initial severity of the study sample, the brevity and simplicity of the intervention, and/or the effects of ongoing occupational stress.

The rate of attrition observed in the present study is higher than clinical trials with CBT-I (10-20%)e.g., [24] and is on par with both self- help programs e.g., [25] and what occurs in clinical practice e.g., [26].

It would be erroneous to assume that failure to complete the study correlated to the subjects' results of using the method. Some of the reasons for not completing the study may have been logistical, such as not enough time, failure of the equipment needed to play the sleep audio recordings, or a work or life crisis that overpowered their willingness to continue with an optional project such as this study.

This said, the intervention produced significant change (and large effects) within a short time frame and did so in the context of a brief self- administered intervention.

The only risk for the SE component of the intervention is related to those that may have an adverse or paradoxical reaction to the induction of relaxation. Generally, this occurs more frequently in individuals with schizophrenia, PTSD, and/or survivors of sexual assault. Whether these, and other Axis 1 or medical disorders, constitute true contraindications remains to be determined.

Results from this study suggest that the SE method may indeed be ideal as a "first step" in a stepped care approach to the management of chronic insomnia. Future studies should be conducted in larger samples under controlled conditions and/or focus on the relative contributions of Stimulus Control, Sleep Hygiene, and the specific components of the SE method, to treatment outcome and the durability of the treatment.

Acknowledgement

Funding was provided by Sleep Easily, Inc. No one associated with Sleep Easily, Inc. interacted with the subjects or had access to the data acquisition or analysis.

References

1. National Sleep Foundation (2014) Sleep Health Index.
2. Morin CM, Belleville G, Bélanger L, Ivers H (2011) The Insomnia Severity Index: psychometric indicators to detect insomnia cases and evaluate treatment response. Sleep 34: 601-608.

3. Okajima I, Komada Y, Inoue D (2011) A meta-analysis on the treatment effectiveness of cognitive behavioral therapy for primary insomnia. Sleep and Biological Rhythms 9: 24-34.
4. Murtagh DR, Greenwood KM (1995) Identifying effective psychological treatments for insomnia: a meta-analysis. J Consult Clin Psychol 63: 79-89.
5. Irwin MR, Cole JC, Nicassio PM (2006) Comparative meta-analysis of behavioral interventions for insomnia and their efficacy in middle-aged adults and in older adults 55+ years of age. Health Psychol 25: 3-14.
6. Morin CM, Culbert JP, Schwartz SM (1994) Nonpharmacological interventions for insomnia: a meta-analysis of treatment efficacy. Am J Psychiatry 151: 1172-1180.
7. Mitchell MD, Gehrman P, Perlis M, Umscheid CA (2012) Comparative effectiveness of cognitive behavioral therapy for insomnia: a systematic review. BMC Fam Pract 13: 40.
8. McClusky HY, Milby JB, Switzer PK, Williams V, Wooten V (1991) Efficacy of behavioral versus triazolam treatment in persistent sleep-onset insomnia. Am J Psychiatry 148: 121-126.
9. Jacobs GD, Pace-Schott EF, Stickgold R, Otto MW (2004) Cognitive behavior therapy and pharmacotherapy for insomnia: a randomized controlled trial and direct comparison. Arch Intern Med 164: 1888-1896.
10. Smith MT, Perlis ML, Park A, Smith MS, Pennington J, et al. (2002) Comparative meta-analysis of pharmacotherapy and behavior therapy for persistent insomnia. Am J Psychiatry 159: 5-11.
11. Morin CM, Colecchi C, Stone J, Sood R, Brink D (1999) Behavioral and pharmacological therapies for late-life insomnia: a randomized controlled trial. JAMA 281: 991-999.
12. Sivertsen B, Omvik S, Pallesen S, Bjorvatn B, Havik OE, et al. (2006) Cognitive behavioral therapy vs zopiclone for treatment of chronic primary insomnia in older adults: a randomized controlled trial. JAMA 295: 2851-2858.
13. Lichstein KL, Wilson NM, Johnson CT (2000) Psychological treatment of secondary insomnia. Psychol Aging 15: 232-240.
14. Edinger JD, Wohlgemuth WK, Krystal AD, Rice JR (2005) Behavioral insomnia therapy for fibromyalgia patients: a randomized clinical trial. Arch Intern Med 165: 2527-2535.
15. Currie SR, Wilson KG, Pontefract AJ, deLaplante L (2000) Cognitive-behavioral treatment of insomnia secondary to chronic pain. J Consult Clin Psychol 68: 407-416.
16. Perlis M, Aloia M, Millikan A, Boehmler J, Smith M, et al. (2000) Behavioral treatment of insomnia: a clinical case series study. J Behav Med 23: 149-161.
17. Jungquist CR, O'Brien C, Matteson-Rusby S, Smith MT, Pigeon WR, et al. (2010) The efficacy of cognitive-behavioral therapy for insomnia in patients with chronic pain. Sleep Med 11: 302-309.
18. Smith MT, Huang MI, Manber R (2005) Cognitive behavior therapy for chronic insomnia occurring within the context of medical and psychiatric disorders. Clin Psychol Rev 25: 559-592.
19. Edinger JD, Olsen MK, Stechuchak KM, Means MK, Margaret D, et al. (2009) Cognitive behavioral therapy for patients with primary insomnia or insomnia associated predominantly with mixed psychiatric disorders: a randomized clinical trial. Sleep 32: 499-510.
20. Savard J, Simard S, Ivers H, Morin CM (2005) Randomized study on the efficacy of cognitive-behavioral therapy for insomnia secondary to breast cancer, part I: Sleep and psychological effects. J Clin Oncol 23: 6083-6096.
21. Perlis ML, Sharpe M, Smith MT, Greenblatt D, Giles D (2001) Behavioral treatment of insomnia: treatment outcome and the relevance of medical and psychiatric morbidity. J Behav Med 24: 281-296.
22. Edinger JD (2009) Is it time to step up to stepped care with our cognitive-behavioral insomnia therapies? Sleep 32: 1539-1541.
23. Espie CA (2009) "Stepped care": a health technology solution for delivering cognitive behavioral therapy as a first line insomnia treatment. Sleep 32: 1549-1558.
24. Morin CM, Vallières A, Guay B, Ivers H, Savard J, et al. (2009) Cognitive behavioral therapy, singly and combined with medication, for persistent insomnia: a randomized controlled trial. JAMA 301: 2005-2015.
25. Ho FY (2014) Weekly brief phone support in self-help cognitive behavioral therapy for insomnia disorder: Relevance to adherence and efficacy. Behav Res Ther 63: 147-156.
26. Morin CM, Benca R (2012) Chronic insomnia. Lancet 379: 1129-1141.

Tourette Syndrome and Non-Coeliac Gluten Sensitivity: Clinical Remission with a Gluten-Free Diet

Rodrigo L[1*], Huerta M[2] and Salas-Puig J[3]

[1]*Gastroenterology Service, Central University Hospital of Asturias (HUCA). Avda. Hospital Universitario, s/n. 33011, Oviedo, Principality of Asturias, Spain*

[2]*Psychiatry Service, Health Mental Center I. Pedro Pablo 42, 33209, Gijon, Principality of Asturias, Spain*

[3]*Neurology Service, Hospital Universitario Central de Asturias (HUCA), c/Celestino Villamil, s. n°, 33006, Oviedo, Spain*

[*]**Corresponding author:** Luis Rodrigo, PhD. Gastroenterology Service, Central University Hospital of Asturias (HUCA). Avda. Hospital Universitario, s/n. 33011. Oviedo, Principality of Asturias, Spain, E-mail: lrodrigosaez@gmail.com

Abstract

Background: Tourette syndrome (TS) is a primary tic disorder, that reaches most commonly medical attention and monitoring, Its etiology remains unknow and there are scant information about the role of associated food intolerance to its presence.

Methods: We analyze the case of a 13 y.o. female, with a long history of 10 years of tics and obsessive-compulsive disorder. She had a family history positive for celiac disease and we studied for her presence, determining serological markers (anti -tissue transglutaminase-2 (tTG), genetic markers of susceptibility (HLA-DQ2 and DQ8) and duodenal biopsies looking for the presence of villous atrophy and or lymphocytic enteritis. IgE specific to wheat, was also done.

Results: The tTG was negative; HLA-DQ8 was positive and there was a moderate lymphocytic enteritis. IgE RAST test for wheat, was also negative. She was diagnosed of non-celiac gluten sensitivity (NCGS) and a gluten-free diet (GFD) was started. A great clinical improvement was observed in few months and after 2.5 years she remains well and completely asymtomatic of her neuro-psychiatric ailments.

Conclusions: This clinical observation opens a new possibility of the existence a causal relationship between the presence of a TS in children with NCGS and by consequence the convenience to start a GFD in these patients. New studies will be needed in order to support this observation.

Keywords: Tourette syndrome; Non-celiac gluten sensitivity; Clinical remission; Gluten-free diet

Introduction

Tourette syndrome (TS) is a primary neurological disorder of unclear origin. It is clinically characterised by the presence of multiple motor and phonic tics that begin in infancy, and which have a duration or more than 1 year. These are associated in most cases with the presence of other problems such as attention deficit hyperactivity disorder (ADHD), obsessive-compulsive disorder (OCD) and other neuropsychiatric disorders.

There are many pharmacological and behavioural treatments that help control the episodes of crisis and the course of the illness but are unable to make them disappear.

We present the case of a young woman with non-coeliac gluten sensitivity (NCGS) who showed an excellent response and clinical remission of neurological and behavioural symptomatology after the establishment of a gluten-free diet (GFD).

Description of the Clinical Case

A 13-year-old female, an only daughter, who had a normal birth after a full-term pregnancy. Both parents are coeliacs.

From the first months of her life, she presented with frequent abdominal pain episodes (infant colic), accompanied by prominent abdominal swelling and accentuated constipation. The digestive symptoms were very intense as a baby, becoming less intense and frequent with age.

They were accompanied by episodes of recurrent dermatitis that had manifested themselves practically since birth, and which were made more acute not only by the application of creams and by contact with metals, but also by environmental heat and exposure to the sun. We consider the possibility of an allergy to nickel and effectively it was confirmed, because the contact patch test was positive. She had suffered from bruxism and restless leg syndrome since infancy.

She presented recurrent episodes of rhinitis and pharyngitis, in conjunction with multiple cutaneous allergic problems, and recurrent outbreaks of urticaria jointly with generalised and highly pruritic processes of atopic dermatitis. She also frequently suffered from headaches, paraesthesias of the legs and low-back pain.

At the age of 3 years, the first episodes of facial tics, especially those involving the eyelids and lips, appeared. The evolution was progressive over time, consisting of simple and more complex motor tics and also phonic tics. The facial tics consisted fundamentally of winks, progressing to include a wide range of gestures, such as tongue movements, puffing and sucking. These were accompanied by cervical tics (rotation and inclination), arm extension and flexion, simultaneously or in different directions, in combination with leaps, flexion and rotation of the trunk, flexion and hyperextension of the fingers, frequent blowing on the hands, etc.

The phonic tics were varied, presenting as guttural sounds, whistles, puffing, throat-clearing, sniffing, and occasional mild stammering. Her sleep was frequently disrupted, with isolated episodes of night terrors, accompanied by considerable distress and anxiety.

The patient's clinical symptomatology had the characteristic pattern of TS, with periods of deterioration mixed with others of mild remission, presenting itself with a varying extent of affectation. She did not have any asymptomatic periods, although she did experience phases of spontaneous remission, during which the tics were less intense or less frequent.

Throughout these years she attended numerous consultations with a wide range of specialists, but failed to receive an accurate diagnosis or, consequently a treatment, that adequately controlled her symptoms.

At age 7 years, she began to present an associated obsessive compulsive disorder (OCD), with an acute bout of obsessive cleanliness, and was then diagnosed for the first time with Tourette syndrome. She was treated with Sertraline (an anti-depressive SSRI) for ten months, but this was poorly tolerated, producing considerable increase in motor activation. In parallel, she had a consultation with a child psychologist, who prescribed ERP (exposure and response prevention) treatment, which was monitored by her and carried out daily by her parents. By this means, remission of the acute pattern was achieved.

At age 9 years, she suffered an acute and very serious flare-up of OCD that required intensive treatment with Risperidone and Clorazepate dipotassium for eight months. This was characterised by the presence of a wide range of obsessions, which interfered notably with the habitual activities of her daily life. The patient's mood was severely affected, giving rise to depressive ideas and isolated suicidal thoughts.

From the first year of her life, her digestion was slow and heavy, accompanied by fluctuating abdominal swelling with a considerable amount of gas. She experienced frequent, significant and uncomfortable epigastric pains with associated reflux. Her intestinal habit was generally normal, with a tendency towards diarrhoea and predominantly soft stools.

At the age of 11 years, studies were done that ruled out an associated coeliac disease (CD), wherein the anti-gliadin antibodies were positive, the anti-transglutaminase tissue antibodies were negative and the genetic markers of susceptibility had the HLA-DQ8 (+). Duodenal biopsies were taken that showed an absence of villous atrophy, along with a 25% increase in intraepithelial lymphocytic infiltrate, compatible with Marsh stage 1. Specific IgE RAST tests, for wheat, gluten and corn, were all negative.

On the basis of all these findings, with the association of a celiac serology negative, with the finding of normal or near normal duodenal biopies with raised intraepithelial lymphocytes and negative IgE serology to wheat, she was diagnosed of Non-Celiac Guten Sensitivity (NCGS) according with the admitted criteria for this entity and placed on a gluten-free diet (GFD). One week after the beginning of this diet, the tics diminished notably and the OCD progressively disappeared. Within a few months, the tics had entirely stopped and the OCD had almost completely disappeared.

Now 13 years old, and after 2.5 years on the diet, the patient is in complete remission from the tics. Since starting the diet she has had occasional flares of the tics and of OCD, but with a clearly lessening tendency and coinciding with involuntary transgressions with gluten or periods of exhaustion or illness.

Currently, several months have passed since the occurrence of any exacerbation. The patient is completely asymptomatic and does not need to take any medication. The flares of atopic dermatitis, which were very acute since birth, have progressively attenuated, to the point where they have now completely disappeared.

In the analytical findings we didn´t found anemia at any moment, and the serum levels of iron, ferritin, folic acid and vitamin B-12 remained always inside normal range. By contrary, we found maintained low serum levels of 25-hidroxi-vit. D during all the study period, despite good exposure to sunlight and performing frequent physical exercise. So, we prescribed oral supplements of vit D, since one year. Anti-gliadin and anti-nuclear antiboides were both positive at a low titer (Table 1)

Parameters	Basal	After 1 year of the onset of a GFD	After 2.5 years of the onset of a GFD
Hemoglobin (g/dl) N= (12-14)	13.7	12.8	12.7
Serum iron (mcg/dl) N= (50-80)	96	24	85
Ferritin levels (ng/ml) N=(10-120)	12.6	34.8	20.3
Folic acid (ng/ml) N> 2.5	9.5	11.0	12.0
25-Hidroxi-Vit. D (ng/ml) N=(30-74)	10.3	11.0	12.8
AGA (IgA) IU/l N= (0-20)	52	24	10
ANA titer IU/l N=(0-1/20)	1/160	1/80	1/80

Table 1: Analytical findings at diagnosis and in the follow-up period after the onset of a GFD (AGA=Antigliadin antibodies; ANA=Antinuclear antibodies).

She has exhibited a maize intolerance for a year, leading to this having to be excluded from her diet. The occasional transgressions with gluten are accompanied by a reactivation of the tics and the OCD, but these are alleviated by the administration of a complex of vitamins B1-B6-B12 for several weeks. Her behaviour is better when she is asymptomatic: her ability to concentrate on her studies and her scholastic performance have improved.

Discussion

Tourette Syndrome (TS) is named after its discoverer, the French neurologist Georges Gilles de la Tourette, who described a series of nine cases with involuntary repetitive reflexes in 1885. TS is a disorder characterised by the presence of recurrent motor and vocal tics, frequently accompanied by various neuropsychiatric disorders. It presents a prolonged clinical course, usually beginning in infancy or childhood, and occurs predominantly in males (3-4 males/1 female)[1].

The failure of the monogenic and multigenic hypotheses to explain the development and transmission of TS has led us to consider the possible influence of a range of environmental factors on its appearance [2].

TS has a prevalence of approximately 1% worldwide, and a study of a large series of children with this syndrome revealed it to be associated with neuropsychiatric disorders in about 90% of them, of which OCD was the most frequent (53%), followed by ADHD (38%) [3].

Clinical diversity and comorbidity are important traits for recognising this process and for planning the most appropriate treatment. Its heterogeneity explains the wide range of aetiological and pathogenic hypotheses generated, including those of an autoimmune nature [4].

A frequent association of various allergic processes with the respiratory system and skin, and a higher frequency of migraines than in the general population have been described [5].

Non-coeliac gluten sensitivity (NCGS) was first described in 1978 on the basis of two isolated clinical cases. The first series of patients with normal duodenal biopsies and gastrointestinal symptoms that disappeared with a gluten-free diet (GFD) was published in 1980 [6].

The diagnostic criteria consist of the appearance of a series of digestive and extra-intestinal symptoms that improve characteristically with a GFD, with habitually negative serology for coeliac disease (CD) (anti-transglutaminase antibodies), with anti-gliadin (+) in 50% of the cases, normal duodenal biopsies or with a moderate increase in intraepithelial lymphocytes and an HLA-DQ2 and/or HLA-DQ8 (+) haplotype in 40% of patients [7].

Currently, the most popular pathogenic hypothesis is that, unlike in CD, in which there is an activation of the adaptive immune response, in NCGS there is only an innate immune response to the injurious agent, through the increased production of IL-15 in the intestinal mucosa, which starts the inflammatory process, spreading it systemically [8].

Although the presence of neurological manifestations in patients with established CD was first described in 1966 it was not until thirty years later that the association of such conditions, such as cerebellar ataxia, with gluten sensitivity in some individuals was confirmed. The existence of extraintestinal manifestations without associated enteropathy is a more recent finding.

The list of neurological processes associated with gluten sensitivity is very long and varied, including repeating headaches, ataxias, polyneuritis, epilepsies and multiple neuroses. Just like the one described here, many of the cases improve notably with the instigation of a GFD [9]. However, it should be pointed out that, to date, we have found no published evidence of its association with TS.

Recent studies support the existence of this new condition, named NCGS, which manifests as intestinal or extraintestinal symptoms that improve or disappear after gluten withdrawal in individuals with normal small-bowel mucosa and negative results on serum antitransglutaminase and antiendomysial antibody testing. Although the clinical value of this concept is under debate, the prevalence of NCGS in the general populationis supposed to be many times higher than that of celiac disease (CD). The lack of an unambiguous definition of NCGS, a major pitfall, is primarily related to the heterogeneous cause of this condition, whose symptoms are presumed to be caused by different mechanisms. If NCGS is an etiologically heterogeneous syndrome, then management options should vary according to the predominant or concomitant underlying pathogenic pathways.

Although challenged with gluten is recommended to confirm the diagnosis, we do not realize it for ethical reasons. However, we appreciate ST clinical relapses related to small and sporadic dietary transgressions unnoticed. So, in these cases a strict GFD is considered mandatory.

The response to the GFD in NCGS is slow and steady, as is the recovery from the intestinal inflammation, which, on average, requires some two years on a strict and continuous GFD. It may be accompanied by other associated dietary intolerances, such as those of lactose, fructose, sorbitol and maize. Dietary transgressions produce relapses not only of digestion but also of the symptoms stemming from TS.

There are doubts about the utility of carrying out screening for gluten intolerance in the general population, but its study is nevertheless recommended in the known risk groups, among which are first-degree relatives. However, the early detection of NCGS is less indicated, because although it is 5-10 times more frequent than CD, its diagnostic criteria are more difficult to establish. Even so, in the face of the persistence of related symptoms, its utility is beyond doubt [10], as we see equally in the case we present here.

References

1. Robertson MM (2012) The Gilles de la Tourette syndrome: the current status. Arch Dis Child Educ Pract Ed 97: 166-175.
2. Deng H, Gao K, Jankovic J (2012) The genetics of Tourette syndrome. Nat Rev Neurol 8: 203-213.
3. Lebowitz ER, Motlagh MG, Katsovich L, King RA, Lombroso PJ, et al. (2012) Tourette syndrome in youth with and without obsessive compulsive disorder and attention deficit hyperactivity disorder. Eur Child Adolesc Psychiatry 21: 451-457.
4. Rotge JY, Aouizerate B, Tignol J, Bioulac B, Burbaud P, et al. (2010) The glutamate-based genetic immune hypothesis in obsessive-compulsive disorder. An integrative approach from genes to symptoms. Neuroscience 165: 408-417.
5. Ghosh D, Rajan PV, Das D, Datta P, Rothner AD, et al. (2012) Headache in children with Tourette syndrome. J Pediatr 161: 303-307.
6. Cooper BT, Holmes GK, Ferguson R, Thompson RA, Allan RN, et al. (1980) Gluten-sensitive diarrhea without evidence of celiac disease. Gastroenterology 79: 801-806.
7. Volta U, De Giorgio R (2012) New understanding of gluten sensitivity. Nat Rev Gastroenterol Hepatol 9: 295-299.
8. Bernardo D, Garrote JA, Arranz E (2011) Are non-celiac disease gluten-intolerant patients innate immunity responders to gluten? Am J Gastroenterol 106: 2201.

Use of Polysomnography and Onabotulinum Toxin Type A (BOTOX®) in the Treatment of Nocturnal (Sleep Related) Bruxism with Associated Craniofacial Pain

Deborah Syna*

Northwest Neurological Specialists PC, Portland, Oregon, USA

***Corresponding author**: Deborah Syna, Northwest Neurological Specialists PC, Portland, Oregon, USA, E-mail: dsyna@comcast.net

Abstract

Objective: Nocturnal bruxism, the repetitive grinding, clenching, and chewing movements of the jaw during sleep, can occur in both children and adults. Case series and anecdotal reports suggest that botulinum toxin type A injection may provide effective treatment of nocturnal bruxism and its sequelae. Open-label trials for patients with nocturnal bruxism indicate that it may confer reduction in pain medication use and migraine headache frequency. This study is an open label, pilot study to establish 'proof of principle' for the use of Onabotulinum toxin A (BOTOX, Allergan) to treat nocturnal bruxism with associated craniofacial pain.

Methods: Five consenting subjects with nocturnal bruxism and craniofacial pain who have tried dental prosthetics, and have failed trials of at least two prophylactic headache medications were enrolled. Four completed the trial. No serious adverse events were experienced by any subject. The primary outcome measure of this study was the change in number of EMG bursts in the temporalis and masseter muscles as measured during nocturnal polysomnography in an accredited sleep laboratory. Polysomnograms were administered once for baseline measurement and at weeks 4, and 8 after injection of 100-150 U of Onabotulinum Toxin A (BOTOX, Allergan) in a fixed site pattern including temporalis and masseter muscles.

Results: Average number of bruxism events decreased through Week 4 after treatment. One of four participants' polysomnograph showed consistent decrease inbruxism events in the weeks following treatment but overall the trends did not reach statistical significance. Secondary outcome measures which demonstrated a trend for improvement included bed partner survey of bruxing activity and sleep interruption, and daily subject craniofacial pain diary. MIDAS scores showed statistical improvement at week 4 after injection. Sleep efficiency and percent rapid eye movement (REM) sleep on polysomnograms demonstrated a trend towards improvement after injection but did not reach statistical significance.

Keywords: Nocturnal bruxism; Sleep bruxism; Migraine; Facial pain; Botulinum toxin; Polysomnography; Oromandibular dystonia; Sleep efficiency; Headache; Parasomnia

Introduction

Case series and anecdotal reports suggest that onabotulinum toxin type A (BOTOX, Allergan) injection may provide effective treatment of nocturnal bruxism and its sequelae. Open-label and placebo controlled trials for patients with nocturnal bruxism indicate that it may reduce bruxing frequency, [1] pain medication use and migraine headache frequency [2].

Bruxism is associated with headaches and migraine [3,4]. Onabotulinum toxin type A has been shown to be safe and effective in the treatment of headache syndromes such as migraine [5,6] and chronic cervical-associated headache [7,8].

Onabotulinum toxin type A (BTX A) has been used to treat a variety of movement disorders including segmental dystonias and oromandibular dystonias, spasticity, muscle spasm, cervical sprain, TMJ syndromes, and bruxism related to a variety of acquired and congenital conditions [9]. Onabotulinum toxin type A is currently FDA approved in the United States for use in intractable migraine, chronic daily headache, and segmental dystonia such as cervical dystonia, but remains "off label" in the treatment of Bruxism.

This pilot study is a "proof of principle trial" using polysomnography to explore the potential of onabotulinum toxin type A in the treatment of sleep related bruxism and associated craniofacial pain and headache.

Background

Bruxism, the repetitive grinding, clenching, and chewing movements of the jaw, can occur as a "parafunctional" (uncommon activity of a specific body part, in this case the jaw) nocturnal behavior in normal children and adults, or as diurnal behavior in those with oromandibular dystonia [10], developmental disorders [11], and traumatic brain injury [12]. Some have postulated a pathophysiological relationship to cranial-cervical dystonia [13,14]. Sleep bruxism can be associated with craniofacial pain, headache, symptoms of temporomandibular joint dysfunction (TMJ), tooth wear, and cosmetically unsightly masseter hypertrophy [15-18].

Methods

This is an open label uncontrolled pilot trial. The protocol was approved by the Western Institutional Review Board. Enrollment in the trial occurred after written informed consent performed by a board certified neurologist. Onabotulinum toxin injections were performed by a board certified neurologist.

Participants

The five study participants ranged from 47 to 72 years of age. Four of the five patients (80%) were female. Participation required: completed minimal criteria for Sleep Bruxism questionnaire and had associated craniofacial pain, score greater than 5 on the Numerical Rating Scale of Pain (NRS), previous trials of dental prosthetics, and prior failed trials of at least two prophylactic headache medications, and stable pharmacological treatment of craniofacial pain, headache and bruxism for one month prior to injection.

Study design

Subjects were enrolled, and prophylactic medications held constant during the first four, pre-treatment, weeks. The primary outcome measure was the change in number of tonic and phasic EMG bursts/hour in the temporalis and masseter muscles as measured during nocturnal polysomnography in an accredited sleep laboratory at baseline pre-injection, and at 4, and 8 weeks after onabotulinum toxin type A injection.

Study interpretations were performed by a neurologist board certified in both neurology and sleep medicine. Participant enrollment and Injections were performed by the principle investigator, a board certified neurologist. The Secondary outcome measures include: daily craniofacial pain diary and daily bed partner self-reports of bruxing activity and sleep interruption, Headache Impact Test (HIT-6), Migraine Disability Assessment Scores (MIDAS), Beck Depression Inventory (BDI-II) at baseline, immediately prior to injection, and four, eight and twelve weeks after injection, and recorded use of prescription pharmaceuticals for prophylaxis and aborting headache, emergency department and urgent care visits.

Treatment procedure

Participants received 100-150 units of onabotulinum toxin type A (10 U/0.1mL, preservative-free, normal saline). Injections were given on day zero (immediately following the 30 day screening period). A fixed-site, bilateral, headache injection paradigm was expanded to include muscles of mastication and was used in the following muscles:

Masseter (bilateral, 10 units each)

Temporalis Superior (bilateral, 10 units each)

Temporalis Inferior (bilateral, 10 units each)

Levator Scapulae (bilateral, 0-20 units each)

Splenius capitus (bilateral, 0- 20 units each)

Frontalis (bilateral, 5 units each)

Procerus muscle (5 units)

Glabellar (bilateral, 2.5-5 units each

Statistical methods

Two-tailed student T-test analyses were performed to compare pre- and post-intervention data. For specific outcomes in which multiple pre-treatment data points were available for each participant (i.e. in which daily assessments were obtained in the 30 days prior to treatment), two-tailed T-tests were performed using the individual's pre-intervention data as baseline for comparison with post-intervention outcomes.

Five subjects (N=5) were involved in the study. Data points for certain outcome measures were not available, because a participant was lost to follow-up or because the participant or his or her bed partner did not self-administer a qualitative assessment.

Results

Of the five subjects enrolled, four were available for assessment of primary outcome after injection. Two participants did not complete self-assessments for secondary outcome measures; bed-partners of three participants provided incomplete reports of audible bruxing and sleep disruption.

Primary outcome measure

The average number of EMG bursts/hour in the temporalis and masseter muscles demonstrated a decreasing trend at Week 4 post injection (mean of 34 events/night to mean 30.4 events). The changes were not statistically significant (p>0.05, n=5) (Figure 1).

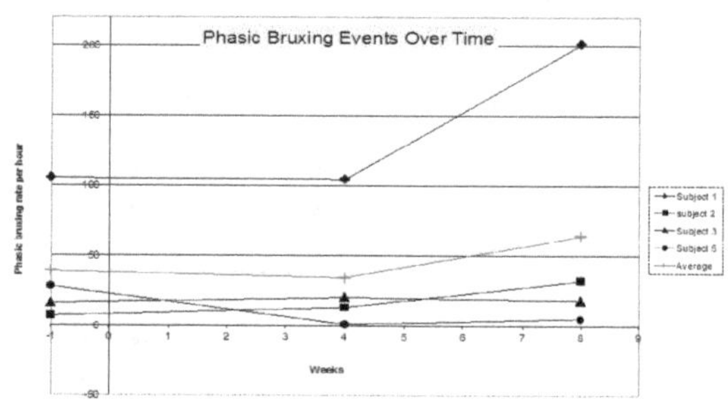

Figure 1: Average number of EMG bursts/HR in the temporalis and masseter muscles during polysomnography demonstrated a decreasing trend at Week 4 post injection (mean of 34 events/night to mean 30.4 events). The changes were not statistically significant (p>0.05, n=5).

Secondary outcome measures

Craniofacial pain: Subjects recorded craniofacial pain using a daily diary of 0 (no pain) to 3 (most severe pain). On average, craniofacial pain decreased during the first eight weeks following injection, from a mean rating of 2.25 to 1.5 over the course of eight weeks, though the change was not shown to be statistical significant (n=4, p>0.05) (Figure 2).

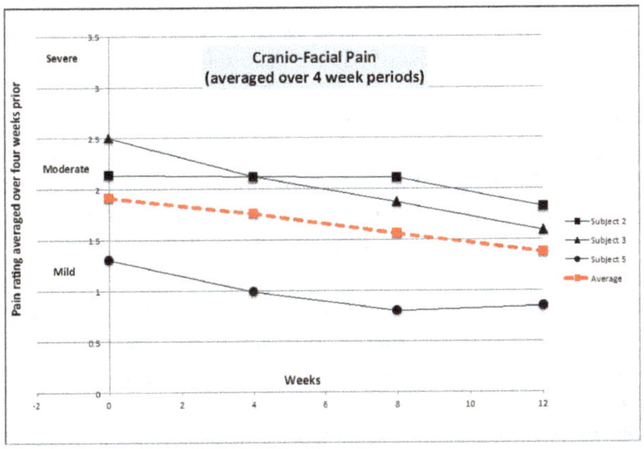

Figure 2: Averaged recorded cranial-facial pain using a daily diary of 0 (no pain) to 3 (most severe pain), over 4 week periods.

Jaw movements and sleep interruptions: Bed partners kept a daily self-reported diary of audible bruxing, and sleep interruption during the study. Per bed partner reports, four of the participants had detectable bruxism events six to seven times per night. Two partners completed the diaries. Both noted audible bruxing, and both noted a decline in these events prior to and after injection.

The average of both reported number of jaw movements and sleep interruptions decreased over the course of eight weeks following treatment. Average jaw movements decreased from 0.83 on Day 0 (averaged over the 30 days prior to treatment) to 0.69 at Week 8 (averaged over the 30 days prior to and including the first day of Week 8). While both subjects showed a decrease in this measure, the average change was not statistically significant (n=2, p>0.05).

Both subjects also experienced a decline in sleep interruptions. The average decreased from 1.7 interruptions per night to 1.3. For subject number 1, the decrease in interruptions between treatment and Week 4 was found to be statistically significant (p=0.035); for subject number 2, the decline in interruptions between Week 4 and Week 8 was found to be statistically significant (p=0.015) (Figure 3).

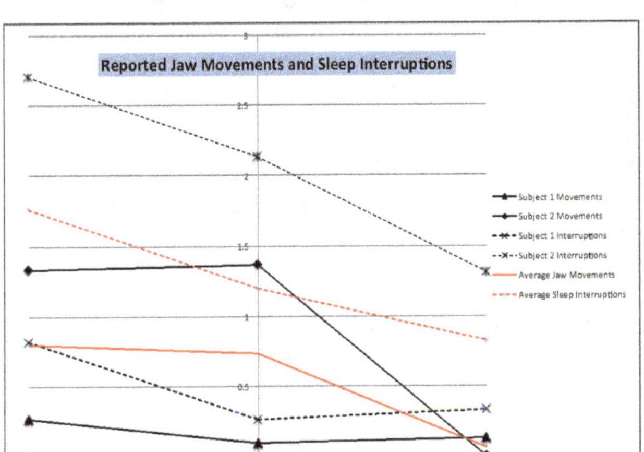

Figure 3: Reports of audible bruxing, and sleep interruption per night, averaged over four week period.

Percent rapid eye movement (REM) sleep increased from an average of 14.2% to 16.6% in the four weeks following treatment, approaching 20%, the expected percent REM sleep in the general population. The change in the participant population, however, did not reach statistical significance (n=4, p>0.05).

Average sleep efficiency increased from 0.76 to 0.81 during the first four weeks after treatment, remaining stable at 0.81 over the next four weeks (Figure 4). The change is not statistically significant but indicates a trend that warrants further study.

These changes may indicate a possible treatment effect, or may be related to first-night effect in the sleep laboratory.

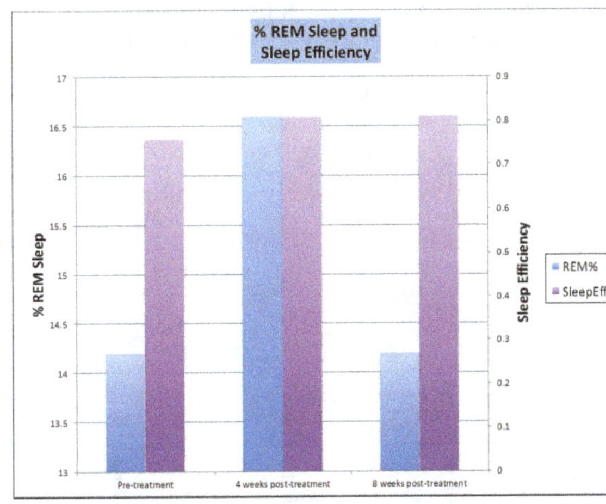

Figure 4: Percent REM sleep increased from an average of 14.2% to 16.6% in the four weeks following treatment. Average sleep efficiency increased from 0.76 to 0.81 during the first four weeks after treatment, remaining stable at 0.81 over the next four weeks. The change is not statistically significant.

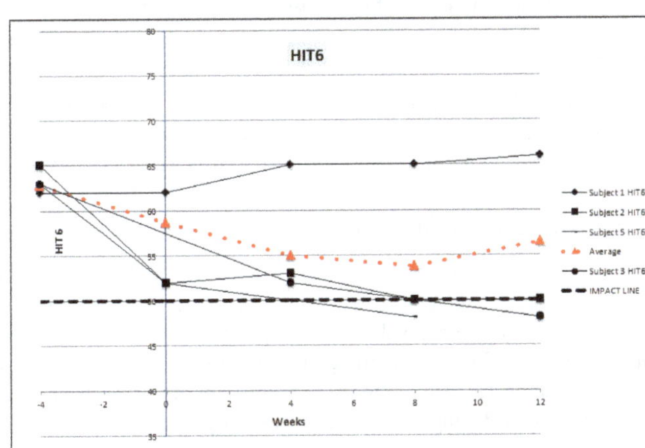

Figure 5: The average HIT-6 score fell after treatment, dropping to 53 points by Week 8; these findings did not reach statistical significance (n=4, p>0.05 for each four week interval).

Headaches and migraine: HIT-6 scores quantify the disability subjects experienced as the result of headaches. Scores were taken at four-week intervals beginning during the pre-treatment phase. Four subjects self-administered the Headache Impact Test (HIT-6) immediately prior to treatment and at four-week intervals thereafter. The average HIT-6 score fell after treatment, dropping to 53 points by Week 8; these findings did not reach statistical significance (n=4, p>0.05 for each four week interval) (Figure 5).

Migraine Disability Assessment Scores range from 0 (no headache-related disability) to 21 and beyond (severe headache-related disability) were obtained for four subjects prior to and following injection at 4 week intervals. While there was notable variability among participants, the average score was 37.5 at Day 0 (prior to treatment) and dropped below 21 to 15.75 by the fourth week. This finding is statistically significant (n=4, p<0.036). Scores remain below 20 for the remainder of the study (n=4, p>0.05) (Figure 6).

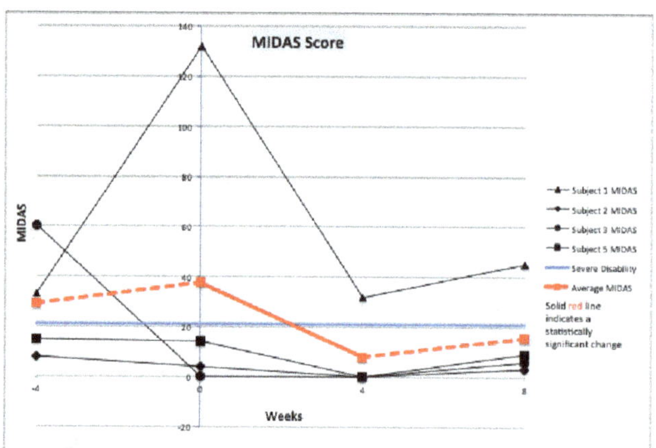

Figure 6: MIDAS average score obtained for four subjects prior to and following injection at 4 week intervals was 37.5 at Day 0 (prior to treatment) and dropped below 21 to 15.75 by the fourth week. This finding is statistically significant (n=4, p<0.036). Scores remain below 20 for the remainder of the study (n=4, p>0.05).

While use of headache prophylaxis did not change following treatment, medications used to abort headaches showed a decline shortly after treatment, followed by a return to pre-treatment levels.

Other secondary outcome measures

The Beck's Depression Inventory II (BDI-II) BID-II scores were obtained during the screening period, on Day 0 (pre-treatment), and subsequent four-week intervals. Average participant scores decreased through the study, though starting and remaining within the "minimal depression" range (0-13). None of the participants were seen at an urgent care facility during the course of the study.

Adverse events

One participant was diagnosed with thyroiditis not attributable to the intervention.

Another participant experienced injection site pain that did not persist or have sequelae

Discussion

Nocturnal or sleep related bruxism, has been considered a parasomnia, and was re-classified as a sleep related movement disorder in 2005 [19]. It can occur in both children and adults [20]. The frequency and duration of bruxism is highly variable night to night, week to week, even year to year [21] potentially limiting the usefulness of intermittent polysomnography to explore a treatment effect on the motor behavior itself. This study's findings are consistent with others that have failed to show a statistically significant treatment response in EMG burst frequency or duration in Masseter and Temporalis recordings four weeks after injection [22]. The use of a portable EMG device has suggested a significant reduction in motor bruxing events after botulinum toxin injections [1] but evaluation of secondary sequelae were limited. Bruxism affects 3-35% of the adult population and 85-90% of the general population report experiencing bruxism in the course of their life time [1,4]. Prevalence estimates vary in part because sufferers are often unaware of the parasomnia [23], confounding diagnosis of associated morbidity [16] such as headache, sleep disruption and craniofacial pain [3]. The etiology of sleep bruxism remains obscure, but is likely centrally mediated [1,20]. This uncontrolled pilot study enrolled subjects who continued to experience chronic daily craniofacial pain despite the use of night guards and prophylactic treatments. This study was limited by small sample size, uncontrolled design, possible sampling error, "first night effect" in the sleep laboratory, and dosage limitations. Despite limitations, the trends indicate a possible treatment effect in bruxing behavior, craniofacial pain, migraine and associated sleep disruptions in subjects who have failed therapy with dental prosthetics, and headache prophylactic medications. Onabotulinum toxin A has shown efficacy for treatment of intractable migraine [6,24] and oromandibular dystonia [25]. As a pilot "proof of principle" trial, the findings support the need for larger, placebo controlled trials investigating the use of onabotulinum toxin type A in the treatment of nocturnal bruxism and it's sequelae. The impact of treatment on sleep disruption and sleep architecture should be further explored.

Conclusion

This uncontrolled pilot trial demonstrated statistical improvement in pain and headache outcome variables and a trend for, but no statistically significant reduction in, polysomnographic EMG bursts in temporalis and masseter muscles after Onabotulinum Toxin A injection in subjects with sleep bruxism who have failed conventional therapy. Larger, placebo controlled trials are indicated.

Disclosures and Acknowledgements

This study was funded by an unrestricted research grant from Allergan, Inc. Thanks are due to Ryan Irvine, Ph.D. for assistance with protocol development, Ina Roy-Faderman Ph.D. for assistance with writing, statistical analysis and graphics, Tiffany Olsen CMA for study coordination, Gerald Rich MD and the Pacific Sleep Center for montage development and sleep study interpretations, and Mathew Brodsky MD and the Pacific Northwest Basal Ganglia Coterie for critical review.

References

1. Lee SJ, McCall WD Jr, Kim YK, Chung SC, Chung JW (2010) Effect of botulinum toxin injection on nocturnal bruxism: a randomized controlled trial. Am J Phys Med Rehabil 89: 16-23.

2. Fross R (2000) Bruxism and Masticatory Myalgias: Use of Botulinum Toxin. Movement Disorders 15: 35.
3. Fernandes G, Franco AL, Gonçalves DA, Speciali JG, Bigal ME, et al. (2013) Temporomandibular disorders, sleep bruxism, and primary headaches are mutually associated. J Orofac Pain 27: 14-20.
4. Bender SD (2014) Orofacial pain and headache: a review and look at the commonalities. Curr Pain Headache Rep 18: 400.
5. Silberstein SD, Stark SR, Lucas SM, Christie SN, Degryse RE, et al. (2005) Botulinum toxin type A for the prophylactic treatment of chronic daily headache: a randomized, double-blind, placebo-controlled trial. Mayo Clin Proc 80: 1126-1137.
6. Brin M (2000) BOTOX for migraine: double-blind, placebo-controlled, region-specific evaluation. Cephalalgia 20: 421: 422.
7. Freund BJ, Schwartz M (2002) Use of botulinum toxin in chronic whiplash-associated disorder. Clin J Pain 18: S163-168.
8. Schwartz M, Freund B (2002) Treatment of temporomandibular disorders with botulinum toxin. Clin J Pain 18: S198-203.
9. Tan EK, Jankovic J, Ondo W (2000) Bruxism in Huntington's disease. Mov Disord 15: 171-173.
10. Sankhla C, Jankovic J, Duane D (1998) Variability of the immunologic and clinical response in dystonic patients immunoresistant to botulinum toxin injections. Mov Disord 13: 150-154.
11. Tan EK, Jankovic J (2000) Tardive and idiopathic oromandibular dystonia: a clinical comparison. J Neurol Neurosurg Psychiatry 68: 186-190.
12. Ivanhoe CB, Lai JM, Francisco GE (1997) Bruxism after brain injury: successful treatment with botulinum toxin-A. Arch Phys Med Rehabil 78: 1272-1273.
13. Watts MW, Tan EK, Jankovic J (1999) Bruxism and cranial-cervical dystonia: is there a relationship? Cranio 17: 196-201.
14. Tan EK, Jankovic J (2000) Treating severe bruxism with botulinum toxin. J Am Dent Assoc 131: 211-216.
15. Molina OF, dos Santos J Jr, Nelson SJ, Grossman E (1997) Prevalence of modalities of headaches and bruxism among patients with craniomandibular disorder. Cranio 15: 314-325.
16. Bailey DR (1990) Tension headache and bruxism in the sleep disordered patient. Cranio 8: 174-182.
17. Clark GT, Takeuchi H (1995) Temporomandibular dysfunction, chronic orofacial pain and oral motor disorders in the 21st century. J Calif Dent Assoc 23: 41-42, 44-6, 48-50.
18. Glaros AG, Rao SM (1977) Effects of bruxism: a review of the literature. J Prosthet Dent 38: 149-157.
19. International Classification of Sleep Disorders (2005) International classification of sleep disorders: diagnostic and coding manual (ICSD-2). 2nd ed. Westchester, IL: American Academy of Sleep Medicine.
20. Bracha HS, Ralston TC, Williams AE, Yamashita JM, Bracha AS (2005) The clenching-grinding spectrum and fear circuitry disorders: clinical insights from the neuroscience/paleoanthropology interface. CNS Spectr 10: 311-318.
21. Lavigne GJ (2000) Sleep bruxism and concomitant motor activity. In MH Kryger, Principles and Practice of Sleep Medicine 773–785.
22. Shim YJ, Lee MK, Kato T, Park HU, Heo K, et al. (2014) Effects of botulinum toxin on jaw motor events during sleep in sleep bruxism patients: a polysomnographic evaluation. J Clin Sleep Med 10: 291-298.
23. Hublin C, Kaprio J, Partinen M, Koskenvuo M (1998) Sleep bruxism based on self-report in a nationwide twin cohort. J Sleep Res 7: 61-67.
24. Blumenfeld AM, Binder W, Silberstein SD, Blitzer A (2003) Procedures for administering botulinum toxin type A for migraine and tension-type headache. Headache 43: 884-891.
25. Hallett M, Albanese A, Dressler D, Segal KR, Simpson DM, et al. (2013) Evidence-based review and assessment of botulinum neurotoxin for the treatment of movement disorders. Toxicon 67: 94-114.

Brainstem Sparing in Human Prion Disease: Sleep and Autonomic Function in a Long Survival Case Report

Alessandro Pincherle[1,2*], Eleonora Tobaldini[3], Lucio Mos[3], Ambra Dominese[2], Vincenzo Patruno[4], Nicola Montano[3], Flavio Villani[2], Fabrizio Tagliavini[2], Giorgio Giaccone[2] and Gabriella Marcon[2-6]

[1]*Neurology Unit, Spitalzentrum Biel, Biel, Switzerland*

[2]*Fondazione IRCCS Istituto Neurologico "Carlo Besta", Milan, Italy*

[3]*Department of Biomedical and Clinical Sciences "L. Sacco", Medicine and Physiopathology Unit, L. Sacco Hospital, University of Milan, Italy*

[4]*Department of Cardiology, San Daniele del Friuli Hospital, Udine, Italy*

[5]*Pneumologia Riabilitativa, Istituto di Medicina Fisica e Riabilitazione "Gervasutta", Udine, Italy*

[6]*Department of Biological and Medical Sciences (DSMB), University of Udine, Italy*

***Corresponding author:** Alessandro Pincherle, Neurology Unit, Spitalzentrum Biel, Biel, Switzerland, E-mail: apincherle@gmail.com

Abstract

Background: The prion diseases are characterized by sleep disruption, with FFI typically characterized also by severe autonomic dysfunction and sympathetic hyperactivity. We report the results of an extensive neurophysiological and autonomic assessment in a CJD patient carrying the D178 mutation with the uncommon homozygosity for valine at codon 129.

Results: A 47years old female presented with a memory impairment followed by progressive cognitive deficits and ataxia. The clinical picture slowly worsened to a state of akinetic mutism in about 2 years, and the patient died six years after the onset of symptoms. Repeated PSG and long-term actigraphic recordings, showed a peculiar, previously undescribed, pattern characterized by conservation of a rudimental circadian and ultradian rhythm, despite dramatic sleep micro-structure deterioration. We also observed a normal autonomic physiological response to orthostatic challenge and normal dynamic autonomic modulation during wake and sleep. The post-mortem brain pathology study, showed that neuronal loss was substantial in the cerebral cortex, diencephalon and thalami, but not in brainstem nuclei.

Conclusions: We hypothesize that, despite a dramatic neurological picture (i.e. akinetic mutism) and a severe sleep micro-structural alteration, the persistence of an autonomic modulation and the persistence of a rudimental circadian and ultradian oscillation, are related to the relatively conserved anatomo-functional integrity of foundamental neuronal systems in the brainstem.

Keywords: Prion; Sleep; Cardiovascular; Autonomic; Actigraphy; Brainstem

Introduction

The prion diseases are a family of rare neurodegenerative disorders that result from the accumulation of a misfolded form of the cellular prion protein termed PrPSc. Although the vast majority of cases are sporadic, 10% to 15% are caused by autosomal dominantly inherited mutations in the prion protein gene (PRNP) and include familial Creutzfeldt-Jakob Disease (CJD), Fatal Familial Insomnia (FFI) and Gerstmann-Sträussler-Scheinker disease (GSS).

The D178N PRNP mutation may result in two distinct phenotypes (i.e. CJD or FFI) specified by the polymorphism at codon 129 of the mutant allele, encoding valine in CJD and methionine in FFI [1].

Sleep disruption, initially considered a peculiar hallmark of FFI, has also been described in sporadic and inherited CJD [2-6]. In addition to profound alterations of the sleep-wake cycle, FFI is typically characterized by progressive disappearance of vegetative and hormonal circadian oscillations and severe autonomic dysfunction with sympathetic hyperactivity [5,7].

Here we report the results of an extensive neurophysiological and autonomic assessment carried out during the six year course of the disease at different time points in a CJD patient carrying the D178N-129V mutation. A detailed post-mortem study allowed us to correlate the clinical findings with the neuropathological evidences.

Case Report

A 47yrs old female presented with a memory impairment followed by progressive cognitive deficits and ataxia. The clinical picture slowly worsened to a state of akinetic mutism in about 2 years, and the patient died for respiratory failure at age 53, six years after the onset of symptoms.

Her father died at age 58 after a two–year history of a similar neurological disorder, and the paternal grandfather died in his 40s after a rapidly progressive dementia. The analysis of PRNP showed that the proband carried the D178N mutation and was homozygous for valine at codon 129. A more detailed clinical history has been already published [6].

The neuropathological examination of the proband [8] showed severe neuronal loss, spongiosis and gliosis in the cerebral cortex, basal ganglia, thalamus and cerebellum and marked myelin loss and tissue rarefaction in the hemispheric white matter, configuring a panencephalopathic form of CJD. Neuronal loss was not evident in brainstem nuclei, including substantia nigra, locus coeruleus, substantia reticularis pontina and inferior olives.

Methods

Sleep and autonomic assessment

Two 24-hours full-Polysomnography (PSG) recording, were performed 12 months and 34 months after the onset of the clinical symptoms.

Actigraphic data were collected with a Zero Crossing Mode (ZCM) 16 Hz sample rate and one-minute fixed epoch length. A total of 31 days in two different periods (32 months and 39 months after the onset of symptoms, respectively) were recorded.

Autonomic assessment included the analysis of heart rate variability (HRV), during wake and sleep, and hormonal circadian oscillations.

For HRV analysis, ECG and respiration traces were extracted from PSG recordings (T1 and T2 respectively) during wake (rest and stand position for 10 minutes) and during different sleep stages.

Two samples of 250 beats were selected during rest and stand for dynamic autonomic response to orthostatic challenge.. Autonomic regulation was evaluated by means of spectral analysis of HRV, based on an autoregressive model [8]. HRV identifies three rhythmic oscillations that characterize heart period time series: very low frequency (VLF), low frequency (LF), marker of sympathetic modulation, and high frequency component (HF, synchronous with respiration and marker of vagal modulation).

Results

Sleep and EEG

The results of the two full-PSG recordings were superimposable. The background wake EEG was characterized by symmetrical 8-8.5 Hz rhythm. Irregular sharp wave complexes (mostly triphasic) were observed isolated or with an irregular 1.5-2.5 seconds periodic pattern, and were attenuated by eyes opening. NREM sleep EEG pattern was characterized by monomorphic low amplitude theta and unstable delta activities, with total absence of vertex waves, spindles and K-complex. Absence slow wave sleep and severe reduction of REM sleep were also observed. Only a rudimental wake-sleep rhythm was detectable with a prevalence of wake during day-time and a prevalence of sleep epochs during the night. Ultradian rhythm was undetectable (Figure 1). Movement and respiratory profiles were unremarkable (data not shown).

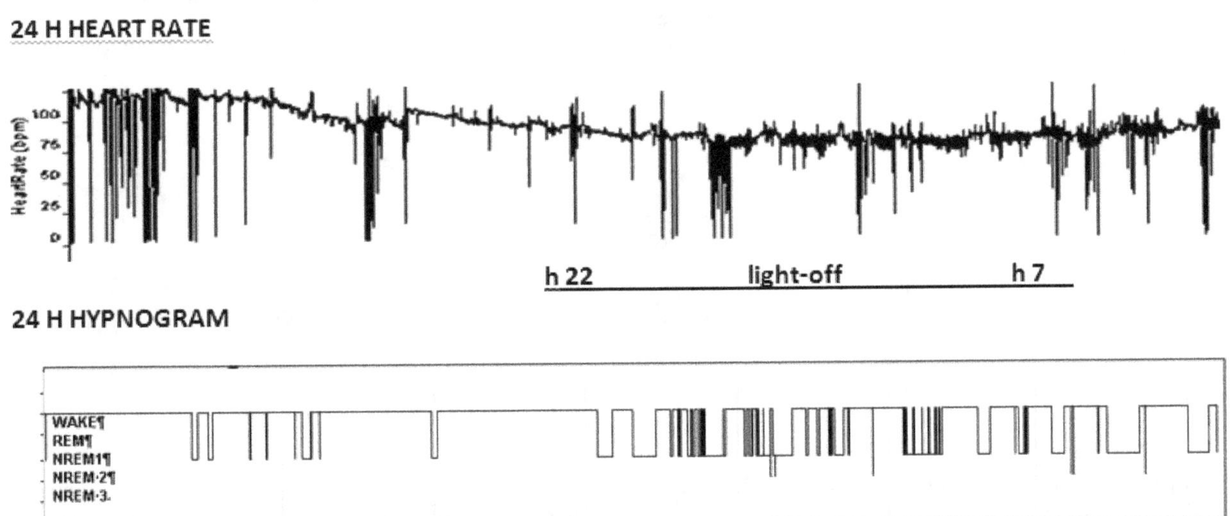

Figure 1: Macrostructual sleep analysis shows absence of NREM-REM cycles, absence of slow wave sleep and severe reduction of REM. A rudimental wake-sleep rhythm is detectable with a prevalence of wake epochs during day-time and a prevalence of sleep epochs during the night. HR is decreased during night-time.

Actigraphic measurements also revealed analogous results: the recording at T1 showed a sleep ratio of 0.66 (Sleep 39.7%, Wake 60.2%) and that of T2 a sleep ratio of 0.63 (Sleep 39%; Wake 61%). A clear prevalence of sleep was observed during night time compared to day time. A peculiar "alternating" pattern was observed during night time (Figure 1).

Autonomic assessment

The orthostatic challenge, performed 54 months after the onset of disease (October 2010) using the rest-stand maneuver, showed an increased heart rate (76 vs 84 bmp) and LFnu, marker of sympathetic modulation (42nu vs 75 nu) during orthostatism, suggesting a normal dynamic autonomic response.

As to sleep analysis, significant differences were observed comparing autonomic control during T1 and T2 and during W and S stages (Figure 2).

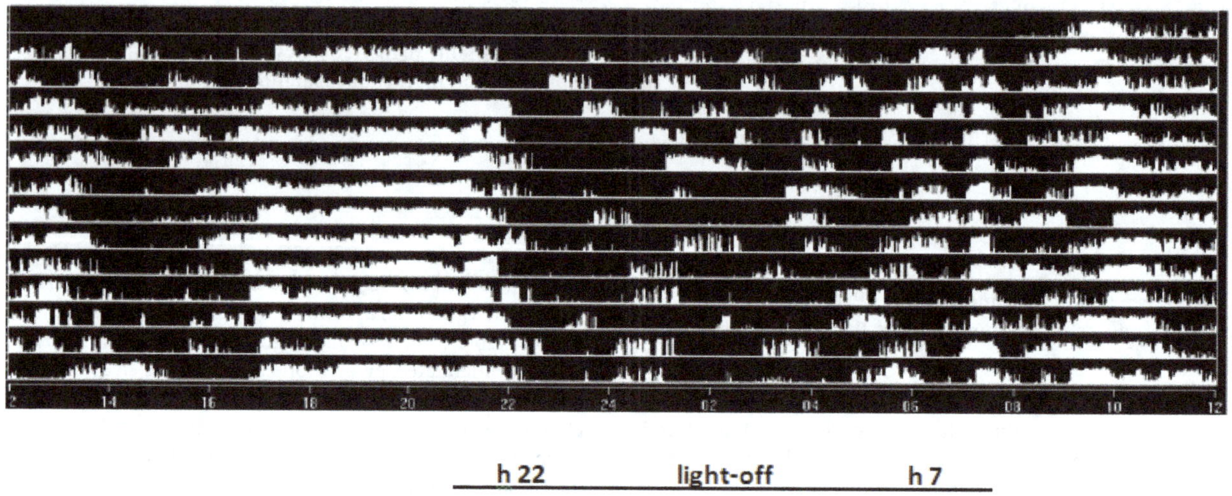

Figure 2: A clear prevalence of sleep is observed during night time compared to day time (circadian oscillation). A peculiar "alternating" pattern is observed during night time (ultradian oscillation).

Comparing T2 to T1, both during W and S, a reduction of total variability and a predominant sympathetic modulation were observed. As to sleep analysis, total power - a global index of autonomic variability - increased from W to S at T1 and T2, mainly due to an increased of VLF component. A predominant parasympathetic modulation during sleep and a predominant sympathetic control during wake were present in both recordings (Figure 3).

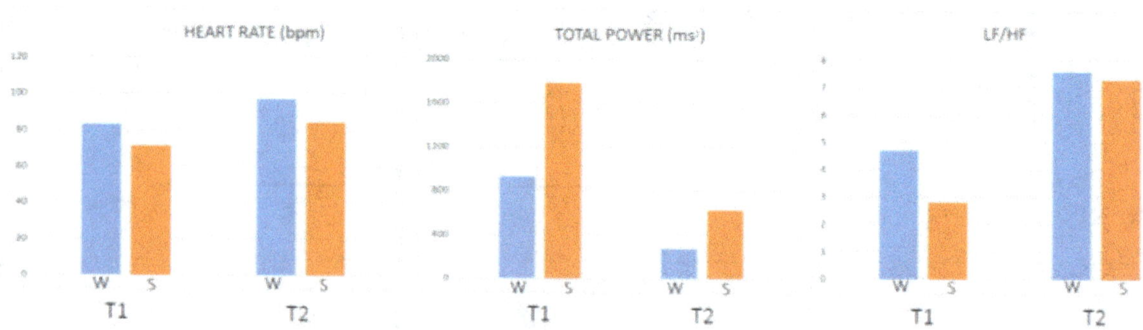

Figure 3: Comparing T2 to T1, both during W and S, a reduction of total variability and a predominant sympathetic modulation is observed. As to sleep analysis, total power increased from W to S at T1 and T2. A predominant sympathetic control during wake is present in both recordings.

Discussion

We have reported the case of a patient affected by a prion encephalopathy, caused by the D178N mutation with the uncommon homozygosity for valine at codon 129, characterized by an exceptionally long survival (6 years after the diagnosis), compared to the faster disease progression commonly observed in CJD. A collaborative study of human transmissible spongiform encephalopathies carried out from 1993 to 2000, showed indeed a median survival time from less than 6 months in sporadic and familial/genetic CJD to around 3 years in the GSS disease [7].

In line with previous evidences in CJD, in our case repeated PSG recordings revealed a severe sleep fragmentation with continuous night transitions between wakefulness and light sleep. This is not surprising since sleep disruption and sleep-wake symptoms are commonly recognized, with a remarkable overlap, both in CJD and FFI. The thalamo-cortical neural networks underling sleep consolidation and organization are indeed altered in prion diseases regardless of the specific etiology [3,9].

Despite the severe sleep microstructural alteration, we founded the persistence of a rudimental circadian sleep-wake rhythm, revealed by the prevalence of sleep epochs during night-time as documented by the PSG study. The long-term actigraphic recordings, similarly showed an atypical actigraphic nocturnal cyclic activity (i.e. rest/sleep periods alternated with wake/activity periods) that may be interpreted as the persistence of an ultradian oscillator, in which REM sleep periods are substituted by periods of wake or pseudo-wake state [10,11]. We hypothesize that the persistence of these rudimental circadian and ultradian oscillations, may be related to the, at least partial, sparing of the brainstem regulating network, with particular relevance of the mesopontine (reticular) cholinergic neurons in the peduncolopontine and laterodorsal tegmental nuclei [12]. In our patient, the post-mortem brain pathology study [8], showed that neuronal loss was substantial in the cerebral cortex, diencephalon and thalami, but not in brainstem nuclei (substantia nigra, locus coeruleus, substantia reticularis pontina and inferior olives), as described in other cases [13].

The brainstem is considered a critical area also for cardiac autonomic modulation and indeed we observed a normal autonomic physiological response to orthostatic challenge, with an increase of sympathetic and a decrease parasympathetic modulation in orthostatism. Several nuclei in the brainstem are critically involved in the autonomic control of cardiovascular functions, through sympathetic and parasympathetic efferent control on the sinus node and are responsible for the oscillatory components of heart rate variability [14,15]. By the contrary FFI, which usually shows a faster disease progression and a severe autonomic failure, is often characterized by widespread and conspicuous brainstem degeneration [16,17].

In conclusion, we can hypothesize that, despite a dramatic neurological picture (i.e. akinetic mutism) and a severe sleep micro-structural alteration, the persistence of an autonomic modulation and the persistence of a rudimental circadian and ultradian oscillator, were related to the relatively conserved anatomo-functional integrity of foundamental neuronal systems in the brainstem. The long survival of our patient carrying the rare VV129-D178 mutation, compared to other CJD forms and FFI, might be the additional consequence.

Acknowledgement

The work was supported by the Italian Ministry of Health, by the Italian Ministry of Education, Universities and Research (PRIN 2008HC7XR8_002).

References

1. Goldfarb LG, Petersen RB, Tabaton M, Brown P, LeBlanc AC, et al. (1992) Fatal familial insomnia and familial Creutzfeldt-Jakob disease: disease phenotype determined by a DNA polymorphism. Science 258: 806-808.
2. Kazukawa S, Nakamura I, Endo M, Hori A, Inao G (1987) Serial polysomnograms in Creutzfeldt-Jakob disease. J Psychiatry Neurol 41: 651-661.
3. Landolt HP, Glatzel M, Blättler T, Achermann P, Roth C, et al. (2006) Sleep-wake disturbances in sporadic creutzfeldt-Jakob disease. Neurology 66:1418-1424.
4. Taratuto AL, Piccardo P, Reich EG, Chen SG, Sevlever G, et al. (2002) Insomnia associated with thalamic involvement in E200K Creutzfeldt-Jakob disease. Neurology 58: 362-367.
5. Lugaresi E, Provini F (2007) Fatal familial insomnia and agrypnia excitata. Rev Neurol Dis 4: 145-152.
6. Dossena S, Imeri L, Mangieri M, Garofoli A, Ferrari L, et al. (2008) Mutant prion protein expression causes motor and memory deficits and abnormal sleep patterns in a transgenic mouse model. Neuron 60: 598-609.
7. Pocchiari M, Puopolo M, Croes EA, Budka H, Gelpi E, et al. (2004) Predictors of survival in sporadic Creutzfeldt-Jakob disease and other human transmissible spongiform encephalopathies. Brain 127: 2348-59.
8. Marcon G, Indaco A, Di Fede G, Suardi S, Finato N, et al. (2014) Panencephalopathic Creutzfeldt-Jakob Disease with Distinct Pattern of Prion Protein Deposition in a Patient with D178N Mutation and Homozygosity for Valine at Codon 129 of the Prion Protein Gene. Brain Pathol 24: 148-151.
9. Montagna P (2005) Fatal familial insomnia: a model di sease in sleep physiopathology. Sleep Med Rev 9:339-353.
10. Bódizs R, Sverteczki M, Mészáros E (2008) Wakefulness-sleep transition: emerging electroencephalographic similarities with the rapid eye movement phase. Brain Res Bull 76: 85-89.
11. Nielsen TA (2000) A review of mentation in REM and NREM sleep: "covert" REM sleep as a possible reconciliation of two opposing models. Behav Brain Sci 23: 851-866.
12. Pace-Schott EF, Hobson JA (2002) The neurobiology of sleep: genetics, cellular physiology and subcortical networks. Nat Rev Neurosci 3: 591-605.
13. Kaatz M, Fast C, Ziegler U, Balkema-Buschmann A , Hammerschmidt B, et al. (2012) Spread of classic BSE prions from the gut via the peripheral nervous system to the brain. Am J Pathol 181: 515-524.
14. Montano N, Gnecchi-Ruscone T, Porta A, Lombardi F, Malliani A, et al. (1996) Presence of vasomotor and respiratory rhythms in the discharge of single medullary neurons involved in the regulation of cardiovascular system. J Auton Nerv Syst 57:116-122.
15. Montano N, Porta A, Cogliati C, et al. (2009) Heart rate variability explored in the frequency domain: a tool to investigate the link between heart and behavior. Neurosci Biobehav Rev 33: 71-80.
16. Manetto V, Medori R, Cortelli P, Montagna P, Tinuper P, et al. (1992) Fatal familial insomnia: clinical and pathologic study of five new cases. Neurology 42: 312-319.
17. Gambetti P, Parchi P, Petersen RB, Chen SG, Lugaresi E (1995) Fatal familialinsomnia and familial Creutzfeldt-Jakob disease: clinical, pathological and molecular features. Brain Pathol 5: 43-51.

Comparison of Risperidone and Melatonin Effects in Methylphenidate Treated Children with Attention Deficit Hyperactivity Disorder for Treatment of Sleep Disorders

Gholami Damian F[1], Mahmoodi Gharaie J[1], Sabzali P[2], Darabi F[3] and Haji Seyed Javadi P*[4]

[1]*Psychiatric, Department of Psychiatry, Roozbeh Psychiatry Hospital, Tehran University of Medical Sciences, Tehran, Iran*

[2]*Psychiatric, Department of Psychiatry Emamhossein Hospital, Shahid beheshti University of Medical Sciences, Tehran, Iran*

[3]*Department of Public Health, Asadabad Medical Sciences Faculty, Hamadan University of Medical Sciences, Hamadan, Iran*

[4]*Psychiatric, Department of Psychiatry, Tehran University of Medical Sciences, Tehran, Iran*

***Corresponding author:** Javadi HSP, Psychiatric, Ruzbeh Hospital, Tehran University of Medical Science, Tehran, Iran, E-mail: p.sedjavadi@gmail.com

Abstract

Objectives: Some studies reported a significant improvement in sleep parameters by melatonin therapy in children with ADHD. Utilizing risperidone along with stimulants is another pharmacologic approach for ADHD treatment. In this study we investigated the effect of melatonin and risperidone on sleep disorders in children with ADHD and compared their effectiveness as well.

Methods & Methods: 29 patient aged 6 years to 12 years old with ADHD were randomly divided into two groups based on file number: either received melatonin (3 mg to 6 mg) combined with Ritalin or received risperidone (0.25mg to 0.5 mg) combined with Ritalin in a single blind randomized clinical trial. Assessments were performed at baseline and were repeated at 2 and 4 weeks after beginning of the treatment.

Results: In risperidone group significant differences has been found in total score of sleep disorders (P=0.000), sleep onset and maintenance score (P=0.000), Sleep-wake transition disorders (P=0.000), but no significant differences in breathing (P=0.104), and hyperhidrosis (P=0.105) and excessive daytime sleepiness score (p=0.065), and in arousal group after 2 weeks (p=0.027) and after 4 weeks (p=0.150). comparison of melatonin group in different weeks (Base line with 2 and 4 weeks after treatment), show significant differences in total score of sleep disorders (P=0.000), sleep onset and maintenance score (P=0.000), Sleep-wake transition disorders (P=0.003), excessive daytime sleepiness (P=0.004), but no significant differences in breathing (P=0.068) and arousal (P=0.218) and hyperhydrosis score (P=0.336).

Conclusion: The results showed the equal effect of risperidone and melatonin. It can be concluded that the risperidone has the same effect of melatonin in the treatment of sleep disorders in children with ADHD.

Keywords: Risperidone; Melatonin; Treated, Sleep disorders

Introduction

Obstructive sleep apnea-hypopnea syndrome (OSAHS) is a common condition characterized by repetitive obstruction of the upper airway resulting in daytime sleepiness due to sleep fragmentation caused by an airway obstruction. There are several papers on the prevalence of OSAHS showing that 7% to 26% of men and 2% to 13% of women have an apnea-hypopnea index (AHI) of more than 15 events per hour [1-5]. In Japan, the prevalence of OSAHS in the male working population has increased over the past decade, being estimated at 22.3% in patients with moderate to severe sleep-disordered breathing (SDB) [6]. It is significantly correlated with cardiovascular morbidity and mortality [7,8]. For patients with moderate to severe OSAHS, standard treatment is the continuous positive airway pressure (CPAP) ventilation. Compliance with and tolerance of CPAP are not always favourable, whose adherence rate is low, being 40% to 83% [9,10]. In Japan, CPAP treatment is not covered by health insurance for OSAHS patients with AHI of less than 20 events per hour. Consequently, one of the oral appliances (OA), prosthetic mandibular advancement (PMA), is a solid alternative to manage patients with mild to moderate OSAHS.

PMA causes protrusion of the mandible and tongue and enlarges and stabilizes the upper airway during sleep. Although the PMA has been shown to be effective for patients with mild to moderate OSAHS, adherence is poor [11,12]. Studies on PMA treatment have indicated that about 75% of patients remained adherent after 12 months of treatment, which may decrease to 50% after 5 years. In the PMA treatment, there are several side effects including tooth pain, pain of the temporomandibular joint (TMJ), gum disease, and dry mouth. Therefore, PMA treatments are not indicated for use in all patients who prefer PMA to CPAP, who do not respond to CPAP, or who show failed treatment attempts with CPAP. It is consequently important to develop other treatment options besides PMA for sleep apnea. A newly developed intraoral pressure gradient therapy system (IPGT), the iNAP® Sleep Therapy System (Somnics Inc., Hsinchu, Taiwan), was introduced as an alternative treatment for OSAHS [13]. The feasibility study explored the abilities and safety of the new device, the iNAP® Sleep Therapy System, for patients with OSAHS in our clinical sleep laboratory using full-night polysomnography.

Materials and Methods

Subjects

Subjects enrolled in this study were from outpatient clinic at the Child and Adolescent Psychiatric Division of Roozbeh Hospital, which is the university hospital of the Tehran University of medical sciences, located in Tehran, Iran. Inclusion criteria were (1) ages between 6 and 12 years old, inclusive; (2) diagnoses of ADHD according to DSMIV criteria (American Psychiatric Association, 2000); (3) receiving ritalin; (4) suffering from sleep disorders. Exclusion criteria included (1) presence of major depressive disorder, bipolar disorder, psychotic disorder, generalized anxiety disorder or other psychotic disorders; (2)Mental Retardation;(3)Drug intolerance;(4) any contraindications to the use of two drugs; (5) BMI above the 85th percentile. Subjects meeting diagnostic criteria for ODD were not excluded because of the high level of comorbidity of ODD in most ADHD populations, being present in around 30% to 60% of children with ADHD [12]. In this study 16 out of 29 ADHD patients had been diagnosed with ODD.

Study design

This study was a 28-day, randomized, single-blind clinical trial and parallel-arm comparison of melatonin and risperidone. The diagnosis of ADHD with or without comorbidity was achieved through clinical interview and CSI-4 (Child Symptoms Inventory-4) questionnaire which is a DSM-IV-referenced rating scale that screens for emotional and behavioral symptoms of childhood disorders.

To assess clinically significant improvement relative to baseline, we used the Clinical Global improvement (CGI-I) scales rated separately for symptoms of mania, depression, and ADHD. The CGI is rated on a 7-point scale that ranges from 1 (very much improved) to 7 (very much worse). Participants with ADHD had to have Scores 2 (much improved) on the CGI. In addition, socio-demographic information was collected from the parents. This research was approved by the Ethics Committee of Tehran University of Medical Sciences and written informed consent was filled with the participant's parents after full description of the study.

Medication schedule

In this study Subjects were randomly (1:1 ratio) allocated to receive either risperidone or melatonin for 4 weeks. Patients were randomized to a group according to the file number that was odd or even. For children who weighed less than 30 kg, melatonin was given at an initial dose of 3 mg at bedtime and for children upper than 30 kg; 3 mg to 6 mg was given. Besides, risperidone was given 0.25 mg to 0.5 mg for treating sleep problems. Parents were called weekly to monitor progress and discuss possible problems.

Assessment of efficacy and side effects

The parents filled in a 26-item sleep questionnaire(Sleep Disturbance Scale for Children)[13]. Assessments were performed at baseline and were repeated at 2 and 4 weeks after beginning of the treatment. Adverse events were recorded throughout the treatment period. Side effects were then compared between the two trial groups.

Data analysis

The two groups were compared using the X2 or Fisher exact test (categorical variables), Independent Sample t test and Repeated Measure ANOVA (continuous variables) using SPSS 20. Statistical significance was determined at $p<0.05$.

Results

Pretreatment patients characteristics

Fifty five patients were screened; 30 ADHD patients were eligible to participate in the study. One of the participants due to hypoglycemia excluded from the study. Afterwards from the remaining 29 patients, 15 were assigned to resperidone and 14 were assigned to melatonin. 10 female (4 and 6 were in the resperidone and melatonin group, respectively) and 19 male (11 and 8 were in the resperidone and melatonin group, respectively) were in the study. There were no statistically significant differences between the genders of two groups according to X2 test.

Patients' quantitative data such as age, body mass index, as well as baseline characteristics were analyzed in two trials before pharmacological intervention. Data analysis showed that there were no significant difference in age (P=0.24), body mass index (P=0.41), total score of sleep disorders (P=0.66), sleep onset and maintenance score (P=0.4), sleep disordered breathing (P=0.67), arousal disorders (P=0.63), sleep-wake transition disorders (P=0.98), excessive daytime sleepiness (P=0.58) and excessive sweating before intervention between two groups (Table 1). There were no significant differences between treatment groups in ODD ratio (P=0.34), and dose of Ritalin effects (P=0.793) in both risperidone and melatonin group.

Comparison of the therapeutic effects (efficacy measure)

The results of SDSC sleep questionnaire were analyzed using ANOVA with repeated measures at baseline, 2 and 4 weeks after the treatment. Data analysis showed that there were no significant difference between two groups in total score of sleep disorders (P=0.339), sleep onset and maintenance score (P=0.212), sleep disordered breathing (P=0.187), arousal disorders (P=0.404), Sleep-wake transition disorders (P=0.858), excessive daytime sleepiness (P=0.349) and excessive sweating (p=0.349).

In a comparison of risperidone group in different weeks(Base line with 2 and 4 weeks after treatment),significant differences has been found in total score of sleep disorders (P=0.000), sleep onset and maintenance score (P=0.000), Sleep-wake transition disorders (P=0.000),but no significant differences in breathing (P=0.104), and hyperhidrosis (P=0.105) and excessive daytime sleepiness score| (p=0.065), and in arousal group after 2 weeks (p=0.027) and after 4 weeks (p=0.150).

Comparison of melatonin group in different weeks (Base line with 2 and 4 weeks after treatment), show significant differences in total score of sleep disorders (P=0.000), sleep onset and maintenance score (P=0.000), sleep-wake transition disorders (P=0.003), excessive daytime sleepiness (P=0.004), but no significant differences in breathing (P=0.068) and arousal (P=0.218) and hyperhydrosis score (P=0.336) (Table 2). No statistically significant differences had been observed between the two groups in any of the side effects (Table 3).

Variables		Resperidone group(N=15)	Melatonin group (N=14)	Statistical analysis
Gender	Female	4	6	χ2(1)=0.840, P=0.359
	Male	11	8	
ge (Mean ± SD)		8.6 ± 1.8	9.5 ± 2.21	t(27)=1.2, P=0.24
Body mass index(Mean ± SD)		27.88 ± 34.33	20.15 ± 6.08	t(27)=-0.83, P=0.41
Total score of sleep disorder(Mean ± SD)		51 ± 9.89	49.57±7.1	t(27)=-0.44, P=0.66
sleep onset and maintenance score(Mean ± SD)		17.27 ± 3.71	18.14 ± 2.8	t(27)=0.71, P=0.48
sleep disordered breathing		3.87 ± 1.68	3.64 ± 1.01	t(27)=-0.43, P=0.67
arousal disorders(Mean ± SD)		3.67 ± 1.29	3.43 ± 1.34	t(27)=-0.49, P=0.63
Sleep-wake transition disorders(Mean ± SD)		11.4 ± 4.29	11.36 ± 4.07	t(27)=-0.03, P=0.98
excessive daytime sleepiness(Mean ± SD)		11.2 ± 4.04	10.43 ± 3.39	t(27)=-0.55, P=0.58
excessive sweating(Mean ± SD)		3.6 ± 2.85	2.57 ± 1.65	t(27)=-1.18, P=0.25

Table 1: Demographic and background data of participant in the study of comparing risperidone and melatonin effect on sleep disorders in children with ADHD.

	Comparison of baseline with second week		Comparison of baseline with fourth week		Comparison of second week with fourth week	
variables	t(14)	P	t(14)	P	t(14)	P
Total Sleep disorder score	5.848	<0.000	9.28	<0.000	2.878	0.013
Disorders of initiating and maintaining sleep	5.983	<0.000	10.001	<0.000	2.447	0.029
Sleep Breathing Disorders	1.989	0.068	2.28	0.04	1	0.336
Disorders of arousal	1.472	0.169	1.295	0.218	1	0.336
Sleep wake Transition Disorder	3.191	0.007	3.702	0.003	1.343	0.202
Disorders of excessive somnolence	2.299	0.01	3.44	0.004	1.735	0.106
Sleep Hyperhydrosis	1	0.336	1	0.336	-	-

Table 2: Comparison of melatonin receiving group in the different weeks.

Side effect	Melatonin group	Riper done group	P-value (Fisher exact test)
Headache	0 (0%)	1 (7.14%)	0.483
Abdominal pain	0 (0%)	2 (14.29%)	0.224
Morning Somnolence	2 (13.33%)	1 (7.14%)	1
Increased appetite	2 (13.33%)	0 (0%)	0.483

Table 3: Analysis of side effects in both risperidone and melatonin group.

Discussion

Attention Deficit-Hyperactivity Disorder (ADHD) is the most common psychological disorder in childhood with estimated prevalence of 5.29% worldwide and 10% in Iran [14,15]. The results of this study indicate that there is no significant difference between risperidone and melatonin in the treatment of sleep disorders in children with ADHD.

The clinician who visit the ADHD children usually focus on improving hyperactivity, attention deficit and impulsiveness. Since the correlation between ADHD and sleep disorder was approved [16,17], it is clear that they should pay enough attention to manage their concomitant sleep disorders.

The effective intervention approaches for ADHD is a combination of different therapeutics strategies including, parent training, cognitive-behavioral and medical therapy by stimulants [18]. Stimulants as the most effective medications for the treatment of ADHD effectively alleviate the symptoms (poor attention, distractibility, hyperactivity and restlessness) [19]. There are a limited number of studies regarding to quality and quantity of sleep in children with ADHD. At present available research results indicate that melatonin can be effective medication in the treatment of insomnia [20].

The results of this study are consistent with the results of previous studies on the effect of melatonin on sleep disorders of ADHD patients. Smits et al. in a double-blind, placebo-controlled study indicated that short-term melatonin administration was relatively safe and significantly more effective than placebo in patients with sleep onset insomnia [21]. Heijden et al. investigated the effect of melatonin treatment on sleep and quality of life. They indicated that melatonin could enhance total asleep time in children with ADHD and chronic sleep onset insomnia [22]. In a double blind randomized clinical trial in Iran with co-administration of melatonin and ritalin significant changes in sleep latency and total sleep disturbance score had been shown in children with ADHD [23].

The effect of risperidone on the quality of sleep has been reported in some studies. For example, Jacobsen [24] reported an improved quality of sleep following treatment with risperidone in affective illness and obsessive-compulsive disorder. In contrast, Daniel et al. [25] reported that patients complained of more insomnia with risperidone and more sedation with clozapine.

It is noteworthy that no statistically significant differences had been observed between the two groups in any of the side effects. Therefore, it can be concluded that the risperidone has the same effect of melatonin in the treatment of sleep disorders in children with ADHD. Since the beneficial effects of melatonin on sleep disorder treatment of patients with ADHD has been proven, the results showed the equal effect of resperidone and melatonin. This prospective follow-up study evaluated a small group of 29 children. A number of issues remain for further investigation. Long-term efficacy and safety of both risperidone and melatonin should be examined in children with ADHD. Additionally, further research is needed with the larger number of subjects and control group to evaluate the clinical impact of risperidone and melatonin.

Limitations

The current research had a number of limitations. It was implemented in 6 years to 12 years. Therefore, these results can be generalized only to adolescent 6 years to 12 years old of Tehran. They could not be generalizable to other geographical areas due to cultural, social, and economic differences.

Acknowledgements

The authors would like to thanks all Roozbeh Hospital authorities and administrators for facilitating data collection. They also express their thanks to all participants who participated in this study.

References

1. Konofal E, Lecendreux M,Cortese S, (2010) Sleep and ADHD. Sleep Med 11: 652-658.
2. Association A.P. Diagnostic and statistical manual of mental disorders DSM-IV-TR Fourth Edition (Text Revision) Author: American Psychiatr. 2000.
3. Owens J, Sangal BR, Sutton KV, Bakken R, JA, et al. (2009). Subjective and objective measures of sleep in children with attention-deficit/ hyperactivity disorder. Sleep Med 10: 446-456.
4. Efron D, Lycett K, Sciberras E (2014) Use of sleep medication in children with ADHD. Sleep Med 15: 472-475.
5. Mark W, Lawrence B, Ronald T, George D, Marian E, et al. (2011) Pediatrics AAO Subcommittee on Attention-Deficit/Hyperactivity Disorder, Steering Committee on Quality Improvement and Management. ADHD: Clinical practice guideline for the diagnosis, evaluation, and treatment of attention-deficit/hyperactivity disorder in children and adolescents. Pediatrics 128: 1007-1022.
6. Stein MA,Weiss M, Hlavaty L (2012) ADHD treatments, sleep, and sleep problems: Complex associations. Neurotherapeutics 9: 509-517.
7. Heijden V, Kristiaan B, Marcel G, Someren EV, Ridderinkhof KR, et al. (2007) Effect of melatonin on sleep, behavior, and cognition in ADHD and chronic sleep-onset insomnia. J Am Acad Child Adolesc Psychiatry 46: 233-241.
8. Weiss MD, Michael BW, Bomben MM, kathleen, Freeman RD (2006) Sleep hygiene and melatonin treatment for children and adolescents with ADHD and initial insomnia. J Am Acad Child Adolesc Psychiatry 45: 512-519.
9. Aman MG, Binder C, Turgay A (2004) Risperidone effects in the presence/absence of psychostimulant medicine in children with ADHD, other disruptive behavior disorders, and subaverage IQ. J Child Adolesc Psychopharmacol 14: 243-254.
10. Leysen JE, Janssen PM, Megens AA, Schotte A (1994) Risperidone: A novel antipsychotic with balanced serotonin-dopamine antagonism, receptor occupancy profile, and pharmacologic activity. J Clin Psychiatry. 55: 5-12.
11. Lind CCK, Carchedi CLR, Staudenmeier LJJ (2005) Atypical Presentations of Atypical Antipsychotics. Psychiatry (Edgmont) 2: 32-39.
12. Biederman J, Newcorn J, Sprich S (1991) Comorbidity of attention deficit hyperactivity disorder with conduct, depressive, anxiety, and other disorders. The Am J Psychiatry 148: 564-577
13. Bruni O, Salvatore O, Vincenzo G, Romoli M, InnocenzI M, et al. (1996) The sleep disturbance scale for children (sdsc) construct ion and validation of an instrument to evaluate sleep disturbances in childhood and adolescence. J Sleep Rrs 5: 251-261.
14. Hendriksen J, Peijnenborgh W, Aldenkamp A, Vles H (2015) Diagnostic overshadowing in a population of children with neurological disabilities: A cross sectional descriptive study on acquired ADHD. Eur J Paediatr Neurol 1-4.
15. Meftagh SD, Najimi A, Mohammadi N, Ghanizadeh A, Rahimi C, et al. (2014) The most effective intervention for attention deficit-hyperactivity disorder: Using continuous performance test. Psychiatria Danubina 26: 165-171.
16. Betancourt F, Leon DJYJ, Jimenez BC (2006) Attention deficit hyperactivity disorder and sleep disorders. Revista de neurologia 42: 37-51.
17. Weiss MD, Salpekar J (2010) Sleep problems in the child with attention-deficit hyperactivity disorder. CNS drugs 24: 811-828.

18. Johnston C, Hommersen P, Seipp C (2008) Acceptability of behavioral and pharmacological treatments for attention-deficit/hyperactivity disorder: Relations to child and parent characteristics. Behav Ther 39: 22-32.

19. Dusan K, Amanda K, Maria G, Lucy C, Cassidy S, et al. (2008) Treatment of adults with attention-deficit/hyperactivity disorder. Neuropsychiatr Dis Treat 4: 389-403.

20. Holvoet E, Gabriëls L (2012) Disturbed sleep in children with ADHD: Is there a place for melatonin as a treatment option. Magazine for psychiatry 55: 349-357.

21. Smits MG, Nagtegaal EE, Heijden J, Anton ML, Kerkhof A, et al. (2001) Melatonin for chronic sleep onset insomnia in children: A randomized placebo-controlled trial. J Child Neurol 16: 86-92.

22. Heijden KBV (2007) Effect of melatonin on sleep, behavior, and cognition in ADHD and chronic sleep-onset insomnia. J Am Acad Child Adolesc Psychiatry 46: 233-241.

23. Mostafavi SA, Mohammadi RM, Hosseinzadeh P, Eshraghian MR, Akhondzadeh S (2012) Dietary intake, growth and development of children with ADHD in a randomized clinical trial of Ritalin and Melatonin co-administration: Through circadian cycle modification or appetite enhancement? Iran J Psychiatry 7: 114-119.

24. Jacobsen FM (1995) Risperidone in the treatment of affective illness and obsessive-compulsive disorder. J Clin Psychiatry 56: 423-429

25. Daniel DG. Different side effect profiles of risperidone and clozapine in 20 outpatients with schizophrenia or schizoaffective disorder: A pilot study. Am J Psychiatry (1995).

Diagnose of Depression in Subjects with Sleep Disorders using Analysis of REM Sleep Electroencephalogram signals

Marzieh Miri[1], **Ali Sheikhani**[1*] **and Khosro Sadeghniiat**[2]

[1]*Biomedical Engineering, Science and Research Branch, Islamic Azad University, Tehran, Iran*

[2]*Tehran University of Medical Science, Tehran, Iran*

[*]**Corresponding author:** Ali Sheikhani, Biomedical Engineering, Science and Research Branch, Islamic Azad University, Tehran, Iran, E-mail: sheikhaniali@yahoo.com

Abstract

By considering the prevalence of depression in subjects with sleep disorders, our purpose is diagnosis of depression in these subjects. Shortened REM latency (i.e, the interval between sleep onset and the occurrence of the first REM period), increased REM sleep duration and increased REM density (i.e., the frequency of rapid eye movements per REM period) have been considered as biological markers of depression, so to diagnose of depression in subjects with sleep disorders we used analysis of EEG signal in REM sleep. The features of frequency and time domains in four channels (C3-C4-O1-O2) and four bands (delta, alpha, beta ,gamma) of REM sleep EEG were compared in 10 depressed (37.5 ± 8.34 years; mean ± standard deviation) and 14 non-depressed (36.6 ± 11.1 years; mean ± standard deviation) subjects with sleep disorders. According to results, most of the significant differences (P<0.05) have related to C3 and O1, in first stage and first period of REM sleep. Our results also show significant increase of beta activity in depressed subjects. Mahalanobis distance has classified 91.7% of the depressed and non-depressed subjects correctly.

Keywords: Depression; Sleep disorder; REM sleep; Sleep EEG signal; Time and frequency analysis

Introduction

Depression is one of the most commonly occurring of the major psychiatric disorders that profoundly affects individuals' thoughts, emotions, sense of self, behaviors, interpersonal relations, physical functioning, biological processes, work productivity, and overall life satisfaction [1]. The prevalence of this disease in the world today is such that the World Health Organization has predicted that by 2020 depression will be the second leading cause of disease worldwide [2,3]. Depression has symptoms like depressed mood, loss of interest and fatigue, tiredness, cognitive dysfunction, i.e., negative view of the self, negative ruminations, loss of appetite and libido, suicidality and sleep problems. Disturbed sleep is reported by up to 90% of depressed subjects and insomnia or hypersomnia are among diagnostic criteria for depression [4]. Depressed patients complain of insomnia (i.e., prolonged sleep latency, frequent awakenings during sleep, early morning awakening), disturbing dreams and nightmares and bad quality of sleep. These symptoms can accompanied with difficulty in maintaining sleep, decrease of total sleep time and quality, abnormalities of REM sleep, changes in the structure of NREM sleep and variables derived from quantitative sleep electroencephalogram (EEG) analysis [5-8].

Many studies have done on the analysis of sleep EEG signals in depressed patient and demonstrated that REM latency (interval between sleep onset and the occurrence of the first REM sleep period) was shorter in patients with depression and correlated inversely with severity of disease [9,10]. However, this is violated in other cases [7,11] or elsewhere stated that REM latency is associated just with primary depression [12]. Also, there is a phasic change in the activity of REM sleep, especially in the first half of the sleep that the severity of this change could be indicative of depression [13]. Gillin et al. using discriminant analysis and by characteristics such as total sleep time, sleep quality, sleep latency, time of early morning awakening and REM sleep, correctly classified 82% of depressed and normal subject [14]. Borbély et al. have reported that a power spectral density of sleep EEG in 0.25 to 2.5 Hz in depressed patients is lower than normal. They also shown that the power density in the entire frequency range (0.25 to 25 Hz) exhibited a decreasing trend over the first three NREM/REM sleep cycles for both groups, but in each cycle depressed people had lower values than controls [6], although this result was breached in later years by Mendelson et al. [7]. Tekell and colleagues in their work demonstrated increase of high frequencies activity in these patients [15]. It was shown that high frequencies and beta are greater in depressed women compared with depressed men, especially in right hemisphere [16]. Some studies shown that alpha activity decreases in depressed subject [17], although some others have reported increase of alpha and beta activity in depressed patients [18]. Liscome et al. by considering gender shown that generally women in both depressed and normal groups had higher delta amplitude than their male counterparts, and this effect was more common in the first REM period. They also shown that depressed men had lower alpha amplitude than depressed women in all three REM periods and also confirmed higher theta amplitude in the depressed women compared with all other groups for each REM period [19]. Armitage and colleagues suggested that depressed girls had lower delta amplitude than healthy girls in the first NREM sleep [20]. Armitage and colleagues in 1995 and 2001 reported that inter-hemispheric coherence decreases in depressed people [17,18]. Knott and colleagues in 2001 using beta and delta inter-hemispheric coherence, beta intra-hemispheric coherence and alpha intra-hemispheric power asymmetry could classify 91.3% of depressed and normal subjects [21].

Palaginii and colleagues [22] have examined the importance of REM sleep in depression and reported that there is a high correlation between the parameters of REM sleep and depression. Yang Li et al. [23] have shown that depressed patients had more regular brain waves during mental arithmetic than rest and so depressed and normal subject are more separable in the rest situation of brain. They could classify 80% of depressed and normal subjects using discriminant analysis. Because of prevalence of depression in the subjects with sleep disorders, the aim of this study has been diagnosed of depression in these subjects, using analysis of REM sleep Electroencephalogram signals.

Materials and methods

Subjects

Twenty four subjects with sleep disorders participated in this study and consent was taken from all of them. By diagnose of psychologist and according to Beck depression inventory (BDI) that was taken from subjects before EEG investigation, 10 persons (37.5 ± 8.34 years; mean ± standard deviation) were depressed with BDI score more than 18 and 14 persons (36.6 ± 11.1 years) were non-depressed with BDI score below 10. These persons only complained of insomnia, hypersomnia, dream and nightmare, excessive daytime sleepiness or poor quality of sleep and none of them had rest leg syndrome (RLS), breathing disorders like apnea or chronic snoring and other sleep disorders. All participants spent one night in the Sleep Disorder Unit of Baharluo Hospital and all of them were medication-free at the time of sleep study for at least 2 weeks.

Polysomnography

Polysomnography includes Electroencephalogram (EEG), Electrooculogram (EOG), Electromyogram (EMG), Electrocardiogram (ECG) and recording of legs movement and breathing signals during sleep. The EEG data that used in this study were collected from C3, C4, O1, and O2 channels referenced to left and right mastoid (A1, A2). Signals were recorded at the sampling frequency of 128 Hz.

Preprocessing

The EEG signals were filtered with 0.5-44 Hz IIR band pass Butterworth filter. Notch filter is also used to remove the 50 Hz frequency. To extract delta, alpha, beta and gamma frequency bands, Butterworth filters with band width of (0.5-4), (8-12 Hz), (14-34 Hz), (36-44 Hz) were used respectively. All of these signal preparations were performed in MATLAB 7.

Sleep staging

In this study, sleep staging has done using EEG of C3, C4, O1 and O2 channels and EOG, based on the Rechtschaffen and Kales criteria [24] by technician of polysomnography and specialist doctor in 30 second epochs of night sleep EEG that was 8 hours on the average. Then all REM sleep stages (set of 30 second epochs of REM sleep with no space) and REM sleep periods (set of REM sleep stages with at least three minutes duration that followed by ≥ 5 consecutive minutes of NREM or wakefulness) have determined in each participants. For statistical purposes, only the first two REM periods and stages were included for analysis because only some of the participants had three or more complete REM periods or stages for the night. Epochs containing movement, breathing or muscle artifacts and NREM sleep or waking epochs were eliminated from the stages or periods of REM sleep. Finally in each person forty-two 30 second epochs, on the average, were saved for later analysis.

Feature extraction

Because of non-stationary nature of EEG signals and existence of artifacts, signals of each channel and in each frequency band first divided to 2 second sections then using Fast Fourier Transform (FFT), power spectrum of each section calculated. Mean, variance, skewness [25], power spectrum threshold and spectrogram threshold criteria [26] for each section calculated and then mean of all section' feature considered as final features. Mean, variance, power and skewness of signals in time domain also considered as features. All features calculated in each frequency band and in four channels. Then magnitude squared coherence (MSC) of EEG signals from different channels in each frequency band determined according to equation (1-2) [26] to measure the degree of coupling between two signals.

$$MSC(f)=\frac{|Pxy(f)|^2}{Pxx(f)Pyy(f)} \qquad (1-2)$$

All features have calculated in first and second stages and first and second periods of REM sleep.

ANOVA statistics test and classification

In this paper, after examining data normality by Levene test, features are evaluated using ANOVA test and those with significant difference (P<0.05) were marked. To classifying depressed and non-depressed subjects that all of them had sleep disorders, Mahalanobis classifier with Leave-one-out cross validation, and for applying significant features, ROC curve were used. All parts of this step performed using the version 20 of SPSS software.

Result

Table 1 shows the Results of ANOVA test for the significant features of the first REM sleep stage.

Features name	Depressed Mean ± Std. Deviation	Non-depressed Mean ± Std. Deviation	P value
C3_gama_power spectrum skewness	0.5697 ± 0.0622	0.5214 ± 0.0314	0.02
C4_delta_ power spectrum skewness	0.9754 ± 0.0154	0.9616 ± 0.0109	0.018

O1_beta_mean amplitude of power spectrum	0.1473 ± 0.0878 (μv^2)	0.0882 ± 0.0458 (μv^2)	0.042
O1_beta_signal variance in time domain	0.1474 ± 0.0878 (μv^2)	0.0880 ± 0.0456 (μv^2)	0.041
O1_beta_signal power in time domain	0.0737 ± 0.0439 (μv^2)	0.0440 ± 0.0228 (μv^2)	0.041
O1_beta_spectrogram threshold	0.1921 ± 0.1237 (μv^2)	0.0821 ± 0.0689 (μv^2)	0.025

Table 1: result of ANOVA test for significant features ($p<0.05$) of first stage of REM sleep

As seen in table, among features of this stage, 6 features had significant difference between groups that most of them are relevant to channel O1. In all these features depressed subjects with sleep disorders had a higher average than non-depressed subjects with sleep disorders.

The result in second stage of REM sleep has shown that only power spectrum skewness in gamma band (mean values and standard deviations of 0.5594 ± 0.0429 and 0.0332 ± 0.5241 respectively for depressed and non-depressed) had significant difference ($p<0.05$) between groups.

Table 2 shows the results of ANOVA test for the significant features of the first period of REM sleep. In the first period, most significant features were related to the C3 channel, and all the values of the skewness had larger mean in the depressed subjects with sleep disorders compared to non-depressed subjects with sleep disorders.

Features name	Depressed Mean ± Std. Deviation	Non-depressed Mean ± Std. Deviation	P value
C3_alpha_ power spectrum threshold	0.1699 ± 0.0333 (μv^2)	0.2025 ± 0.0406 (μv^2)	0.049
C3_gama_ power spectrum skewness	0.5674 ± 0.0630	0.5240 ± 0.0331	0.039
C4_delta_ power spectrum skewness	0.9748 ± 0.0141	0.9620 ± 0.0113	0.022
O1- Beta- spectrogram threshold	0.1842 ± 0.1301 (μv^2)	0.0614 ± 0.0338 (μv^2)	0.016

Table 2: Result of ANOVA test for significant features ($p<0.05$) of first period of REM sleep

By studying the features in second REM sleep period coherence between O1 and O2 in delta band (mean values and standard deviations of 0.83903 ± 0.20813 and 0.50441 ± 0.39057 respectively for depressed and non-depressed) significantly ($P<0.05$) was more in depressed subjects.

Among the calculated features in the delta and alpha bands, the mean amplitude of the power spectrum at all studied phases of REM sleep and in all four channels C3, C4, O1, and O2 has always been lower in depressed subjects. Checking the power of these bands in time domain also shown the same result, and in most of the cases depressed subjects had lower delta and alpha power but because of greater scattering of these features in non-depressed subjects, no significant difference was shown. The calculation of the mean amplitude of gamma band power spectrum has shown that this feature in the first stage and first period of REM sleep is always more in depressed subjects. The same result was achieved for power of this band in time domain, but because of greater scattering of these features in depressed subjects no significant differences have been shown.

The best classification result using significant features has been obtained 91.7% (sensitivity=90%, specificity=92.9%) , using "power spectrum skewness in gamma band of channel C3 in first stage of REM, power spectrum skewness in delta band of channel C4 in first period of REM, spectrogram thresholds criteria in beta band of channel O1 in first stage and first period of REM and coherence between O1 and O2 in delta band of second period of REM" with area under ROC curve 0.736, 0.764, 0.821, 0.836 and 0.761 respectively.

Discussion

In this study using processing of REM sleep EEG signal, depression was diagnosed among people with sleep disorders. For this purpose, features of frequency and the time domains were extracted and using Mahalanobis classification, two groups were separated by an appropriate accuracy.

The studying of delta band features has shown that activity of this band in depressed subjects with sleep disorders always was lower, although the difference was not significant. Similar findings have been reported in [19] and in some other researches, decrease of delta activity in first cycle of sleep or in NREM sleep of depressed people also was expressed [6,20]. The results of studying mean amplitude of power spectrum and power of signals in time domain in alpha band revealed that activity of this band has been lower in depressed patients but these differences only approached significance ($P=0.05$) in first period of REM in channel C3. This is in contradiction with the results of Armitage (2001), which states that alpha activity is greater in depressed people [18]. However their results have related to NREM and total sleep cycle while our results are related to REM sleep and are in accordance with Liscombe's findings [19]. Mean amplitude of power spectrum, power of signals in time domain and threshold of spectrogram of signal in beta band have shown that depressed subjects had higher values and these features had significant differences in first stage of REM in channel O1. The gamma activity in most of the case was higher in depressed subjects but has showed no significant differences in this study. These findings are in agreement with results of [15,19] which reported increase of beta and gamma activity in depressed subjects.

The results showed that skewness of power spectrum in gamma band of channel C3 and in delta band of channel C4 in some stages and periods of REM sleep were significantly higher in depressed group. Studying the coherence between signals in different channels and in different frequency bands reported that inter-hemispheric coherence between C3 and C4 in beta band and total signal although was not significant, but is always lower in depressed subjects and is in agreement with findings of [17,18,21]. Inter-hemispheric coherences between O1 and O2 in all bands were always higher in depressed subjects and had significant difference in delta band of second REM sleep. Using "skewness" and "spectrogram threshold criteria" and "coherence" together, improved the accuracy of classification and at best, mahalanobis classifier with leave-one-out cross validation has separated 91.7% of depressed and non- depressed subjects that in compared with [14,21,23] is a better result. The results of this study indicate that features extracted from REM sleep could classified depressed and non-depressed as well as NREM sleep.

Despite one of the problems of people who referred to sleep disorder clinics is depression, but as far as we know, depression was not diagnosed by analysis of their sleep signals and this research is the first study in this regard. Due to the limitations of the study, the results have obtained by studying the small number of subjects, so the larger population is needed to confirm them. As a future work, it is suggested to study the different age ranges and distinct gender groups with larger populations. Different sleep disorders can also be separately examined.

Acknowledgement

This research has been supported by Islamic Azad University, Science and Research branch-Tehran-Iran and sleep disorder clinic of Baharlou hospital. We express our appreciation to personnel of sleep disorder clinic of Baharlou hospital for cooperation in collecting data of depressed people with sleep disorders.

References

1. Hankin BL (2006) Adolescent depression: Description, causes, and interventions. Epilepsy & Behavior 8: 102–114.
2. Carvalho A, Moraes H, Silveira H, Ribeiro P, Piedade RA, et al. (2011) EEG frontal asymmetry in the depressed and remitted elderly: is it related to the trait or to the state of depression? J Affect Disord 129: 143-148.
3. Geneva (1992) International statistical classification of diseases and related health problems. World Health Organization (WHO).
4. Palagini L, Baglioni C, Ciapparelli A, Gemignani A, Riemann D (2013) REM sleep dysregulation in depression: state of the art. Sleep Med Rev 17: 377-390.
5. Landolt HP, Gillin JC (2005) Similar sleep EEG topography in middle-aged depressed patients and healthy controls. Sleep 28: 239-247.
6. Borbély AA, Tobler I, Loepfe M, Kupfer DJ, Ulrich RF, et al. (1984) All-night spectral analysis of the sleep EEG in untreated depressives and normal controls. Psychiatry Res 12: 27-33.
7. Mendelson WB, Sack DA, James SP, Martin JV, Wagner R, et al. (1987) Frequency analysis of the sleep EEG in depression. Psychiatry Res 21: 89-94.
8. Armitage R, Roffwarg HP, Rush AJ, Calhoun JS, Purdy DG, et al. (1992) Digital period analysis of sleep EEG in depression. Biol Psychiatry 31: 52-68.
9. Kerkhofs M, Hoffmann G, De Martelaere V, Linkowski P, Mendlewicz J (1985) Sleep EEG recordings in depressive disorders. J Affect Disord 9: 47-53.
10. Hubain P, Le Bon O, Vandenhende F, Van Wijnendaele R, Linkowski P (2006) Major depression in males: effects of age, severity and adaptation on sleep variables. Psychiatry Res 145: 169-177.
11. Kravitz HM, Avery E, Sowers M, Bromberger JT, Owens JF, et al. (2011) Relationships between menopausal and mood symptoms and EEG sleep measures in a multi-ethnic sample of middle-aged women: the SWAN sleep study. Sleep 34: 1221-1232.
12. Kupfer DJ (1976) REM latency: a psychobiologic marker for primary depressive disease. Biol Psychiatry 11: 159-174.
13. Kupfer DJ, Bulik CM, Grochocinski V (1984) Relationship between EEG sleep measures and clinical ratings of depression. A revisit. J Affect Disord 6: 43-52.
14. Gillin JC, Duncan W, Pettigrew KD, Frankel BL, Snyder F (1979) Successful separation of depressed, normal, and insomniac subjects by EEG sleep data. Arch Gen Psychiatry 36: 85-90.
15. Tekell JL, Hoffmann R, Hendrickse W, Greene RW, Rush AJ, et al. (2005) High frequency EEG activity during sleep: characteristics in schizophrenia and depression. Clin EEG Neurosci 36: 25-35.
16. Armitage R, Hudson A, Trivedi M, Rush AJ (1995) Sex differences in the distribution of EEG frequencies during sleep: unipolar depressed outpatients. J Affect Disord 34: 121-129.
17. Armitage R (1995) Microarchitectural findings in sleep EEG in depression: diagnostic implications. Biol Psychiatry 37: 72-84.
18. Armitage R, Hoffmann RF (2001) Sleep EEG, depression and gender. Sleep Med Rev 5: 237-246.
19. Liscombe MP, Hoffmann RF, Trivedi MH, Parker MK, Rush AJ, et al. (2002) Quantitative EEG amplitude across REM sleep periods in depression: preliminary report. J Psychiatry Neurosci 27: 40-46.
20. Armitage R, Emslie GJ, Hoffmann RF, Rintelmann J, Rush AJ (2001) Delta sleep EEG in depressed adolescent females and healthy controls. J Affect Disord 63: 139-148.
21. Knott V, Mahoney C, Kennedy S, Evans K (2001) EEG power, frequency, asymmetry and coherence in male depression. Psychiatry Res 106: 123-140.
22. Palagini L, Gemignani A, Guazzelli M (2012) Significance of REM sleep in Depression: Effects on Neurogenesis. J Sleep Disord Ther 1: 3.
23. Yang Li, Yingjie Li, Tong S, Tang Y, Zhu Y (2007) more normal EEGs of depression patients during mental arithmetic than rest. Proceedings of NFSI & ICFBI, IEEE.
24. A.Rechtschaffen, A.A. Kales (1968) a Manual of Standardized Terminology, Techniques and Scoring for Sleep Stages of Human Subjects. U.S. Department of Health, Education, and Welfare, Washington DC.
25. Remond A (1973) Handbook of electroencephalography Clinical neurophysiology. Elsevier Scientific publishing company - Amesterdam, The Netherlands.
26. Sheikhani A, Behnam H, Mohammadi MR, Noroozian M, Mohammadi M (2012) Detection of abnormalities for diagnosing of children with autism disorders using of quantitative electroencephalography analysis. J Med Syst 36: 957-963.

Association of Childhood Asthma and Pediatric Obstructive Sleep Apnea

Chien-Heng Lin[1,2], Wei-Ching Lin[3-5], Cheng-Li Lin[4,5] and Liang-Wen Hang[6,7*]

[1]*Division of Pediatric Pulmonology, China Medical University Children's Hospital, Taichung, Taiwan*
[2]*Department of Biomedical Imaging and Radiological Science, College of Health Care, China Medical University, Taichung, Taiwan*
[3]*Department of Radiology, College of Medicine, School of Medicine, China Medical University, Taichung, Taiwan*
[4]*College of Medicine, China Medical University, Taichung, Taiwan*
[5]*Management Office for Health Data, China Medical University Hospital, Taichung, Taiwan*
[6]*Department of Respiratory Therapy, College of Health Care, China Medical University*
[7]*Sleep Medicine Center, Department of Pulmonary and Critical Care Medicine, China Medical University Hospital*

Abstract

Background and objective: Asthma is a risk factor for obstructive sleep apnea (OSA) in adult patients. However, the relationship between pediatric OSA and childhood asthma remains unclear. Here, we conducted a large-scale population-based cohort study for evaluating our hypothesis that childhood asthma is a risk factor for pediatric OSA.

Methods: From 2000 to 2007, children with and without asthma who were frequency matched by age, sex, urbanization level, comorbidities, and baseline year were enrolled from the Taiwan National Health Insurance Research Database (NHIRD). We compared pediatric OSA risk between asthma and non-asthma cohorts by using multivariable Cox regression analysis.

Results: We observed a significant relationship between asthma and OSA. In total, we included 305094 children with asthma and 305094 without asthma. The overall incidence rate ratio of OSA was 3.56-fold higher in the asthma cohort than in the non-asthma cohort (566 *vs.* 249 per 1000 person-year). After adjustment for potential risk factors, the adjusted hazard ratio (HR) of OSA was 1.82 [95% confidence interval (CI)=1.56-2.13]. Regardless of sex, the asthma cohort had a higher OSA risk than the non-asthma cohort did. Patients with asthma, excluding particular comorbidities, had a significantly increased OSA risk. Compared with those without asthma, patients with asthma who had more medical visits for asthma per year (particularly>5 visits per year) had a higher subsequent OSA risk (adjusted HR, 10.1, 95% CI=8.13-12.6).

Conclusion: This nationwide retrospective cohort study demonstrated that childhood asthma may increase subsequent pediatric OSA risk.

Keywords: Asthma; ICD-9-CM code; National Health Insurance Research Database; Population-based study; Obstructive sleep apnea

Abbreviations: CI: Confidence Interval; HR: Hazard Ratio; ICD-9-CM: International Classification of Diseases, Ninth Revision, Clinical Modification; NHIRD: National Health Insurance Research Database; OSA: Obstructive Sleep Apnea

Introduction

Pediatric obstructive sleep apnea (OSA) is a sleep disorder characterized by repeated episodes of apnea and hypopnea. The upper airway obstruction resulting from adenotonsillar hypertrophy, neuromuscular disease, and craniofacial abnormality usually causes pediatric OSA [1]. The major symptom of pediatric OSA is snoring or mouth breathing during sleep, affecting approximately 3% to 12% of the pediatric population [2,3].

Early diagnosis and treatment of OSA is crucial because of associated comorbidities, and untreated OSA can lead to serious complications and consequences, such as failure to thrive, behavioral and neurocognitive dysfunction, metabolic syndrome, and pulmonary hypertension [1,4,5]. Numerous studies have investigated male sex, age, obesity, and nasal disease as risk factors for subsequent OSA [2-5].

Asthma is the most common chronic respiratory inflammatory disease in childhood and has various comorbidities such as overweight, allergic rhinitis, dysfunctional breathing, depressive disorders, and, perhaps, gastro esophageal reflux disease (GERD) [6]. Children with asthma often have poor sleep quality, which contributes to the nocturnal deterioration of symptoms [7].

Several authors have reported a relationship between asthma and OSA [8-14]. The prevalence of OSA is higher among patients with adult asthma; OSA symptoms, which further deteriorate asthma symptoms, are commonly observed in the asthmatic population; thus, treating OSA can improve asthma symptoms [9-12]. Recent studies have shown that adult patients with asthma have a significantly higher risk of OSA [14,15]. However, a large-scale population-based cohort study evaluating the risk factors for OSA in pediatric patients with asthma has not been performed.

We hypothesized that childhood asthma is a risk factor for pediatric OSA. Therefore, we conducted a population-based retrospective

***Corresponding author:** Liang-Wen Hang, MD, Sleep Medicine Center, Department of Pulmonary and Critical Care Medicine, China Medical University Hospital, No. 2, Yuh-Der Road, Taichung-404, Taiwan,
E-mail: d2292@mail.cmuh.org.tw

cohort study by using data from the Taiwan National Health Insurance Research Database (NHIRD) for investigating the relationship between asthma and subsequent OSA risk.

Methods

The Taiwan National Health Insurance (NHI) program is a compulsory insurance program for Taiwanese citizens, and 99% of Taiwan's 23 million residents were enrolled in 1998 [16]. The NHIRD contains all reimbursement claims data from the Taiwan NHI program, including beneficiary registries, medical records, and registries for drug prescriptions and other medical services [17,18].

The NHIRD includes all claims data for children aged ≤ 18 years from 2000 to 2008; these data were a selected sample of half of all insured children. Detailed information on half of all the insured children has been provided in previous high-quality studies. To protect patient privacy, the Taiwan government eliminated original identification numbers and encrypted all personal identification information before releasing the database for research. The medical records were compiled on the basis of International Classification of Diseases, Ninth Revision, Clinical Modification (ICD-9-CM) codes. This study was approved by the Ethics Review Board of China Medical University and Hospital in Taiwan (CMUH104-REC2-115).

Study participants

The asthma cohort included patients<18 years with asthma (ICD-9-CM codes 493 and 494) diagnosed from 2000 to 2007, with the date of asthma diagnosis as their index date. For each child with asthma, we selected simultaneously one child without asthma matched by age (within a 1-year interval), sex, urbanization level, and year of asthma diagnosis. Children with pre-existing OSA (ICD-9-CM codes 327.23, 780.51, 780.53, and 780.57) were excluded. Tonsillectomy and adenoidectomy before a diagnosis of OSA were all excluded. All children were followed up from the index date until the date of OSA diagnosis, withdrawal of insurance, death, or 31 December 2008.

The type of medical visit is defined as medical visit for asthma. The baseline comorbidities considered were GERD (ICD-9-CM codes 530.11 and 530.81), craniofacial abnormalities (ICD-9-CM code 756.0), neuromuscular abnormalities (ICD-9-CM codes 330-337), prematurity (ICD-9-CM codes 764 and 765), genetic syndrome (ICD-9-CM code 758), laryngomalacia or tracheomalacia (ICD-9-CM codes 748.3 and 519.19, respectively), diabetes (ICD-9-CM code 250), hypertension (ICD-9-CM codes 401-405), hyperlipidemia (ICD-9-CM code 272), obesity (ICD-9-CM code 278), rhinitis (ICD-9-CM codes 472-477), chronic sinusitis (ICD-9-CM code 473), and adenotonsillar hypertrophy (ICD-9-CM codes 474.10, 474.11, and 474.12).

Statistical analysis

The chi-square test was used for examining the distribution of demographic data between asthma and non-asthma cohorts. Continuous data were presented as mean ± standard deviation (SD) and examined using the Student t test. We calculated the overall, age-specific, sex-specific, urbanization level-specific, and comorbidity-specific incidence density rates of OSA (per 100000 person/year) in each cohort.

The multivariate Cox proportional hazards model was used for calculating the hazard ratios (HRs) and 95% confidence intervals (CIs) of developing OSA in association with asthma. The multivariable models were simultaneously adjusted for age, sex, urbanization level, and comorbidity. Further analysis was performed for assessing the dose response on OSA risk according to the average frequency of medical visits for asthma. All data analyses were conducted using the Statistical Analysis System software (Version 9.3 for Windows; SAS Institute, Inc., Cary, NC, USA). P<0.05 was considered significant for a 2-tailed test.

Results

We included 305,094 children in the asthma cohort and 305094 children in the nonasthma cohort. In the asthma cohort, 37.5% children were aged<3 years and 58.9% were boys. The mean age of children in both cohorts was 4.71 years. More than half of the children lived in urbanized areas. The prevalence of GERD, neuromuscular abnormalities, prematurity, genetic syndrome, laryngomalacia or tracheomalacia, diabetes, hypertension, hyperlipidemia, obesity, rhinitis, chronic sinusitis, and adenotonsillar hypertrophy was higher in the asthma cohort than in the nonasthma cohort (P<0.05). The mean follow-up period in the asthma and nonasthma cohorts was 5.22 years (SD=2.30) and 5.19 years (SD=2.31), respectively. The Kaplan–Meier plots in Figure 1 show that the 9-year cumulative incidence of OSA was greater in the asthma cohort than in the nonasthma cohort (log-rank test, P<0.001) (Figure 1).

The overall incidence of OSA in the asthma and nonasthma cohorts was 3.56 and 1.57 per 10000 person-years, respectively (Table 2). In total, 194 (34.3%) and 79 (31.78%) patients underwent tonsillectomy and adenoidectomy in the asthma and nonasthma cohorts, respectively. After adjustment for age, sex, urbanization level, and comorbidities, children with asthma were associated with an increased OSA risk compared with those without asthma [adjusted HR (aHR)=1.82, 95% CI=1.56-2.13]. The age-specific aHRs of OSA were higher for all age subgroups in both cohorts. After stratification by sex, the relative OSA risk was higher in both the girls (aHR=2.03, 95% CI=1.47-2.80) and boys (aHR=1.78, 95% CI=1.49-2.13) of both cohorts. The OSA risk was higher among those of all urbanization levels in both cohorts (Table 1). After stratification by comorbidity, the relative OSA risk was higher in the asthma cohort than in the nonasthma cohort for both patients without (aHR=1.84, 95% CI=1.50-2.26) and with comorbidity

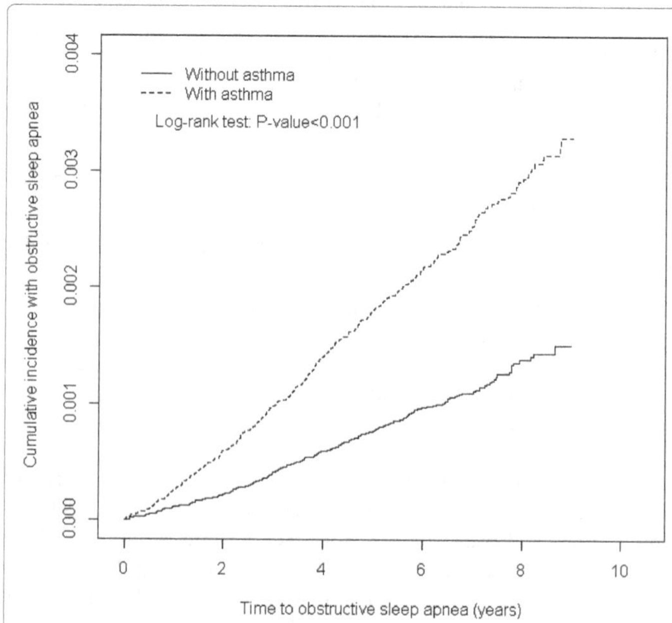

Figure 1: Kaplan–Meier analysis of the cumulative incidence of obstructive sleep apnea for the asthma cohort compared with the non-asthma cohort.

Variables	Non-Asthma		Asthma		p-value
	(N=305094)		(N=305094)		
	n	(%)	n	(%)	
Age, years, mean (SD)*	4.71	-3.61	4.71	-3.59	0.68
Stratified age, years					
<3	114542	-37.5	114542	-37.5	0.99
03-Jun	112712	-36.9	112712	-36.9	
06-Dec	60613	-19.9	60613	-19.9	
≥ 12	17227	-5.65	17227	-5.65	
Sex					
Girl	125556	-41.2	125556	-41.2	0.99
Boy	179538	-58.9	179538	-58.9	
Urbanization level†					
1 (highest)	89154	-29.2	89154	-29.2	0.99
2	92889	-30.5	92889	-30.5	
3	55357	-18.1	55357	-18.1	
4 (lowest)	67694	-22.2	67694	-22.2	
Comorbidity					
GERD	167	-0.05	371	-0.12	<0.001
Craniofacial abnormalities	75	-0.02	80	-0.03	0.69
Neuromuscular abnormalities	683	-0.22	961	-0.31	<0.001
Prematurity	2446	-0.8	4598	-1.51	<0.001
Genetic syndrome	196	-0.06	271	-0.09	0.001
Laryngomalacia/tracheomalacia	216	-0.07	472	-0.15	<0.001
Diabetes	170	-0.06	266	-0.09	<0.001
Hypertension	110	-0.04	146	-0.05	0.02
Hyperlipidemia	69	-0.02	155	-0.05	<0.001
Obesity	207	-0.07	391	-0.13	<0.001
Rhinitis	61858	-20.3	138067	-45.3	<0.001
Chronic sinusitis	4286	-1.4	12799	-4.2	<0.001
Hypertrophy of tonsil with adenoid	526	-0.17	742	-0.24	<0.001

Chi-square test and *Student t-test comparing children with and without asthma; †The urbanization level was categorized by the population density of the residential area into 4 levels, with level 1 as the most urbanized and level 4 as the least urbanized.

Table 1: Demographics of children with and without asthma.

(aHR=1.77, 95% CI=1.40-2.25). Table 3 shows that the aHR of OSA increased to 10.1 (95% CI=8.13-12.6) for patients with asthma with>5 medical visits for asthma per year compared with that for patients without asthma (P for trend<0.0001). In addition, similar trends were observed for both girls and boys.

Discussion

On the basis of the literature review, this is the first population-based case-control study to demonstrate an increased pediatric OSA risk in children with asthma compared with that in those without asthma. We observed that this association was independent of other risk factors, such as age, sex, urbanization level, and comorbidity (adjusted for HR). In addition, these patients with asthma seeking medical visits more often 5 times per year for asthma have increased OSA risk.

In children, OSA often results from adenotonsillar hypertrophy, neuromuscular diseases, and craniofacial abnormalities [1], whereas in adults, it results from velopharyngeal narrowing and obesity [19]. Teodorescu et al. reported that patients aged 30 years to 60 years with self-reported asthma had the risk of developing OSA [15]. Shen et al. reported that patients aged>20 years have a significantly higher risk of OSA than the general population does [14]. The adjusted relative risk of OSA was 1.39 (95% CI=1.06-1.82) and 2.51 (95% CI=2.19-2.89) in the studies by Teodorescu et al. and Shen et al. respectively. We used the same NHI database as that used in the study by Shen et al. moreover, our study included patients aged<18 years [15]. The adjusted relative risk was 1.82 (95% CI=1.56-2.13) in our study, and we did not observe the combined effects of comorbidities on pediatric OSA risk. However, comorbid conditions such as GERD, rhinitis, and obesity are more crucial risk factors for OSA in adult patients with asthma compared with the general population [14].

In our study, we observe that asthma is the primary risk factor for sequent OSA and three mechanisms may explain why childhood asthma increases OSA risk. First, the systemic inflammation may affect the strength or force generation of respiratory muscles, including the upper airway dilator muscles, and then destabilize the central breathing controller [20]. Second, the deformable pharyngeal airway duration inspiration and the active contraction of respiratory muscles during forced exhalation in an asthma attack could promote the collapse of the upper airway at night [21]. Third, corticosteroid therapy may affect the pharyngeal airway and render pharyngeal dilators more floppy, thus reducing their ability to protect the upper airway patency during sleep [22,23]. More clinical trials or animal studies should be performed to confirmed these mechanisms or pathophysiology.

In our study, children with asthma had a higher incidence of subsequent OSA when the frequency of medical visits per year was more than two, and the hazard ratios increase when the medical visits

	Non- Asthma			Asthma			Adjusted HR† (95% CI)
Variables	Event	Person-years	IR	Event		IR	
All	249	1583683	1.57	566	1591841	3.56	1.82(1.56, 2.13)***
Stratified age							
<3	93	618282	1.5	219	623819	3.51	2.07(1.61, 2.65)***
03-Jun	113	577969	1.96	232	578804	4.01	1.57(1.24, 1.98)***
06-Dec	39	333522	1.17	99	334865	2.96	1.96(1.33, 2.90)***
≥ 12	4	53910	0.74	16	54353	2.94	3.48(1.12, 10.8)***
Sex							
Girl	56	647225	0.87	135	650604	2.07	2.03(1.47, 2.80)***
Boy	193	936458	2.06	431	941238	4.58	1.78(1.49, 2.13)***
Urbanization level‡							
1 (highest)	101	460372	2.19	202	462735	4.37	1.68(1.31, 2.16)***
2	59	480489	1.23	172	483187	3.56	2.22(1.63, 3.02)***
3	39	287940	1.35	101	289272	3.49	2.07(1.41, 3.03)***
4 (lowest)	50	354883	1.41	91	356647	2.55	1.48(1.03, 2.12)*
Comorbidity§							
No	164	1286744	1.27	214	896016	2.39	1.84(1.50, 2.26)***
Yes	85	296940	2.86	352	695825	5.06	1.77(1.40, 2.25)***

IR: incidence rate, per 10, 000 person-y; Adjusted HR†: adjusted for age, sex, urbanization level; comorbidities such as GERD, craniofacial abnormalities, neuromuscular abnormalities, prematurity, genetic syndrome, laryngomalacia or tracheomalacia, diabetes, hypertension, hyperlipidemia, obesity, rhinitis, chronic sinusitis, and adenotonsillar hypertrophy; ‡The urbanization level was categorized by the population density of the residential area into 4 levels, with level 1 as the most urbanized and level 4 as the least urbanized; Comorbidity§: Patients with any of the comorbidities, including GERD, craniofacial abnormalities, neuromuscular abnormalities, prematurity, genetic syndrome, laryngomalacia or tracheomalacia, diabetes, hypertension, hyperlipidemia, obesity, rhinitis, chronic sinusitis, and adenotonsillar hypertrophy were classified as the comorbidity group; *P <0.05, **P <0.01,***P <0.001.

Table 2: Risk of obstructive sleep apnea compared with children without asthma and stratified by demographics in Cox proportional hazards regression.

Average frequency for medical visit, per years	Event	Person-years	IR	Adjusted HR† (95% CI)
		All		
None	249	1583683	1.57	1.00(Reference)
≤ 3	384	1469305	2.61	1.36(1.15, 1.60)***
04-May	46	54496	8.44	4.31(3.13, 5.93)***
>5	136	68040	20	10.1(8.13, 12.6)***
p for trend				<0.001
		Girl		
None	56	647225	0.87	1.00(Reference)
≤ 3	86	606104	1.42	1.42(1.00, 2.01)*
04-May	11	20269	5.43	5.40(2.79, 10.4)***
>5	38	24230	15.7	15.6(10.1, 24.1)***
p for trend				<0.001
		Boy		
None	193	936459	2.06	1.00(Reference)
≤ 3	298	863201	3.45	1.34(1.11, 1.62)**
04-May	35	34226	10.2	3.88(2.70, 5.60)***
>5	98	43810	22.4	8.46(6.57, 10.9)***
p for trend				<0.001

IR: Incidence rate, per 10000 person-y; Adjusted HR†: adjusted for age, sex, urbanization level, and comorbidities such as GERD, craniofacial abnormalities, neuromuscular abnormalities, prematurity, genetic syndrome, laryngomalacia or tracheomalacia, diabetes, hypertension, hyperlipidemia, obesity, rhinitis, chronic sinusitis, and adenotonsillar hypertrophy; *P <0.05, **P <0.01,***P <0.001.

Table 3: Risk of obstructive sleep apnea according to average frequency of medical visits for asthma per year in Cox proportional hazards regression.

increase. The same phenomenon was noted in the study of Shen et al. showed that the more medical visits per year for asthma, the more risk of subsequent OSA in adults [14]. Teodorescu et al. reported that the association between asthma and OSA was significantly dose dependent on the duration of asthma [15]. Julien et al. also reported that obstructive sleep apnea-hypopnea was significantly more prevalent among patients with severe compared with moderate asthma [24]. In our study, we did not know if the severity of asthma is the risk of subsequent OSA, but only know that the frequency of medical visits per year, which meaning the poor control of childhood asthma, increases the risk of subsequent OSA.

The strength of the current study is the precise analysis of the future OSA risk in children with asthma on the basis of a large population database with a minimal selection bias. Although differences in comorbidities between asthma and non-asthma cohorts were significant, we adjusted the data for various comorbidities, such as GERD, craniofacial abnormalities, neuromuscular abnormalities, prematurity, genetic syndrome, laryngomalacia or tracheomalacia, diabetes, hypertension, hyperlipidemia, obesity, rhinitis, chronic sinusitis, and adenotonsillar hypertrophy; we observed that the asthma cohort still had a higher OSA risk than the non-asthma cohort did, even after propensity score matching. Our results demonstrate that childhood asthma increases subsequent OSA risk with or without comorbidities.

However, our study has some limitations that should be addressed. First, the diagnoses of asthma and OSA were made on the basis of ICD-9-CM codes, and serum laboratory data on IGE or specific I_gE as well as the results of the pulmonary function test and polysomnography were not available. However, the diagnoses of asthma and OSA in children mainly depend on the detailed medical history and not on the results of the pulmonary function test and polysomnography, respectively. In addition, we enrolled only patients that were diagnosed at least twice within a year for increasing the validity and accuracy of diagnosis. The NHIRD covers a highly representative sample of Taiwan's general population because the reimbursement policy is universal and operated by a single buyer, the Taiwan government. All insurance claims are scrutinized by medical reimbursement specialists and subjected to peer review according to standard diagnosis criteria. When specialists or physicians misdiagnose diseases or miscode diagnoses, they are criticized and the revision of diagnosis code will be made by reviewers. Therefore, the diagnoses of asthma and OSA in this study were highly reliable.

Additionally, information on the severity of asthma and OSA is unavailable in the NHIRD; therefore, we could not evaluate the correlation between the severities of these two diseases. Furthermore, information on other confounding factors, such as oral or inhaled steroid use and body mass index, which may be related to subsequent pediatric OSA risk, was unavailable in our study. Therefore, further prospective and case–control studies with larger cohorts and expanded diagnostic testing are warranted.

Conclusion

In conclusion, the risk of OSA was significantly higher in sexes, all age groups, and all urbanization levels in patients with asthma compared to patients without asthma, even with and without comorbidities. In addition, children with>5 medical visits per year for asthma have increased subsequent OSA risk. Further studies evaluating the mechanism of childhood asthma that increases pediatric OSA risk are warranted.

Acknowledgments

This study is supported in part by Taiwan Ministry of Health and Welfare Clinical Trial and Research Center of Excellence (MOHW104-TDU-B-212-113002); China Medical University Hospital, Academia Sinica Taiwan Biobank, Stroke Biosignature Project (BM104010092); NRPB Stroke Clinical Trial Consortium (MOST 103-2325- B-039 -006); Tseng-Lien Lin Foundation, Taichung, Taiwan; Taiwan Brain Disease Foundation, Taipei, Taiwan; Katsuzo and Kiyo Aoshima Memorial Funds, Japan; and CMU under the Aim for Top University Plan of the Ministry of Education, Taiwan. The funders had no role in study design, data collection and analysis, decision to publish, or preparation of the manuscript. No additional external funding received for this study.

Conflict of Interest

The authors declare no conflict of interest.

Author Contributions

Chien-Heng Lin, Wei-Ching Lin and Liang-Wen Hang conceptualized and designed the study, drafted the initial manuscript, and approved the manuscript. Cheng-Li Lin conducted the initial analysis, reviewed and revised the manuscript, and approved the final manuscript. Liang-Wen Hang coordinated and supervised data collection, critically reviewed the manuscript and approved the final manuscript.

References

1. Chen J, Edman JC, Koltai PJ (2004) Obstructive sleep apnea in children. Am Fam Physician 69: 1147-1155.
2. Ferreira AM, Clemente V, Gozal D, Gomes A, Pissarra C, et al. (2000) Snoring in portuguese primary school children. Pediatrics 106: E64.
3. Hultcrantz E, Lofstrand-Tidestrom B, Ahlquist-Rastad J (1995) The epidemiology of sleep related breathing disorder in children. Int J Pediatr Otorhinolaryngol 32: 563-566.
4. Qubty WF, Mrelashvili A, Kotagal S, Lloyd RM (2014) Comorbidities in infants with obstructive sleep apnea. J Clin Sleep Med 10: 1213-1216.
5. Oscar SC, Leila KG, Ehab D, David G (2008) Pediatric obstructive sleep apnea: Complications, management, and long-term outcomes. Proc Am Thorac Soc 5: 274-282.
6. de Groot EP, Duiverman EJ, Brand PL (2010) Comorbidities of asthma during childhood: Possibly important, yet poorly studied. Eur Respir J 36: 671-678.
7. Fagnano M, Bayer AL, Isensee CA, HernandezT, Halterman JS (2011) Nocturnal asthma symptoms and poor sleep quality among urban school children with asthma. Acad Pediatr 11: 493-499.
8. Alkhalil M, Schulman E, Getsy J (2009) Obstructive sleep apnea syndrome and asthma: What are the links? Clin Sleep Med 5: 71-78.
9. Teodorescu M, Consens FB, Bria WF, Coffey MJ, McMorris MS, et al. (2006) Correlates of daytime sleepiness in patients with asthma. Sleep Med 7: 607-613.
10. Ekici A, Ekici M, Kurtipek E, Keles H, Kara T, et al. (2005) Association of asthma-related symptoms with snoring and apnea and effect on health-related quality of life. Chest 128: 3358-3363.
11. Salles C, Terse-Ramos R, Souachado A, Cruz AA (2013) Obstructive sleep apnea and asthma. J Bras Pneumol 39: 604-612.
12. Guilleminault C, Quera-Saalva MA, Powell N, Riley R, Romaker A, et al. (1988) Nocturnal asthma: Snoring, small pharynx and nasal CAPA. Eur Respir J 1: 902-907.
13. Ciftci TU, Cifci B, Guven SF, Kokturk O, Turktas H (2005) Effect of nasal continuous positive airway pressure in uncontrolled nocturnal asthmatic patients with obstructive sleep apnea syndrome. Respir Med 99: 529-534.
14. Shen TC, Lin CL, Wei CC, Chen CH, Tu CY, et al. (2015) Risk of obstructive sleep apnea in adult patients with asthma: A population-based cohort study in Taiwan. PLoS One 10: e0128461.
15. Teodorescu M, Barnet JH, Hagen EW, Palta M, Young TB, et al. (2015) Association between asthma and risk of developing obstructive sleep apnea JAMA 313: 156-164.
16. Database NHIR (2015) Taiwan.
17. Lin JN, Lin CL, Lin MC, Lai CH, Lin HH, et al. (2015) Risk of leukaemia in children infected with enterovirus: A nationwide, retrospective, population-based, Taiwanese-registry, cohort study. Lancet Oncol 16: 1335-1343.
18. Wei CC, Lin CL, Shen TC, Kao CH (2015) Neonatal jaundice and risks of childhood allergic diseases: a population-based cohort study. Pediatr Res 78: 223-230.
19. Rabelo FA, Küpper DS, Sander HH, Santos Júnior Vd, Thuler E, et al. (2013) A comparison of the Fujita classification of awake and drug-induced sleep endoscopy patients. Braz J Otorhinolaryngol 79: 100-105.
20. Reid MB, Lännergren J, Westerblad H (2002) Respiratory andlimb muscle weakness induced by tumor necrosis factor-alpha: involvement of muscle myofilaments. Am J Respir Crit Care Med 166: 479-484.
21. Grotberg JB (1994) Pulmonary flow and transport phenomena. Ann Rev Fluid Mech 26: 529-571.

22. Lakser OJ, Dowell ML, Hoyte FL, Chen B, Lavoie TL, et al. (2008) Steroids augment relengthening of contracted airway smooth muscle: Potential additional mechanism of benefit in asthma. Eur R Espir J 32: 1224-1230.

23. Teodorescu M, Xie A, Sorkness CA, Robbins J, Reeder S, et al. (2014) Effects of inhaled fluticasone on upper airway during sleep and wakefulness in asthma: A pilot study. J Clin Sleep Med 10: 183-193.

24. Julien JY, Martin JG, Ernst P, Olivenstein R, Hamid Q, et al. (2009) Prevalence of obstructive sleep apnea-hypopnea in severe versus moderate asthma. J Allergy Clin Immunol 124: 371-376.

Permissions

All chapters in this book were first published in JSD&T, by OMICS International; hereby published with permission under the Creative Commons Attribution License or equivalent. Every chapter published in this book has been scrutinized by our experts. Their significance has been extensively debated. The topics covered herein carry significant findings which will fuel the growth of the discipline. They may even be implemented as practical applications or may be referred to as a beginning point for another development.

The contributors of this book come from diverse backgrounds, making this book a truly international effort. This book will bring forth new frontiers with its revolutionizing research information and detailed analysis of the nascent developments around the world.

We would like to thank all the contributing authors for lending their expertise to make the book truly unique. They have played a crucial role in the development of this book. Without their invaluable contributions this book wouldn't have been possible. They have made vital efforts to compile up to date information on the varied aspects of this subject to make this book a valuable addition to the collection of many professionals and students.

This book was conceptualized with the vision of imparting up-to-date information and advanced data in this field. To ensure the same, a matchless editorial board was set up. Every individual on the board went through rigorous rounds of assessment to prove their worth. After which they invested a large part of their time researching and compiling the most relevant data for our readers.

The editorial board has been involved in producing this book since its inception. They have spent rigorous hours researching and exploring the diverse topics which have resulted in the successful publishing of this book. They have passed on their knowledge of decades through this book. To expedite this challenging task, the publisher supported the team at every step. A small team of assistant editors was also appointed to further simplify the editing procedure and attain best results for the readers.

Apart from the editorial board, the designing team has also invested a significant amount of their time in understanding the subject and creating the most relevant covers. They scrutinized every image to scout for the most suitable representation of the subject and create an appropriate cover for the book.

The publishing team has been an ardent support to the editorial, designing and production team. Their endless efforts to recruit the best for this project, has resulted in the accomplishment of this book. They are a veteran in the field of academics and their pool of knowledge is as vast as their experience in printing. Their expertise and guidance has proved useful at every step. Their uncompromising quality standards have made this book an exceptional effort. Their encouragement from time to time has been an inspiration for everyone.

The publisher and the editorial board hope that this book will prove to be a valuable piece of knowledge for researchers, students, practitioners and scholars across the globe.

List of Contributors

Jeffrey J Stanley
Department of Neurology, Michael S. Aldrich Sleep Disorders Center, University of Michigan, Ann Arbor, Michigan, USA
Department of Otolaryngology, Head and Neck Surgery, University of Michigan, Ann Arbor, Michigan, USA

John Palmisano
Department of Neurology, Michael S. Aldrich Sleep Disorders Center, University of Michigan, Ann Arbor, Michigan, USA
Department of Oral & Maxillofacial Surgery, University of Michigan, Ann Arbor, Michigan, USA

Steven Hoshal and Lizabeth Binns
Department of Neurology, Michael S. Aldrich Sleep Disorders Center, University of Michigan, Ann Arbor, Michigan, USA

Louise O'Brien
Department of Neurology, Michael S. Aldrich Sleep Disorders Center, University of Michigan, Ann Arbor, Michigan, USA
Department of Oral & Maxillofacial Surgery, University of Michigan, Ann Arbor, Michigan, USA
Department of Obstetrics & Gynecology, University of Michigan, Ann Arbor, Michigan, USA

Monika Sharma and Samhita Panda
Department of Sleep Medicine, Sir Ganga Ram Hospital, New Delhi, India

Khurshid A Khurshid and Mark S Gold
Department of Psychiatry & McKnight Brain Institute, University of Florida College of Medicine, USA

Marlene Oscar-Berman
Departments of Psychiatry, Neurology, and Anatomy & Neurobiology, Boston University School of Medicine, and Boston VA Healthcare System, USA

Rajendra D Badgaiyan
Department of Neuroimaging and Psychiatry, University of Buffalo College of Medicine, USA

Kenneth Blum
Department of Addiction Research & Therapy, Malibu Beach Recovery Center, USA
Department of Nutrigenomics, IGENE, LLC, Austin, Texas, USA
Dominion Diagnostics, LLC, North Kingstown, Rhode Island, USA
Department of Clinical Neurology, PATH Foundation NY, USA

Ozge oral Tapan, Begum Gorgulu, Kemal Can Tertemiz, Aylin Ozgen Alpaydin, Ibrahim Oztura, Oya Itil and Baris Baklan
Department of Chest Disease, Dokuz Eylul Universitesi Tip Fakultesi, Turkey

Yun Kyung Park
Department of Neurology, College of Medicine, Konyang University Hospital, Korea

Su Jung Choi
Department of Neurology, Neuroscience Center, Samsung Biomedical Research Institute, Samsung Medical Center, Sungkyunkwan University School of Medicine, Seoul, Korea

Eun Yeon Joo
Department of Neurology, Neuroscience Center, Samsung Biomedical Research Institute, Samsung Medical Center, Sungkyunkwan University School of Medicine, Seoul, Korea
Department of Health Sciences and Technology, SAIHST, Sungkyunkwan University, Seoul, Korea

Sharon Valente
Greater Los Angeles Healthcare System, Los Angeles, CA, USA

Shittu RO, Odeigah LO and Sule AG
Department of Family Medicine, Kwara State Specialist Hospital, Nigeria

Issa BA and Olanrewaju GT
Department of Behavioral Sciences, University of Ilorin Teaching Hospital, Nigeria

Sanni MA
Department of Hematology, Kwara State Specialist Hospital, Nigeria

Aderibigbe SA
Department of Epidemiology and Community Health, University of Ilorin Teaching Hospital, Nigeria

Annie Vallières
École de psychologie, Université Laval, Québec, Québec, Canada
Laboratoire Psycho Socio Culturel du sommeil, Centre de recherche de l'Institut universitaire en santé mentale de Québec, Québec, Québec, Canada

Monica Roy, Emmanuelle Bastille-Denis, Sonia Claveau and Tarek Simon
École de psychologie, Université Laval, Québec, Québec, Canada
Laboratoire Psycho Socio Culturel du sommeil, Centre de recherche de l'Institut universitaire en santé mentale de Québec, Québec, Québec, Canada

Elhadd K and Bharambe V
Specialist Registrar in Neurology, Walton Centre for Neurology and Neurosurgery, United Kingdom

Larner AJ
Consultant Neurologist, Walton Centre for Neurology and Neurosurgery, United Kingdom

Ilona Quaak, Marijke de Cock and Margot van de Bor
Department of Health and Life Sciences, Faculty of Earth and Life Sciences, VU University, De Boelelaan 1085, 1081 HV Amsterdam, The Netherlands

Michiel de Boer
Department of Health Sciences, Faculty of Earth and Life Sciences, VU University, De Boelelaan 1085, 1081 HV Amsterdam, The Netherlands

Jayne Roberts
Department of Medicine, Austin Health and Northern Health, University of Melbourne, Parkville, Victoria, Australia

David J Berlowitz
Department of Medicine, Austin Health and Northern Health, University of Melbourne, Parkville, Victoria, Australia
Institute for Breathing and Sleep, Austin Hospital, Heidelberg, Victoria, Australia

Jo Spong
Institute for Breathing and Sleep, Austin Hospital, Heidelberg, Victoria, Australia

Enzo Iacomino
ENT Department, Hospital "San Salvatore", L'Aquila, Italy

Martina Pagliarella
Department of Biotechnological and Applied Clinical Sciences, University of L'Aquila, Italy

Franco Pestilli
Expert in Orthodontic Technique, freelancer, Italy

Giovanni Falisi
Department of Life, Health and Environmental Sciences, University of L'Aquila, Italy

Vittorio Bisogni
Department of Pneumology, Hospital "San Pietro Fatebenefratelli", Rome, Italy

Navneet Sharma, Justin Lee, Irini Youssef, Moro O Salifu and Samy I McFarlane
Department of Medicine, Divisions of Endocrinology and Nephrology, New York, USA

Gail A Welsh, Mary O Whipple, Ann Vincent, Laura L Loehrer and Dietlind L Wahner-Roedler
Division of General Internal Medicine, Mayo Clinic, Rochester, Minnesota, USA

Eric J Olson
Division of Pulmonary and Critical Care Medicine, Mayo Clinic, Rochester, Minnesota, USA

Stephen S Cha
Division Biomedical Statistics and Informatics, Mayo Clinic, Rochester, Minnesota, USA

Kader Semra Karataş
Department of Psychiatry Internal Medical Sciences, Rize Training and Research Hospital, Recep Tayyip Erdogan University, Rize, Turkey

Mustafa Bilici
Psychology Department, Sabahattin Zaim University, Istanbul, Turkey

Zerrin Pelin
Somnus Sleep Disorders Center, Neurology, Istanbul, Turkey

Florim Delijaj
Department of Public Health and Caring Sciences (IFV), Uppsala Centre for Clinical Research Sormland (CKFD), Eskilstuna and Department of Primary Care, Tunafors Family Center, Sormland County Council, Sweden

Gustaf Levin
Department of Surgery, ENT Clinic in Eskilstuna, Sormland County Council, Sweden

Eva Lindberg
Department of Medical Sciences, Respiratory, Allergy and Sleep Research, Uppsala University, Sweden

Eugen Wang
Department of Surgery Sciences, Uppsala University and Center for Clinical Research, Sormland, Uppsala University, Eskilstuna, Sweden

Oommen Nainan
Graded Specialist-Orthodontics & Dentofacial Orthopedics, Naval Institute of Dental Sciences, India

Jayan B
Department of Dental Surgery, Armed Forces Medical College, India

Chopra SS
Classified Specialist-Orthodontics & Dentofacial Orthopedics, Corps Dental Unit, India

Mukherjee M
Classified Specialist-Periodontology, Military Dental centre, India

Lois E Krahn
Sleep Medicine, Mayo Clinic Arizona, Phoenix, Arizona, USA

Eve R Rogers
Sleep Medicine, Columbus, Ohio, USA

Geerdink M and Beersma DGM
Department of Chronobiology, GeLifes, University of Groningen, The Netherlands

Hommes V
Philips Consumer Lifestyle, Drachten, The Netherlands

Gordijn MCM
Department of Chronobiology, GeLifes, University of Groningen, The Netherlands

Eusebi Chiner, Jose N Sancho-Chust, Esther Pastor, Pedro Landete, Cristina Senent and Patricia Pérez-Ferrer
Pneumology Section, Hospital Universitario San Juan de Alicante, Alicante, Cta Alicante-Valencias/n. 03550, Sant Joan d'Alacant, Spain

Ivana Meyer Prado, Marcela Oliveira Brant, Sheyla Márcia Auad, Saul Martins Paiva, Isabela Almeida Pordeus and Junia M Serra-Negra
Department of Pediatric Dentistry and Orthodontics, Federal University of Minas Gerais, Belo Horizonte, Brazil

Pennie S Seibert and Christian G Zimmerman
Physician Research Services at Saint Alphonsus Regional Medical Center, Boise, Idaho, USA

Jennifer Valerio, Codieann Dehaas, Danielle Nebeker and Fred Grimsley
Physician Research Services at Saint Alphonsus Regional Medical Center, Boise, Idaho, USA
Boise State University, Boise, Idaho, USA

Najafipour Hamid
Physiology Research Center, Institute of Neuropharmacology, Kerman University of Medical Sciences, Kerman, Iran

Sabahi Abdolreza
Religion and Medicine Research Center and the Department of Psychiatry, Kerman University of Medical Sciences, Kerman, Iran

Mirrashidi Fatemeasadat
Cardiovascular Research Center, Institute of Basic and Clinical Physiology sciences, Kerman University of Medical Sciences, Kerman, Iran

Afshari Mahdi
Department of Community Medicine, Zabol University of Medical Sciences, Zabol, Iran

Haghdoost Ali Akbar
Research Center for Modeling in Health, Institute of Future Studies in Health, Kerman University of Medical Sciences, Kerman, Iran

Kenji Tsunoda
Physical Fitness Research Institute, Meiji Yasuda Life Foundation of Health and Welfare, Tokyo, Japan
Department of Occupational Therapy, School of Healthcare, Ibaraki Prefectural University of Health Sciences, Ibaraki, Japan

Kazushi Hotta
Department of Occupational Therapy, School of Healthcare, Ibaraki Prefectural University of Health Sciences, Ibaraki, Japan

Hirotaka Mutsuzaki
Department of Orthopaedic Surgery, Ibaraki Prefectural University of Health Sciences, Ibaraki, Japan

Kaori Tachibana
Department of Physical Therapy, School of Healthcare, Ibaraki Prefectural University of Health Sciences, Ibaraki, Japan

Yukiyo Shimizu
Department of Rehabilitation Medicine, University of Tsukuba Hospital, Ibaraki, Japan

Takashi Fukaya
Department of Physical Therapy, Faculty of Health Sciences, Tsukuba International University, Ibaraki, Japan

Eiji Ikeda
Faculty of Education, Art and Science, Yamagata University, Yamagata, Japan

Naruki Kitano
Institute of Health and Sport Sciences, University of Tsukuba, Ibaraki, Japan

Yasuyoshi Wadano
Department of Rehabilitation Medicine, Ibaraki Prefectural University of Health Sciences, Ibaraki, Japan

Thibaut Gentina, Catherine Lamblin, François Jouniaux and François Codron
Hôpital Privé La Louvière, Générale de Santé, Lille, France

Elodie Gentina
Skema Business School - Université de Lille, MERCUR Research, France

Aiman Tulaimat
Cook County Health and Hospital Systems, Division of Pulmonary, Critial Care, and Sleep Medicine, USA

Ziso B and Larner AJ
Cognitive Function Clinic, Walton Centre for Neurology and Neurosurgery, Liverpool, United Kingdom

Anqiong Ji
Department of Management, Chengdu University of Traditional Chinese Medicine, Chengdu, P.R. China

Rufang Wang
Department of Management, Chengdu University of Traditional Chinese Medicine, Chengdu, P.R. China
Department of Psychiatry & Health Behavior, Medical College of Georgia, Augusta University, Augusta, GA, USA

Xi Han
Department of Neurosurgery, Huashan Hospital, Fudan University, China

Chengguang Huang, Mingkun Yu and Lijun Hou
Department of Neurosurgery, Second Military Medical University, China

Ping Sheng and Yan Dong
Department of Neurosurgery, Second Military Medical University, China
Neuroscience center, Second Military Medical University, China

Diana Maier
Independent Researcher and Quality and Performance Improvement Consultant, Denver, United States

Jonathan Savelle
Independent Researcher and Statistical Consultant, Cheyenne, United States

Valerie Vidana
Independent Researcher and Data Organization Specialist, Boulder, United States

Richard Shane
Founder and Manager, Sleep Easily LLC, Boulder, United States

Rodrigo L
Gastroenterology Service, Central University Hospital of Asturias (HUCA). Avda. Hospital Universitario, s/n. 33011, Oviedo, Principality of Asturias, Spain

Huerta M
Psychiatry Service, Health Mental Center I. Pedro Pablo 42, 33209, Gijon, Principality of Asturias, Spain

Salas-Puig J
Neurology Service, Hospital Universitario Central de Asturias (HUCA), c/Celestino Villamil, s. n°, 33006, Oviedo, Spain

Deborah Syna
Northwest Neurological Specialists PC, Portland, Oregon, USA

Alessandro Pincherle
Neurology Unit, Spitalzentrum Biel, Biel, Switzerland
Fondazione IRCCS Istituto Neurologico "Carlo Besta", Milan, Italy

Ambra Dominese, Flavio Villani, Fabrizio Tagliavini and Giorgio Giaccone
Fondazione IRCCS Istituto Neurologico "Carlo Besta", Milan, Italy

Eleonora Tobaldini, Lucio Mos and Nicola Montano
Department of Biomedical and Clinical Sciences "L. Sacco", Medicine and Physiopathology Unit, L. Sacco Hospital, University of Milan, Italy

Vincenzo Patruno
Department of Cardiology, San Daniele del Friuli Hospital, Udine, Ital

Gabriella Marcon
Fondazione IRCCS Istituto Neurologico "Carlo Besta", Milan, Italy
Department of Biomedical and Clinical Sciences "L. Sacco", Medicine and Physiopathology Unit, L. Sacco Hospital, University of Milan, Italy
Department of Cardiology, San Daniele del Friuli Hospital, Udine, Italy
Pneumologia Riabilitativa, Istituto di Medicina Fisica e Riabilitazione "Gervasutta", Udine, Italy
Department of Biological and Medical Sciences (DSMB), University of Udine, Italy

Gholami Damian F and Mahmoodi Gharaie J
Psychiatric, Department of Psychiatry, Roozbeh Psychiatry Hospital, Tehran University of Medical Sciences, Tehran, Iran

Sabzali P
Psychiatric, Department of Psychiatry Emamhossein Hospital, Shahid beheshti University of Medical Sciences, Tehran, Iran

Darabi F
Department of Public Health, Asadabad Medical Sciences Faculty, Hamadan University of Medical Sciences, Hamadan, Iran

Haji Seyed Javadi P
Psychiatric, Department of Psychiatry, Tehran University of Medical Sciences, Tehran, Iran

Marzieh Miri and Ali Sheikhani
Biomedical Engineering, Science and Research Branch, Islamic Azad University, Tehran, Iran

Khosro Sadeghniiat
Tehran University of Medical Science, Tehran, Iran

Chien-Heng Lin
Division of Pediatric Pulmonology, China Medical University Children's Hospital, Taichung, Taiwan
Department of Biomedical Imaging and Radiological Science, College of Health Care, China Medical University, Taichung, Taiwan

Wei-Ching Lin
Department of Radiology, College of Medicine, School of Medicine, China Medical University, Taichung, Taiwan
College of Medicine, China Medical University, Taichung, Taiwan
Management Office for Health Data, China Medical University Hospital, Taichung, Taiwan

Cheng-Li Lin
College of Medicine, China Medical University, Taichung, Taiwan
Management Office for Health Data, China Medical University Hospital, Taichung, Taiwan

Liang-Wen Hang
Department of Respiratory Therapy, College of Health Care, China Medical University
Sleep Medicine Center, Department of Pulmonary and Critical Care Medicine, China Medical University Hospital

Index

www.ingramcontent.com/pod-product-compliance
Lightning Source LLC
LaVergne TN
LVHW060609210926
848485LV00005B/1393